D0470627

The Writing Lab Approach
to Language Instruction
and Intervention

The Writing Lab Approach to Language Instruction and Intervention

by

Nickola Wolf Nelson, Ph.D., CCC-SLP
Western Michigan University, Kalamazoo

Christine M. Bahr, Ph.D., ATP
St. Mary-of-the-Woods College, Indiana

and

Adelia M. Van Meter, M.S., CCC-SLP
Western Michigan University, Kalamazoo

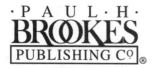

·P A U L·H·
BROOKES
PUBLISHING Co.®

Baltimore • London • Sydney

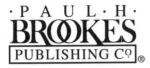

Paul H. Brookes Publishing Co.
Post Office Box 10624
Baltimore, Maryland 21285-0624

www.brookespublishing.com

Copyright © 2004 by Paul H. Brookes Publishing Co., Inc.
All rights reserved.

"Paul H. Brookes Publishing Co." is a registered trademark of Paul H. Brookes Publishing Co., Inc.

Typeset by Integrated Publishing Solutions, Grand Rapids, Michigan.
Manufactured in the United States of America by
Sheridan Books, Fredericksburg, Virginia.

Case studies are derived from the authors' actual experiences. In most cases, pseudonyms have been given and identifying details have been changed. Real names are used by permission.

Purchasers are granted permission to photocopy materials in the appendices to Chapters 4 and 15. None of the forms may be reproduced to generate revenue for any program or individual. Photocopies may only be made from an original book. You will see the copyright protection at the bottom of each photocopiable page.

The development of the writing lab approach was supported by the U.S. Department of Education, Office of Special Education and Rehabilitative Services Grant No. H180G20005, Grant No. HO29B10245, Grant No. HO29B40183, and Grant No. H324R980120. However, no official endorsement by the federal government should be inferred.

Library of Congress Cataloging-in-Publication Data

Nelson, Nickola.
    The writing lab approach to language instruction and intervention/Nickola Wolf Nelson, Christine M. Bahr, and Adelia M. Van Meter.
      p.   cm.
    Includes bibliographical references and index.
    ISBN 1-55766-673-3
    1. Language and languages—Study and teaching.   2. Composition (Language arts).   3. Language laboratories.   I. Bahr, Christine M., 1958– II. Van Meter, Adelia M.   III. Title.
    P53.27.N45 2004
    418'.0071—dc21
                                               2003057701

British Library Cataloguing in Publication data are available from the British Library.

Contents

Extended Contents

About the Authors

Nickola Wolf Nelson, Ph.D., CCC-SLP, Professor, Department of Speech Pathology and Audiology, Associate Dean for Research in the College of Health and Human Services, 1903 West Michigan Avenue, Western Michigan University, Kalamazoo, Michigan 49008

Dr. Nelson received her bachelor's, master's, and doctoral degrees from Wichita State University. She is the author of *Childhood Language Disorders in Context: Infancy Through Adolescence, Second Edition* (1998, Allyn & Bacon), and *Planning Individualized Speech and Language Intervention Programs, Second Edition* (1989, PRO-ED), as well as numerous articles and chapters on classroom-based language intervention and related topics. Dr. Nelson began her professional career as a school clinician in Kansas and also served as a speech-language consultant specialist for Berrien County Intermediate School District in Michigan. She has been a member of the faculty at Western Michigan University since 1981. Dr. Nelson and her husband live on a lake in Three Rivers, Michigan. They enjoy gardening, boating, and entertaining their children, grandchildren, and extended families on the lake.

Christine M. Bahr, Ph.D., ATP, Associate Professor and Chair, Department of Education, St. Mary-of-the-Woods College, 221 Hulman Hall, St. Mary-of-the-Woods, Indiana 47876

Dr. Bahr received her bachelor's degree in special education from Fontbonne College in St. Louis, Missouri. Her master of science degree in educational administration and supervision is from Southern Illinois University, and her doctorate in special education and instructional systems technology is from Indiana University. Dr. Bahr began her professional career as a teacher of students with severe disabilities in St. Louis County Special School District. She was on the faculty of Western Michigan University from 1988 to 1998. Her presentations and publications address uses of assistive technology as a means of promoting participation of students with special needs in the general education curriculum. She and her husband live in Terre Haute, Indiana. They enjoy attending their four children's sporting events and musical activities, camping, and visiting relatives from coast to coast.

Adelia M. Van Meter, M.S., CCC-SLP, Faculty Specialist II, Department of Speech Pathology and Audiology, Western Michigan University, Kalamazoo, Michigan 49008

Ms. Van Meter is Clinic Coordinator at the Charles Van Riper Language, Speech, and Hearing Clinic. Her bachelor's and master's degrees are from the University of Michigan. Ms. Van Meter has presented widely and is co-author of a number of articles on language assessment and intervention in curriculum-based contexts. She began her professional career in the University of Michigan's C.S. Mott Children's Hospital in Ann Arbor. She has been affiliated with Western Michigan University since 1992. Ms. Van Meter, her husband, and their two daughters live in Kalamazoo, Michigan. They enjoy swimming, traveling, hiking, and entertaining each other with stories.

ABOUT THE CONTRIBUTOR

Kathryn Kinnucan-Welsch, Ed.D., is Associate Professor and Chair of the Department of Teacher Education at the University of Dayton in Dayton, Ohio. Her bachelor of arts degree is from the University of Illinois, and her master of arts and doctorate in education degrees are from Western Michigan University. Dr. Kinnucan-Welsch has published and presented extensively on professional development of practicing teachers, particularly in the area of early literacy instruction. She began her career as a Title I Reading Specialist and is currently working with Literacy Specialists in a statewide literacy professional development initiative in Ohio. She has been at the University of Dayton since 1997. Dr. Kinnucan-Welsch lives in Springboro, Ohio, and enjoys spending time in Michigan and Ohio with her four grown children, gardening, and traveling.

Acknowledgments

This book is the culmination of 10 years of joint research and clinical intervention projects. The collaboration started when Dr. Bahr and Dr. Nelson became Co-Principal Investigators and Ms. Van Meter became Project Supervisor for a 3-year technology and literacy research project funded from 1992 to 1995 by the U.S. Department of Education, Office of Special Education and Rehabilitative Services (Grant No. H180G20005). The project was called Linking Text Processing Tools (LTPT) to Student Needs. In that project, the three authors worked with elementary and middle school students referred from the Kalamazoo area for an after-school program that was held twice a week in a computer lab housed in the College of Education at Western Michigan University. Although most of the students had labels of learning disability and written language goals on their individualized education programs, there was one child with Down syndrome and several students with speech-language impairments.

Our work in this experience was aided by a number of undergraduate students in special education who assisted in data collection and by graduate students in speech-language pathology who were participating in a personnel preparation project known as Project COLLABORATE, which was directed by Dr. Nelson and co-directed by Dr. Michael Clark and Donna Oas. This project also was funded by the U.S. Department of Education, Office of Special Education and Rehabilitative Services (Grant No. HO29B10245).

At the conclusion of the LTPT research project, Dr. Nelson and Ms. Van Meter continued to develop the writing lab approach, with consultation from Dr. Bahr, from 1995 to 1997 as a component of a Language-Based Homework Lab within the Charles Van Riper Language Speech and Hearing Clinic. That clinical experience was implemented at, and with partial support from, the University Unified Clinics in the College of Health and Human Services at Western Michigan University. The children and adolescents who participated in the homework lab were elementary and middle school students who were referred by their parents and teachers for a variety of language, communication, and academic difficulties.

During the 1997–1998 school year, we conducted an after-school writing lab at King Westwood Elementary School. This lab, which was held in the school library using computers rolled in from nearby classrooms, targeted computer-supported expository writing for fourth- and fifth-graders who had been referred by their teachers as needing extra help. During these experiences, the graduate students in speech-language pathology who were learning to implement the model were supported by traineeships from Project CONNECT, co-directed by Dr. Nelson and Dr. Clark, which also was funded by the U.S. Department of Education, Office of Special Education and Rehabilitative Services (Grant No. HO29B40183).

The three co-authors collaborated again from 1998 to 2002 to conduct a Writing

Lab Outreach Project with support from an early childhood grant from the U.S. Department of Education, Office of Special Education and Rehabilitative Services (Grant No. H324R980120). In that project, we worked in partnership with administrators and teachers of the Kalamazoo Public Schools, as well as with professionals from a number of outreach sites. The goals of the project were to include students with disabilities in the actual writing process instruction activities of general education classrooms, to work with "development teams" in our partner school district to fine tune the model, and to teach "outreach teams" in other school districts how to implement the model in their own settings. Being supported by an early childhood grant, this work was based in first-, second-, and third-grade classrooms. It was implemented by including children with disabilities in general education classroom-based and computer-lab writing process activities, in collaboration with teacher volunteers in three different elementary schools in Kalamazoo—Milwood Elementary, Washington Writer's Academy, and Spring Valley Center for Exploration. During the summers, we held summer school programs and outreach institutes in each of these schools. The participants in these summer institutes were general and special education teachers and speech-language pathologists from around the region and across the country (Texas and Ohio), some of whom worked in secondary school programs.

Although this work would not have been possible without the tangible support we received from the U.S. government, Western Michigan University, and Kalamazoo Public Schools, we point out that the views expressed in this book are our own. Neither our sponsors nor our collaborative partners are responsible for any of the opinions or errors that might be contained herein.

Special acknowledgments go to a few graduate students who worked with us particularly closely to organize Writing Lab Outreach Project activities, provide support for teachers and students, and code written language samples. In the order of their participation, they are Carrie Nagayda, Anna Putnam, Karey Hill, Melanie Lynam, Carrie Kopitzki, Kristen Kopacz, and Amanda Luna-Bailey. They kept us organized (as much as possible) and provided creative input. Another former graduate student and research assistant in special education, Kim Van Loo, assisted Dr. Bahr in cataloguing text-processing programs and building the taxonomy of software features explained in Section II. Jolaina Jackson assisted with this work as well. We also benefited from the contributions of Joyce Gard, Office Assistant in the Western Michigan University Department of Speech Pathology and Audiology, who managed our budgets, handled contracts with participants, and ordered software for the schools.

In addition, we want to acknowledge the special contributions of three people to the actual writing of the book. First is Kara McAlister, a former graduate student, who conducted her master's thesis research by interviewing the students who participated in our first writing lab about their perceptions of writing process instruction. Ms. McAlister's work on student attitudes toward a computer-based writing process instructional approach led to a publication (McAlister, Nelson, & Bahr, 1999), excerpts from which appear in Chapter 13. After graduating with her master's degree from Western Michigan University, Ms. McAlister went on to develop writers' workshops collaboratively with special and general education teachers in the Chicago public schools. Based on these experiences, she provided us with written examples, which have informed the suggestions in this book in a number of places, particularly Chapters 4 and 13. Ms. McAlister is a doctoral student at the University of Illinois at Chicago.

A second friend and colleague, Dr. Janet Sturm, read Chapter 11 in a draft stage and provided feedback. Dr. Sturm was on the faculty of the University of North Carolina at Chapel Hill when she read the manuscript, but she now is Assistant Professor at Central Michigan University.

The third special contributor, Dr. Kathryn Kinnucan-Welsch, worked with us in implementing the summer institutes and evaluating the teacher outcomes. She also provided special consultation to one of our outreach teams who developed their inclusive writing lab activities in Dayton. Dr. Kinnucan-Welsch's research focuses on helping teachers develop their skills as reflective practitioners and active researchers, continually modifying their practices based on evidence from their own practice. Our work, and sections of this book, have benefited from her special wisdom, her writings, and her interviewing skill, as well as her respect for the professionalism of classroom teachers and the roles they play in educating all children.

Everyone who has contributed to this endeavor has left a mark on it, in the mini-lessons they created, the projects they implemented, the stories they developed, the scaffolding they provided, the case studies they presented, and the workshops they taught or attended. They have our deep, deep appreciation. We hope that they will recognize their influence within the pages of this book.

As this phase of our work draws to a close, the three of us also want to acknowledge our appreciation for each other. It has been a partnership of mutual respect and support through a variety of experiences and life changes. We also want to acknowledge our spouses and children—Larry, David, Nicky, and Clayton Nelson and grandchildren Jessica, Justin, and Jess Jr.; Michael, Joseph, Justin, Emily, and Ryan Bahr; Pete, Emile, and Ellen Van Meter. Our families have supported our work through thick and thin, have put up with absences when we were working at our computers across the room or at conferences across the country, and have added to our understanding of written language development. Without our families' support, this book would not have come to fruition. It also would not have been possible without the patient support of our editor, Elaine Niefeld, and the other staff of Paul H. Brookes Publishing Co., especially our book production editor, Janet Betten.

Finally, we want to acknowledge the most important contributors to this work. They are the students—students with disabilities, students without disabilities but with wobbly language skills, second-language learners, typical students, gifted students—who have participated in the computer-supported writing process activities through which we developed the writing lab approach. They and their parents have allowed this book to be illustrated with real-life examples. Their stories are sprinkled throughout. These students are real people who provided our strongest motivation for writing this book. Their stories, both the ones they wrote and the ones they lived, have inspired us, as we hope they will inspire our readers. It is to them that we dedicate this book.

The following pages contain a list of individuals who have worked with us at various times in developing the writing lab approach. We appreciate the contributions of these individuals and apologize to any individuals whose names we may have forgotten to include.

1993–1998

Graduate Student Clinicians

Susan Armstrong
Cassandra Baer
Jennifer Baker
Kelly Beens
Jill Burgess
Chris Bursian
Jennifer Crouse
Beth Crow
Diana Drooger
Dan Finstrom
Monica Gillum
Roberta Grimstad
Rachel Hauser
Shawn Herron
Melissa Hoffmann
Jennifer Irvine
Jolaina Jackson
Jennifer Jankowski

Laura Johnson
Tricia Johnson
Mary Kimball
Stacey Kinney
Becky Little
Kara McAlister
Carrie McCarter-Barnes
Jennifer McCune
Nikki McDonnell
Amy McJames
Carolyn Moore
Catharine Nagayda
Wendy Popkes
Katie Sechrist
Jennifer Shephard
Karen TenHarmsel
Tameka Tyson
Kim Van Loo

Sue Vugteveen
Heather Weinert

Graduate Assistants

Kelli Beckman
Kristee Guy
Jolaina Jackson
Sarabdeep Singh
Joani Triezenberg
Kim Van Loo

Data Collectors

Karen Callens
Amy Cravero
Julie Crockatt
Nancy Nolan

1998–2002

Kalamazoo Public School Administrators

Dr. Janice Brown
Dr. Pat Coles-Chalmers
Cindy Green
Dr. Kay Royster

Patricia Williams
Audrey Fitzgerald
Yvonne Payton

Consultants

Dr. Kathryn Kinnucan-Welsch
Dr. Candace Bos
Dr. Janet Sturm
Kara McAlister

Sponsors of Intensive Outreach Workshops

Sally Disney—*Hamilton County, OH, Special Service Center*
Dr. Maureen Staskowski—*Macomb, MI, Intermediate School District*

1998–1999

Graduate Assistants

Carrie Nagayda
Anna Putnam

Milwood Elementary School Development Team Members

Carl Czuchna
Sharon Lawson
Roger Fleming

Greg Socha
Pam Ward
Kathy Palmer

Outreach Teams

Team 1

Benton Harbor, MI
Shelley Griffin
Toni Doswell

Team 2

Bridgman, MI

Shirley Cole
Shirley Hoag

Team 3

Patterson-Kennedy Elementary, Dayton, OH
Cheryl Zinck
Molly Spears
Heidi Riffle
Debbie Tauber
Joan Morgan

Team 4
Northeastern Elementary,
Kalamazoo, MI
Lisa Barkovich
Wilma Virkus

Team 5
Upper Elementary,
Kalamazoo, MI
Heidi Nestell
Flo Thole

Team 6
Edison School,
Kalamazoo, MI
Nikki Jenkins
Marsha Bettison

1999–2000

Washington Writers'
Academy Development
Team Members

Barbara Witzak
Dawn Chamberlain
Anne Lape
Christy Roth
Kathy Sandow
April Widner
Beverly Wilson
Sylvia Washington
Charlene Cromwell

Graduate Assistants

Karey Hill
Anna Putnam
Melanie Lynam

Outreach Teams

Team 7
Comstock, MI
Laura Jane Van Niman
Shawn McMeekan
Janet DeZwaan

Team 8
San Antonio, TX
Karen Biggerstaff

Team 9
Amarillo, TX
Mary Ann Ellis

Team 10
Kalamazoo, MI
Irma Johnson

2000–2001

Spring Valley Center
for Exploration
Development Team
Members

Kevin Campbell
Angela Neaton
Shirley Schostarez
Karie Hokenmaier

Graduate Assistants

Karey Hill
Carrie Kopitzki
Kathy Enslen

Outreach Teams

Team 11
Battle Creek, MI
Carol Sewell

Team 12
Arcadia Elementary,
Kalamazoo, MI
Fran Bartocci
Tracy Wilson

Team 13
Central High School,
Kalamazoo, MI
Fannie Charles

Lynel Hackley
Linda Lee

Team 14
Lincoln Elementary,
Dayton, OH
Elizabeth Damico
Maura Fitsgerald

Team 15
Parkwood Elementary,
Kalamazoo, MI
Susan Dragt
Kristin Vankirk
Mindy McNulty

2001–2002

Spring Valley Center
for Exploration
Development Team
Members

Kevin Campbell
Laura Zigmont

Upper Elementary
Patty Buckingham

Michelle Keene
Jennifer Garrow
Dawn Hosler
Sarah Corwin

Second Grade
Julie Jones
Beth Vargas
Cheryl Wright

Graduate Assistants

Carrie Kopitzki
Amanda Luna-Bailey
Kristen Kopacz

*To all of the children and adolescents,
families, teachers, special service providers, and
graduate students who influenced this book*

Introduction

The mission of the writing lab approach is to foster language knowledge and skills among all students (including those with disabilities) that are sufficient to support them in their communicative interactions—whether listening, speaking, reading, or writing—in inclusive academic and social contexts. The purpose of this book is to foster the development of interdisciplinary writing lab teams who will adopt the mission and adapt the methods of the writing lab approach, making it their own, with the result that students for whom they share ownership will achieve success as learners and literate language communicators.

Our mission is consistent with a renewed commitment around the world to help all people become literate. Literacy and power concerns are not just Third World issues. In projecting health care needs for the 21st century, G. Reid Lyon, Ph.D., Chief, Child Development and Behavior Branch, National Institute of Child Health and Human Development, NIH, estimated that reading would be a "formidable challenge" for 60% of the children entering schools in the United States, with 20%–30% of those children finding literacy development to be the primary challenge of their academic careers (1998, p. 2).

In this book, we support the literacy learning process and educators who facilitate it by describing computer-supported writing process instruction as a means to language and literacy development. We call this a writing lab approach in order to emphasize the importance of computers and individualized assessment and instructional practices. It is a dynamic approach that allows for considerable flexibility to fit varied collaborative contexts.

The ideal writing lab includes opportunities for students to use an actual computer laboratory or transportable laptops, with sufficient stations for all students in a class. Modifications are possible, however. Although far from ideal, many of the writing lab components could be implemented in classrooms with only a few computers at the back of the room.

The writing lab approach is intended to be curriculum-based and inclusive, but we have implemented writing labs in many other contexts, including after-school university- and school-based clinics and summer programs. The essence of this approach is not where it is implemented, but how it is implemented—that is, with an integrated implementation of the three key components: writing process instruction, computer supports, and inclusive practices. As noted previously, the mission of the writing lab approach is to help all students—both with and without special education needs—to connect listening, speaking, reading, writing, and thinking. The intended outcomes are literate language, effective listening and linguistic expression, and the self-confidence to continue to grow.

The primary audience for this book is the group of educators who share responsibility for helping all school-age children become literate. We use the terms *educa-*

tors and *instructors* interchangeably to refer both to general education classroom teachers and specialists. Among the specialist group, we include speech-language pathologists, special education teachers, reading specialists, and others concerned with educating children with special needs. Parents and students are part of the target audience as well. Our intention is that teams of professionals and family members will use the book as they plan their versions of a writing lab approach in their own educational settings. In addition, we hope that undergraduate and graduate students in technology and language and literacy courses (both general and special education) will find the book meaningful as they prepare to turn theory into practice in their own work.

The writing lab approach can be used with students across all ability levels and ages. In this book we focus particularly on meeting the needs of students having difficulty learning spoken and written language—some of whom have been assigned special education labels, but not all. A major strength of the writing lab approach is that it can be appropriately challenging for all authors—from beginner to expert. Just as we refer to all professionals as educators or instructors, we refer to all school-age writers as students or authors. Our examples come from our work with student authors from early elementary school to high school.

The book is organized into three sections, which correspond to the three major components of the writing lab model as shown in Figure I.1. Section I addresses the writing processes part of the model. Section II describes computer supports, and Section III focuses on inclusive, collaborative practices.

Stories of change are woven throughout the book. These are drawn from the work of students who have participated in our varied computer-supported writing lab experiences. The case studies, often set apart in boxes, demonstrate how to use the integrated elements of the approach to plan intervention and to facilitate and monitor change for individual students. They also provide evidence for the changes that the writing lab approach can foster.

In Section I, Chapter 1 introduces the writing lab model, emphasizing a writing process approach to instruction and the values and BACKDROP principles that motivate all decision-making and activities. These principles, which are woven throughout the book, are balance, authentic audience, constructive learning, keep it simple, dynamic, research and reflective practice, ownership, and patience. Most of the chapters in this book can be read in any order, but we recommend reading Chapter 1 first and returning to it after initiating the writing lab approach. This will help to keep the values and principles in their central place as other aspects of the lab are developed.

Chapter 2 describes the language skills the writing lab is intended to promote. It provides a primer on the five systems of language—phonology, morphology, syntax, semantics, and pragmatics. It also introduces our system of categorizing language levels for assessment and intervention. This system is designed to help instructional teams think about language targets at the discourse level, sentence level, word level (including spelling), writing conventions level, and for other spoken communication abilities. The language target areas are treated in greater depth in later chapters. For example, Chapter 5 describes how to scaffold growth within each of these target areas. Chapter 15 (Section III) describes how to analyze individual students' current levels of performance, based on written language samples, using the same organization for characterizing language targets. Chapter 16 describes how to establish instructional goals, objectives, and benchmarks, again using the same framework of language and communication targets.

Chapter 3 focuses on students with and without disabilities who can benefit from a writing lab approach. It links their needs to the opportunities of writing process instruction for all students. The review of literature in Chapter 3 is organized to illuminate what is known about effects of disabilities on each stage of the writing process. It also discusses the needs of students who are second-language learners.

Chapter 4 describes the actual procedures for setting up a writing lab and establishing a daily routine. It also describes other aspects of writing lab organization and implementation—identifying and planning projects within the regular curriculum, using the computer lab, designing minilessons, providing author notebooks, establishing peer and teacher conferencing routines, and maximizing the effectiveness of author chair and other presentation opportunities.

Section I ends with two chapters focused on the critical individualized instructional technique of scaffolding. Skillful scaffolding on the part of the instructional team is key to providing intervention that allows the writing lab to be therapeutic for those who need it and educational for all.

Chapter 5 introduces the basics of scaffolding and its relationship to executive functioning and self-regulation. This chapter describes scaffolding as a set of strategically implemented techniques (framing, focusing, feeding back, and guiding) that instructors use to help students make sense of cues they have previously missed, and to conceive of themselves as authors with good ideas. This chapter ends with a series of profiles that characterize some students at different stages of development—paper wadder, fragile beginner, avoider, reluctant writer, perfectionist, quick to finish, risk taker, and independent learner. It offers suggestions for scaffolding students with each of these profiles.

Chapter 6 continues the discussion on scaffolding. It first focuses on scaffolding techniques for supporting each stage of the writing process—planning and organizing, drafting, revising, editing, publishing, and presenting. Then, it describes scaffolding techniques for addressing language development targets at the discourse level, sentence level, word level, writing conventions level, and for spoken communication.

Section II introduces a taxonomy of features for supporting all stages of the writing process. The first five chapters describe software and computer access features that support students as they engage in each of these recursive stages. Features are introduced and described, with examples of software that offer each feature. The chapters of Section II then provide considerations for use of each feature, including research evidence where available. These chapters also provide teaching tips, based on our experience and reports of our colleagues, regarding ways to introduce many of the features and to take advantage of the learning opportunities they offer.

Chapter 7 reviews features that support planning and organizing. These include idea generation tools that are both graphics based and text based. Organizational aids also are discussed relative to their graphics-based and text-based features.

Chapter 8 reviews features that support drafting. These include picture symbols, word prediction and other word list tools, abbreviation expansion and macros, collaborative writing, and speech recognition software.

Chapter 9 reviews features that support revising and editing. These include standard editing tools, such as cut-and-paste, delete, and insert. Such tools generally are quite familiar to adults who use word processors, but they need to be introduced systematically, along with their vocabulary, to students who are first learning to use word processing software. Other features covered in Chapter 9 are spelling checkers, homonym checkers, grammar checkers, and on-screen manuals. Chapter 9 ends with a discussion of speech synthesis. Speech synthesis is a particularly important feature for students with limited reading abilities. It provides feedback for revising and editing, but speech synthesis also might play important roles in supporting other stages of the writing process.

Chapter 10 describes software features that support publishing. First, Chapter 10 describes desktop publishing features, including basic features, book formatting, and alternative publishing formats. Then, it describes features that support desktop presentation of published works. These include multimedia options, electronic book formatting, and publishing on the web.

Chapter 11 describes keyboarding, including features of instructional programs and considerations for their use. It also describes specialized access for students with motor, sensory, or cognitive disabilities.

Chapter 12 closes Section II by suggesting ways that educators can use the information in the previous five chapters to make software selection decisions. It describes the basics of locating text-processing software and examining it for the features that were reviewed in the previous chapters. A form is provided to summarize the evaluation results. This allows writing lab teams to keep track of the features of the software programs they are considering. Chapter 12 also recommends that decision making include a process designed to match software features to individual students' needs.

Section III is designed to give readers information that will enable them to develop collaborative teams that function well. The chapters in this section also discuss the tools for conducting formal and informal individualized assessments, establishing goals and objectives, and measuring and documenting change. Section III ends with a chapter that presents both qualitative and quantitative evidence of the changes a writing lab approach can foster.

Chapter 13 focuses on supporting inclusion through collaboration, using the case study of a student to illustrate levels of inclusion from visitor to resident. It presents the perspectives of writing lab teams, using quotations from interviews held by our project evaluator, Dr. Kathryn Kinnucan-Welsch, with many of the educators who have worked with us in developing the writing lab approach. Chapter 13 also presents the voices of middle school students who described their perceptions of writing lab activities in interviews conducted by another special contributor, Kara McAlister, as part of her master's thesis research.

Chapter 14 describes formal and informal assessment processes. It includes a table with most of the available formal assessment tools that focus on the assessment of written language development. It also offers a review of commonly used methods for scoring written language samples—holistic, analytic or trait scoring (with rubrics), and quantitative measures. This chapter ends with descriptions of a variety of informal assessment methods, including portfolio samples and written language probes, with directions for gathering such probes.

Chapter 15 presents an assessment tool we have designed for analyzing written language probes. It starts with analysis of writing processes. Then, it describes techniques for analyzing written products at discourse, sentence, and word levels, and for writing conventions. The assessment process also includes methods for analyzing spoken communication in writing lab contexts. Where available, developmental progressions are summarized in tables to guide assessment and intervention planning. Chapter 15 uses a narrative probe case example to illustrate these procedures, but it also considers how similar methods could be used to analyze other forms of discourse, or to analyze portfolio samples gathered during curricular activities.

Chapter 16 focuses on the process of establishing individualized goals, objectives, and benchmarks for guiding instruction and marking progress. Using case examples, it describes how to take the information from the assessment process and weave it into a comprehensive plan. The chapter ends with a procedure and a form for engaging students in evaluating their own written products.

Chapter 17 provides two types of evidence to support the effectiveness of the writing lab approach. It provides qualitative case study evidence from students with special needs to demonstrate the progress that can be made when students with varying degrees and types of disability are engaged in a writing lab approach. It also presents the quantitative evidence from a series of three probes gathered across the school year in a group of third-grade classrooms in one inner-city school in which we worked.

Taken as a whole, this book should get any team started in adapting the writing lab approach to a variety of settings. We have planned the book to serve as a resource with the intention that individuals and teams will read the chapters and sections as they need them and return to them for refreshers after they implement the approach in their own settings. Throughout the book are stories written by and about the children and adolescents who have participated in our work. Through these stories, we hope to have communicated the joy of making a difference in students' lives. We think our readers will agree that the writing lab approach aproach is a far cry from the sterile and boring drills of years past. We have found students' original ideas and language to be a constant source of joy when providing intervention and instruction in this manner, but it is the students' improved language and literacy outcomes that cause us to share our experiences and evidence and to recommend these practices to you.

REFERENCE

Statement of Dr. G. Reid Lyon before the Senate Committee on Labor and Human Resources, 105th Cong. (1998, April 28) (testimony of G. Reid Lyon). Also available on-line: http://www.nichd.nih.gov/publications/pubs/jeffords.htm

Using the Writing Lab Approach to Provide Instruction

I

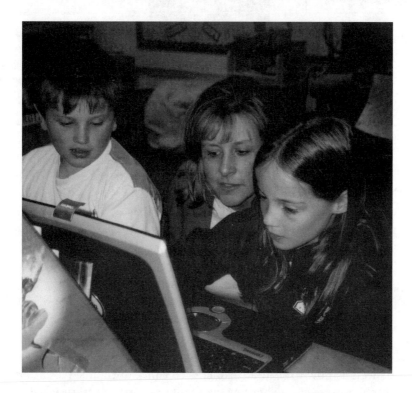

One of the greatest challenges facing educators is helping all children learn to read and write. Children who historically have been isolated from the power of literacy because of poverty or disability are now being included in initiatives aimed at helping all children learn and become literate. As part of this effort, special educators and other special service providers, such as speech-language pathologists (SLPs), are seeking new ways to address the needs of students with disabilities. The writing lab approach involves a set of educational activities that are equally and appropriately challenging for the brightest, most capable students and for students with the most dramatic special needs.

Section I introduces the writing lab approach and provides background for understanding the writing process approach, school-age students with special language and

Computer-Supported Writing Lab Model

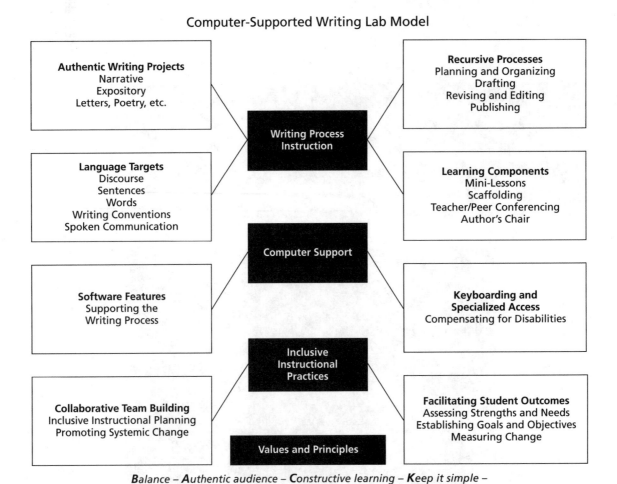

Authentic Writing Projects
Narrative
Expository
Letters, Poetry, etc.

Recursive Processes
Planning and Organizing
Drafting
Revising and Editing
Publishing

Writing Process Instruction

Language Targets
Discourse
Sentences
Words
Writing Conventions
Spoken Communication

Learning Components
Mini-Lessons
Scaffolding
Teacher/Peer Conferencing
Author's Chair

Computer Support

Software Features
Supporting the
Writing Process

Keyboarding and Specialized Access
Compensating for Disabilities

Inclusive Instructional Practices

Collaborative Team Building
Inclusive Instructional Planning
Promoting Systemic Change

Facilitating Student Outcomes
Assessing Strengths and Needs
Establishing Goals and Objectives
Measuring Change

Values and Principles

*Balance – Authentic audience – Constructive learning – Keep it simple –
Dynamic – Research and reflective practice – Ownership – Patience*

Figure I.1. Major components of the writing lab approach. (From Nelson, N.W., Van Meter, A.M., Chamberlain, D., & Bahr, C. [2001]. The speech-language pathologist's role in a writing lab approach. *Seminars in Speech and Language, 22*(3), 211; adapted by permission.)

learning needs, and the comprehensive language and communication skills that are targeted with the writing lab approach. This section also describes how to set up a writing lab, as well as how to scaffold students to think of themselves as authors and how to scaffold them to reach higher levels of language and communication functioning.

The writing lab approach includes three major components (see Figure I.1):

- Writing process instruction

- Computer support

- Inclusive instructional practices

The three major components of the approach also provide the organizational structure of the three major sections of the book. Section I addresses writing process instruction; Section II focuses on computer supports; and Section III tells how to optimize inclusive, individualized, collaborative practices.

A writing process approach is ideal for helping all students acquire literate language and certainly is not unique to special education. Writers' workshops are already common and accepted within general education classrooms across grade levels. The variation we describe in this book is unique because of its focus on using a writing process approach for meeting the individualized needs of students with disabilities while appropriately challenging typically developing students. This approach systematically integrates computer use for supporting all stages of the writing process and uses collaborative practices in classrooms and computer labs to foster the participation and inclusion of all students. The approach also is clearly within the purview of general education, yet is ripe with opportunities for special educators and SLPs to work directly with students on their individualized education program (IEP) goals in general education classrooms. It is designed for implementation in inclusive environments, but elements of the approach can be adapted and integrated into other service delivery models.

Chapter 1 introduces the writing lab approach and the inclusive computer-supported writing-process instructional components, including the BACKDROP principles that underlie the other activities and decisions that make up the writing lab approach. BACKDROP is an acronym for *b*alance, *a*uthentic audience, *c*onstructive learning, *k*eep it simple, *d*ynamic, *r*esearch and reflective practice, *o*wnership, and *p*atience. We recommend reading Chapter 1 first and returning to it after reading and implementing aspects of the other chapters in order to reap its important messages to the fullest. Most of the other chapters can be read in any order.

Chapter 2 provides a primer on the five systems of language—phonology, morphology, syntax, semantics, and pragmatics—for those who are less familiar with them or would like to review them. Chapter 2 also introduces our system of categorizing language levels for assessment and intervention—discourse-level, sentence-level, word-level (including spelling), writing conventions, and other spoken communication abilities. It is an introduction to areas that are treated in greater depth in Chapter 15, which describes our recommended procedures for language sample analysis.

Chapter 3 introduces the written language needs of school-age students with language-learning disabilities and other disabilities who need and can benefit from a writing lab approach. It links their needs to the opportunities of writing process instruction for all students. It also discusses students whose special learning needs stem from second-language learning.

Chapter 4 describes the actual procedures for setting up a writing lab and establishing a daily routine. It also describes other aspects of writing lab organization and implementation—identifying and planning projects within the general curriculum, using the computer lab, designing minilessons, providing author notebooks, establishing peer and teacher conferencing routines, and maximizing the effectiveness of author chair and other presentation opportunities.

Chapters 5 and 6 discuss scaffolding as the key technique of individualized instruction and intervention. Chapter 5 introduces the basics of scaffolding and how it relates to concepts of executive functioning and self-regulation. It also discusses scaffolding techniques for framing, focusing, giving feedback to, and guiding students to make sense of cues that they have previously missed and to conceive of themselves as authors with good ideas. Chapter 5 ends with a series of profiles that characterize some students— paper wadder, fragile beginner, avoider, reluctant writer, perfectionist, quick to finish, risk taker, and independent learner—accompanied by suggestions about how to scaffold their transitions toward becoming confident learners. Chapter 6 first focuses on scaffolding techniques for supporting each of the stages of the writing process—planning and organizing, drafting, revising, editing, and publishing and presenting. Then, it describes scaffolding techniques for addressing language development targets at the discourse level, sentence level, word level, and writing conventions level, as well as for spoken communication.

In summary, Section I describes the contexts of writing process instruction and how it can bridge gaps and extend language skills both for children who are typical learners and for children with language development difficulties. It provides the overview of the writing lab approach and how to implement it with regard to setting up the lab, designing projects, making the most of the learning contexts, and using scaffolding discourse to address individualized students' needs. Essentially any of the goals that can be targeted in traditional language and communication therapy, as well as any of the goals that can be targeted in general curricular requirements for written language use, can be addressed with the writing lab approach. The chapters in this section introduce the procedures for doing so, both at the classroom and individual levels.

Overview of the Writing Lab Approach

Some children breeze through school, communicating effectively and learning to read and write on schedule. Others struggle. Many students who struggle with school do so because of inadequate language abilities or abilities that are mismatched to the language demands of schooling. In this chapter, we introduce the writing lab approach as a method for helping all students develop their language and communication abilities to become more successful at school. Readers should note that writing lab approach is not capitalized. This is not an approach that requires abandoning all else, carving out a part of preexisting curriculum to make room for the writing lab, and following a set of procedures step by step. Rather, it is a way for general educators and special service providers to work together within the existing curriculum to address their mutual goals and help all of their students become literate and acquire communicative competence.

This chapter provides an overview of the writing lab approach and describes the BACKDROP principles on which collaborative teams base their plans and daily decisions as they implement the approach. These values and principles form the essence of the approach and make it flexible and adaptable to a variety of instructional contexts.

COMMUNICATION ABILITY AND CLASSROOM PARTICIPATION

Education both depends on and teaches communication. Students whose language skills support their learning come to the classroom with major advantages. Written language proficiency is a direct goal of schooling, particularly of the language arts areas of reading and writing. Spoken language also is a powerful force in determining a student's school and social success. Most of the activities of schooling are based on an implicit assumption that children come to school knowing spoken language and that they will be able to use that language to learn other things. Students with inadequate spoken language abilities are at risk for educational underachievement and academic failure.

Students with inadequate communication abilities and special education needs also are at risk for lower acceptance by their peers. It is ironic that students who have difficulty fitting in with their classmates are the ones who are often pulled out to work on the skills that are problematic for them. Pulling students with disabilities out of the classroom for decontextualized "fixing" exercises does little to address their isolation from the core learning enterprise. They miss opportunities to learn from and to interact with their fellow students. Equally important, their fellow students miss opportunities to learn from them. It also is not acceptable to keep students with disabilities included full time in general education experiences without special supports. Students who are present but not intellectually engaged reap few advantages from being in the classroom. The wide variety of students who can benefit from a writing lab approach is described in Chapter 3.

WHY USE THE WRITING LAB APPROACH?

Many researchers have noticed that sustained writing rarely occurs in general education classrooms; they have lamented its absence and have recommended that student authors emulate real authors (Cooper & Odell, 1977; Emig, 1971, 1977). That is, students who are learning to write should be real authors writing about their own ideas for an authentic audience (Hayes & Flower, 1980). A number of educators have subsequently interpreted the writing process for students in general education (Atwell, 1987; Calkins, 1983, 1990, 1994; Graves, 1983, 1994; Muschla, 1993) and special education (Bos, 1988; Erickson & Koppenhaver, 1995; Harris & Graham, 1996; Isaacson, 1989; MacArthur, Schwartz, & Graham, 1991a, 1991b; Mather & Roberts, 1995).

Writing process instruction now is a frequent feature of general education classrooms. The concept of a writers' workshop evokes for many educators a picture of students busy at their desks and/or computer stations, periodically communicating with peers and teachers about how well they are meeting their personal authorship goals. Teachers move about the room to help students by scaffolding their written and spoken language production. Students have a sense of ownership and goal direction as they work on individual projects within activities that are structured to a greater or lesser extent by their teachers. This picture, however, does not always include students with language-learning disabilities and other special education needs. Traditionally, such students have been pulled out of their classrooms, especially during language arts instruction, to receive language intervention services in separate speech-language therapy rooms and special education classrooms.

The frequent use of writing process instruction by general education teachers coincides with the widespread implementation of national- and state-level high-stakes testing. Many statewide tests, in fact, use a focus on writing processes and written language products to measure student progress and evaluate schools and school systems. Testing practices, although sometimes controversial, contribute to teachers' motivations to modify their classroom practices and to devote more planning and instructional time to helping all students acquire higher-level written language and critical thinking skills.

Along with forces influencing general education teachers toward more frequent use of writing process instruction, the Individuals with Disabilities Education Act (IDEA) Amendments of 1997 (PL 105-17) indicated for the first time that special education instruction must be designed to keep students with disabilities active in the general education curriculum. That is, a student's IEP must include "a statement of measurable annual goals, including benchmarks or short-term objectives, related to meeting the child's needs that result from the child's disability to enable the child *to be involved in and progress in the general curriculum*" (Sec. 614[a][1][A]; italics added).

Even prior to the implementation of IDEA 1997, special educators and SLPs had been urged to get "out of the broom closet and into the classroom" (Simon, 1987) and to be more relevant to their students' classroom- and curriculum-based needs (e.g., Deno, 1989; Merritt & Culatta, 1998; Nelson, 1989, 1990). Although special service providers share with parents the goal of making a difference in students' lives and helping students achieve meaningful outcomes that lead to school success, many remain uncertain about how to accomplish these goals.

The writing lab approach is designed to take advantage of the existing climate that values high levels of written language use and devotes classroom time to writing and small group interactions. It makes no sense to provide classroom-based service delivery if it means that special service providers serve primarily as classroom aides standing at the back of the classroom, participating with students only intermittently, while teachers lecture at the front. In contrast, the writing lab approach offers many opportunities for individualized work and small group activities, both in the classroom and in the computer lab, so that special educators and SLPs can work with students with disabilities in ways that help them become full members of their general education classes, learn better ways of interacting with their fellow students, and learn what their fellow students are learning.

The time is right for such an approach. Teachers are more welcoming than ever of classroom-based assistance if it can address existing goals and improve the written language abilities of all students. The writing lab approach is not an add-on or another curriculum for already stressed educators to implement. Rather, it provides opportunities for a team of educators, with parental support, to come together in a collaborative enterprise to address mutual goals.

WRITING PROCESS INSTRUCTION

Writing process instruction includes recursive writing processes, authentic writing projects, language targets, and learning components.

Recursive Writing Processes

In the context of writing process instruction, students are guided to reflect on where they are in the writing process and how well they are communicating to their audiences in writing. They learn to move deliberately through the recursive stages of the writing process, including planning, organizing, drafting, revising, editing, publishing, and presenting.

By focusing on writing processes and not just products, the writing lab approach encourages students to think of writing as a communicative event with a real audience of peers, parents, and others, not just an exercise that will be graded by teachers. Teachers also assume a nontraditional role. Rather than serving primarily to evaluate, correct, and grade, teachers facilitate, mentor, and collaborate with students. Teachers focus on helping students acquire new processes that will yield better products over time. The focus for students shifts from producing a transitory product for a grade to producing a published product that will be understood and appreciated by multiple readers. These characteristics are desirable features of a writing process approach whether it occurs within general or special education contexts—or both.

In this view, writing process instruction can vary along a continuum from mostly child centered to mostly teacher directed. We use the term *writing lab* to include both ends and many variations along the continuum. Essential features of writing process instruction in the writing lab approach include

- Focus on writing processes at least as much as written products

- Recursive movement among the processes of planning, organizing, drafting, revising, editing, publishing, and presenting

- Degree of student choice—if not full choice of topic and genre, at least choice as to how ideas are expressed within a particular project framework

- Clear sense of audience and of authorship as authentic communication

- Scaffolding tailored for achieving individualized objectives with measurable outcomes within the general education curriculum

Others may prefer such terms as *writers' workshop* to convey a similarly constructed set of learning experiences. Writers' workshops, however, often carry connotations of students beginning with free writing and having full control over topic, genre, and when and how they publish (Atwell, 1987; Calkins, 1986, 1994; Graves, 1983, 1994). In other words, they are completely student centered. Although the writing lab concept is compatible with writers' workshops and thrives in classrooms of teachers who have been trained to use a writers' workshop approach, it also can be introduced in classrooms in which teachers are worried about losing time for addressing the teacher-directed aspects of the curriculum.

In any case, the environment associated with writers' workshops should be encouraged. It involves establishing a classroom culture in which authors

- Choose their own topics

- Write for extended periods of time on the same piece

- Focus first on expressing their ideas and later on correctness—all for the sake of communicative effectiveness

- Engage in peer editing within a community of authors

- Reflect on uses of language to convey literal meanings but also to express ideas, communicate feelings, and trigger responses in readers

- Write for real audiences, including teachers, peers, and others

- Reflect on whether their language accomplishes its intended purposes

- Gain increasing control over how to allocate their time and other author choices

- Decide how long to work on a piece and when it is done

- Anticipate publication and participate in deciding how to format their documents

All of these elements, including those of choice and ownership, are valued and encompassed within our broader definition of *writing lab*. Although writing lab projects may have fewer degrees of choice in order to be consistent with a school's general education curriculum specifications, they still involve choice. For example, when a school's curriculum dictates completion dates for the production of a portfolio of poetry or a science fair project, students still can select their own topics and make choices about how to proceed.

Authentic Writing Projects

The two major factors that make writing projects authentic are *purpose* and *audience*. It is important for teams to build a sense among students that they are working on their own projects for real communicative purposes rather than completing assignments for a grade.

Encouraging student choice and ownership does not necessarily mean that students should exercise complete free choice in deciding what kind of projects they will work on. The writing lab approach is designed to be compatible with general education in the broad sense. All aspects of the curriculum present opportunities to work on authentic writing projects, and a degree of student choice can be built into any of them. Activities can be planned to further the objectives of the language arts curriculum but also those of science and social studies. Stories, reports, essays, letters, poems, and other discourse genre all present language-learning and communication opportunities.

Section I touches on the language demands and opportunities associated with varied genres (Chapter 2), strengths and difficulties experienced by students with disabilities in working with varied discourse genres (Chapter 3), suggestions for deciding on genres and planning projects (Chapter 4), scaffolding techniques for developing self-regulation and independence as authors (Chapter 5), and scaffolding techniques for encouraging development within varied genres (Chapter 6). In Section III, Chapter 13 addresses the relationship-building aspects of helping students discover the joys of authentic communication for an appreciative audience of their instructors, parents, and peers.

Language Targets

Chapter 2 introduces language targets at the levels of discourse, sentences, words, writing conventions, and spoken communication. Chapter 2 also relates language targets to language systems that children generally learn naturally, but which may require specialized instruction for students with disabilities. It provides a primer for the five systems generally used by language specialists to characterize language: phonology, morphology, syntax, semantics, and pragmatics. It also shows how to capitalize on the reciprocal relationships between spoken and written language to help students improve their skills across modalities and contexts. Chapter 6 describes scaffolding techniques for all levels of language targets.

In Section III, Chapter 15 describes individualized assessment techniques for analyzing probe samples and establishing individualized language targets. Chapter 16 elaborates on goal setting and shows how the writing lab approach can produce change among the language targets for individual students. Chapter 17 provides evidence from stories of change and group outcome data that the approach is effective.

Learning Components

The learning activities of the writing lab approach are conducted with students in general and special education classrooms working side by side at their desks or computer stations, with adults stopping by and helping them to reflect on their written language in order to improve it. Students with special education needs are included in all writing lab activities (a topic covered more fully in Chapter 13). Although these students may receive relatively more attention from their special service providers, students should not have adult instructors or assistants constantly hovering over them or they will not develop independent skills to carry over to other times and places.

Author chair, peer conferencing, computers, and joint reflection on drafted language can enhance language learning in the school-age years for learners with diverse abilities. Author chair is an activity where one student sits in front of the class to share his or her work, and peers have an opportunity to provide feedback on the work. Peer conferencing involves students exchanging their work and asking one another questions about areas that can be clarified. Students use computers to help them choose topics and organize their ideas, type in their work, add graphics or sounds, and print out their finished products. Joint reflection involves the teacher helping the student to evaluate the work, but the student decides what changes to make.

Although individualized needs may vary, all students share the need for approval of their ideas and guidance for growth. The computer-supported writing process fosters change for all students because it provides much-needed approval while challenging students in an individualized and strategic way. The outcome of the writing lab approach is that a child has a set of integrated cognitive, linguistic, and social skills that transfer readily to other academic and communicative contexts. Writing lab activities foster growth in spoken language for social interaction purposes, contribute to written language acquisition, and emphasize reciprocal spoken–written language relationships.

Group minilessons, for example, develop specific aspects of written and spoken language use. Author groups and peer conferencing work on spoken and written language communication skills. Author chair and other presentation experiences develop reading skills and self-esteem for student authors and listening, commenting, and questioning skills for student audience members.

Author notebooks are an important activity in the writing lab approach. Students create notebooks that include lab schedules and other organizational supports, as well as group minilesson handouts and individualized minilesson pages. The group minilesson handouts serve as print-based guides for building independent strategy use, and the individualized minilesson pages support personalized practice and review of targeted written and spoken language patterns. Students also store their drafts of works in progress in their author notebooks. These drafts are dated to show change and used in author groups for making handwritten edits. Conferencing records, completed with students to help them internalize stages of the writing process and to develop their skills for planning and evaluating their work, also are stored in the author notebook.

Early in the writing lab process, teachers negotiate with students to write classroom and individualized goals and objectives using "kid language" to assist students in developing personal ownership for instructional targets. A copy of these goals and objectives is included in the author notebook.

The writing lab approach has many classroom organizational supports, including

- Predictable routines, with alternatives for students at varying stages of the process, aimed at increasing independence and time on task

- Extended time to write, with at least 2–3 full hours per week devoted to the process

- Tools for writing and illustrating one's work, both computer supported and otherwise

- Posted references and other resources, including word walls and other environmental supports for student authors

Other features of the writing lab approach include computer software supports for all stages of the writing process, along with instructional strategies for helping students learn how to use them and design modifications for making less than optimal computer availability conditions work (topics covered in Section II). In addition, general and special education teachers, SLPs, paraprofessionals, and volunteers (e.g., parents, higher grade-level schoolmates, university students, community members) work as an interdisciplinary team on collaborative goals.

COMPUTER SUPPORTS

Computers clearly have changed the way people live, work, and play. During recent decades, exponential growth has occurred in the availability of computers in schools. In 1983, fewer than half of all elementary schools owned a computer, and the majority of schools had fewer than five to serve the entire student body (Becker, 1985). By the mid-1990s, nearly all schools in the United States were using computers (Ely, 1993), and approximately one computer was available for every nine students. The ratio continued to improve through the late 1990s, and by the end of the 20th century, computers were more prevalent than televisions in classrooms. In fact, they are becoming the most widely available type of instructional technology (Simonson & Thompson, 1997). It is not difficult to imagine that soon every child will have access to a computer for a significant portion of each school day.

The increasing availability of computers for students sets the stage to use computers as a central tool for helping school-age students with and without disabilities to develop their language skills through the writing process (Zeni, 1990). Computers can support weaker writers to improve the quality of their writing, add to the sense of playfulness in writing, and provide support for knowledge-building communities (Bangert-Drowns, 1993; Daiute, 1989, 1990; Scardamalia & Bereiter, 1994). Simply providing computer supports, however, is not enough. Computer use and word processing alone do not lead to improvements in written language. Effective instructional practices also are needed (Harris & Graham, 1996; Isaacson & Gleason, 1997; MacArthur, 2000; MacArthur, Graham, & Schwartz, 1993).

Many variables influence how authors perform with word processors (Erickson, 1992). It takes more than simply putting a student in front of a computer to get him or her to write, but computer software features can be highly motivating to students who initially are reluctant to write (see Chapter 5). They also can be used to support students with special needs and to compensate for sensory or physical disabilities (see Chapter 11).

Software Features for Supporting Writing Processes

Writing process approaches certainly can be implemented without computers, but in Section II, we show how computer software features can support all stages of the writing process. Throughout this book, we highlight the learning opportunities computers can provide. Most important, while working together at computers, educators focus jointly with students on students' own language. This provides opportunities to work on any objective that might have been targeted with more traditional language intervention approaches. Computer-based presentations and interactions also provide a context for peer interactions in which peers learn from each other (Daiute & Dalton, 1993; MacArthur, 2000).

When instructors mediate how students use computers, computer software features can serve as a tool to support students to higher levels of independent language and thinking, acting almost as a human scaffold might, but leaving students more immediately independent (see Chapters 5 and 6). By this, we mean that a combination of mediator input and software options can be used to frame cues, focus the students' attention, compensate for difficulties, and feed back information strategically. For example, a speech synthesis feature can feed back information that a student can use in revising and editing. Students' authentic efforts to make a written product clear and interesting creates a need for arriving at a stimulating topic, organizing the information effectively to achieve a purpose, selecting appropriate vocabulary and syntax to convey the ideas while drafting, and monitoring and editing correct uses of spelling and writing conventions while writing. Chapters 7–10 describe computer software features and instructional tips for helping students take advantage of those features.

Keyboarding and Specialized Access

Teachers and administrators express a range of perspectives on the importance of students learning keyboarding skills during the elementary years. No one doubts that it is a good idea. It is just a question of how to deal with limited instructional time and limited access to the school's computer lab. This situation may change as more schools are able to make computers readily available on a regular basis to all students. In her synthesis of early research on computer-supported composition, revision, and quality, Erickson (1992) noted that it takes extended time for students to become proficient with keyboarding, but that keyboarding requires more than knowing where the letter keys are located. Learning general word processing procedures and commands for inserting, deleting, moving, and reorganizing gives students access to the full capabilities of computer software for making the writing process easier. Our experience has shown that even primary students in first- through third grade can learn these features with only a few trials. Thus, students in early elementary grades can take advantage of many keyboarding features even though they are not yet proficient typists.

Computers hold special potential for meeting the written language needs of students with physical, cognitive, and learning disabilities (e.g., Blischak, 1995; Hunt-Berg, Rankin, & Beukelman, 1994; MacArthur, 1996; MacArthur, Schwartz, & Graham, 1991b; Sturm, Rankin, Beukelman, & Schutz-Muehling, 1997; Wood, Rankin, & Beukelman, 1997). Computers and computer software serve as the basic "pencil" for students who have limited motor abilities but who can activate a single switch (Beukelman & Mirenda, 1998). Becoming literate is an essential aspect of gaining access to education, social interaction (including the ability to generate completely unique messages), and the rewards of schooling and distance communication for students with cognitive and physical disabilities (Koppenhaver, Coleman, Kalman, & Yoder, 1991; Koppenhaver & Yoder, 1993; Light & McNaughton, 1993). Computers are an essential tool for helping all students benefit from the writing lab approach.

INCLUSIVE COLLABORATIVE PRACTICES

Students experiencing unusual difficulties with the literate language demands of schooling (see Chapter 3 for a review) come to the attention of various instructional specialists. For some, the general education teacher first notices the problem. Other children receive services from SLPs before they come to school (Catts, Hu, Larrivee, & Swank, 1994). Many students with special language and learning needs receive services from special educators and SLPs during their elementary and secondary school years. Some children who are referred for assessment do not qualify for intervention services even though their general education teachers are convinced that language and organization weaknesses are at the root of many of their academic difficulties (Constable, 1987; Sternberg, Okagaki, & Jackson, 1990). Others may receive services from Title I teachers or other general education instructional specialists, such as reading teachers.

The challenge is to provide supportive instruction for all students who need it, without offering a patchwork of isolated approaches in separate places that are confusing to students and less effective than a coordinated effort might be. When professionals collaborate across disciplines to provide integrated services to students and to support each other, students benefit from coordinated team efforts focused on helping them integrate disconnected spoken and written language fragments into higher levels of thinking and communicating.

Collaborative Team Building

The writing lab approach uses a transdisciplinary method of collaborative team building. This approach involves role release, as team members from one profession learn to implement some of the roles and methods of another. For example, in one team the general education classroom teacher might assist the SLP to acquire skill with whole class organization. The SLP, in turn, might show the general education teacher how to take advantage of oral–written language connections to scaffold invented spelling or how to get a reluctant talker to make contributions to group discussions. The team's special education teacher might offer assessment and intervention information about students on the shared caseload. All might learn from the team's occupational therapist how to apply positioning and handwriting strategies.

The success of this effort depends, in part, on the sense of common ownership among a team of professionals for educating all children, with and without disabilities, and the absence of turf protection. In Chapter 13, we describe approaches for achieving inclusive collaborative service delivery and show how turning points can occur when general educators begin to see students with disabilities as true members of the class and when students with disabilities also begin to see *themselves* as true members of the class. It is our interdisciplinary goal to promote sharing across territorial boundaries and to encourage professionals to interact with and learn from each other in the context of inclusive, collaborative computer-supported writing process labs for the benefit of all students.

Facilitating Student Outcomes

Shared understanding of the specialized needs of students with language difficulties can be established best on a foundation of shared understanding of the general education curriculum and shared expectations for developing spoken and written language within it. The "special" nature of this form of language intervention (or "special" education) lies more in its deliberate intentionality and intensity than in any uniqueness of the procedures it entails.

Chapters 14 and 15 describe strategies for assessing the language and communication strengths and needs of students with and without disabilities in the contexts of the writing lab approach. Chapter 16 describes how to write goals and objectives that promote language learning and address other goals in the IEPs of students with disabilities. Chapter 17 provides group outcome data and individual stories of change. Together, they illustrate the comprehensive processes of goal setting and instruction, and they provide evidence of the changes the writing lab approach can foster.

VALUES AND "BACKDROP" PRINCIPLES

Rather than following a set of prescribed steps, implementing the writing lab approach involves basing decisions on a set of guiding values and principles. The values of *respect* and *trust* provide the support for student-to-instructor, student-to-student, and

Table 1.1. "BACKDROP" principles

Balance
- Mediating the learning process requires balancing several competing needs.
- Accepting students where they are while scaffolding them to reach higher levels is critical for maximizing measurable outcomes.
- Assisting students to shift their focus between whole and part helps them become skilled, effective communicators in both written and spoken language.
- Keeping targeted objectives in mind while looking flexibly for teachable moments is the essence of individualized instruction.
- Curriculum-prescribed and student-centered activities and outcomes should be kept in balance.

Authentic audience
- Awareness of an interested audience is an essential element of good communication.
- Students need opportunities to write for authentic purposes and audiences.
- Teachers should show primary interest in a student's ideas and secondary interest in technical skill and correctness.
- Peers act as important primary audience members who can help each other evaluate their degree of communicative success.
- Parental and community values are important, and concerns about topic choices and technical correctness should be addressed.

Constructive learning
- Making sense with language and making learning stick both require active, reciprocal involvement in the construction of meaning.
- Constructivist instruction is designed intentionally to mediate experiences so that students can make discoveries on their own with scaffolding.
- In a constructivist approach, students learn to
    Organize their thoughts
    Select words to represent their meanings
    Become more observant of their world and its words
    Become sensitive to the ideas and needs of their fellow authors

Keep it simple
- Integrated instructional practices present wonderful learning opportunities, but also create danger of cognitive overload.
- Teachers learning new instructional methodologies might start with fewer collaborative partners and simpler writing projects.
- Planning should include consideration of cognitive load of students.

Dynamic
- The implementation of the writing lab model should remain dynamic.
- By using the BACKDROP principles to guide them, instructional teams can avoid the pitfalls of a static approach, which may become mundane and boring to teachers and students alike.
- Dynamic implementation keeps the model responsive to varying conditions, strengths, and needs.

Research and reflective practice
- Basing the implementation of the model on research keeps it fresh and maximizes the effectiveness.
- Existing literature supports the effectiveness of the writing lab model.
- Action research conducted by instructional teams while implementing the model can maximize its effectiveness for them.
- Reflective practitioners keep journals and analyze data in order to reflect on what works and what does not work and to improve their practice.

Ownership
- Authors should have ownership for their ideas, decisions, and personal goals.
- Self-generation of topics is possible for all students.
- Authors should have a sense of control and responsibility about writing decisions.
- Success occurs when student authors share with each other as much as with their instructors.

Patience
- Long-term payoffs justify interim patience.
- Focusing on process as well as product yields better communicators as well as better products, even though it takes more time.
- Granting students true ownership often leads to testing in the short run, but to better critical thinking, independent learning, and responsibility for personal choices in the long run.
- Collaborating across discipline boundaries is challenging and sometimes frustrating for all partners, but the long-term benefits are worth the effort.

collaborative team relationships. The eight guiding principles serve as a backdrop for the many decisions instructional teams have to make every day in the context of inclusive, computer-supported writing lab experiences.

Developing a writing lab is an evolutionary process with many stages and variations. The authors, with the support of the U.S. Department of Education, developed this approach in collaboration with administrators, classroom teachers, special educators, and SLPs in the Kalamazoo Public Schools (Nelson, Van Meter, Chamberlain, & Bahr, 2001), and in after-school laboratories and summer institutes where instructional teams came together from several states and grade levels (including high school). Each participant brought new ideas and unique talents to the process. Throughout this book, the activities we suggest are designed to get groups started or to get them to rethink current practices, but there is no one right way to implement the writing lab approach. Instructional teams that are dynamic and flexible while remaining guided and intentional can tailor instruction to integrate special intervention within the general curriculum across grade levels and settings.

The principles outlined in Table 1.1 provide the guidance for making instructional choices and evaluating the approach's effectiveness. To make these principles easier to remember, they are represented by the acronym BACKDROP—balance, authentic audience, constructive learning, keep it simple, dynamic, research and reflective practice, ownership, and patience.

Balance Principle

As we work with students in our own writing labs, we are often struck by the need to balance competing demands. On the one hand, we believe that building better and happier language users and writers requires an accepting attitude on the part of instructors, who delight in students' unique expressions of ideas and who encourage students to follow their own constructive pathways to make independent decisions. On the other hand, we know that students with special language and learning needs may not grow as fast or venture down developmental pathways as far as their typically developing peers unless they receive explicit instruction. The essence of education for all students is to provide adult mediation designed to challenge them to grow while supporting them in the process so that all may rise to higher challenges (Tharp & Gallimore, 1989).

In today's high-pressure educational environment, teachers face extreme demands to meet particular curriculum requirements, to prepare students for high-stakes district- and statewide testing, and to be accountable for measurable outcomes (Vaughn, Klingner, & Hughes, 2000). If a writing lab approach is to work for all students, the educational team must respond to such external pressures on teachers while addressing individual needs of students.

A writing process approach to language intervention involves establishing a classroom culture in which students feel safe to try out new skills and strategies while maintaining a routine that helps them structure their time and use it wisely. The process must allow students to gain a sense of control over their writing, but it must also challenge them to learn new skills that they might not otherwise attempt on their own. It must help them see writing as an opportunity to produce whole discourse while instructing them directly in the linguistic elements missing from their knowledge and skills. An example of possible results when students are encouraged to take risks in a safe environment is illustrated in Box 1.1.

Box 1.1.   Implementing the Balance Principle

Marcus, a fourth grader, was participating in Computers Researching Exploring Writing (CREW) Lab, an after-school writing lab we offered in his elementary school. The lab was held in the school library. Although only a few computers were in the library, we collected others from nearby classrooms and rolled them in two times per week when the students stayed after school for lab. In this writing lab, we targeted expository language exclusively after collaborating with the fourth- through sixth-grade teachers, who were concerned about their students' abilities to handle expository writing on upcoming statewide tests.

Marcus was referred by his teacher for help on his written language. He was a personable, gentle child with an engaging smile and a kind spirit. Although Marcus was not identified as having a disability, his teacher and mother reported problems with attention, self-regulation, and both spoken and written language. Marcus's mother and teacher had requested he be included in the writing lab because they were concerned that reading and writing were holding him back academically, especially in the area of comprehension. They expressed a desire for Marcus to show greater motivation to improve his skills and independent ability to complete his assignments.

Marcus needed both acceptance of where he was and expectation to attempt higher-level skills. He also needed a balance of intervention targets across a range of language levels and strategies. With his SLP, Marcus established a page of goals for his author's notebook, which appears in Table 1.2. All of these goals could be targeted within the balanced activities of the writing lab.

Table 1.2.   Marcus's goals

1. I will organize myself. I will set 3–5 things I'll get done every day. I will write them down and check them off when I am done.
2. I will work on my writing—I will write paragraphs using sentences that go together:
    One beginning sentence (What is this paragraph going to be about?)
    At least three sentences (facts) from my notes.
    One closing sentence.
   I will put periods and exclamation points at the end of my sentences (at the end of each idea).
   I will put capitals on the beginning of my sentences.
3. I will work on my reading
   Before I read
    I will look at pictures and writing under them.
    I will read the titles.
    I will ask myself, "What will this be about?"
   While I read
    I will read over or ask somebody when I don't understand what I read.
   After I read
    I will stop after each paragraph and ask myself, "What did I read?"
4. I will work on my listening.
   I will look at people every time they are talking.
   I will ask somebody when I don't understand directions.

Authentic Audience Principle

The authentic audience principle takes into account the role that audience plays in any communicative event. Effective speakers and writers make choices about what to say based on assumptions about the informational needs and stylistic preferences of their audiences (Grice, 1975). When instructional teams design writing experiences to have authentic communicative purposes and audiences, they can use these elements to help students become more reflective writers.

Peer conferencing, author groups, and formal presentations for parents and others all offer opportunities for instructors to scaffold students to higher levels of communicative competence. Teachers, peers, and parents act as authentic audience members to help students acquire this sensitivity and to move forward, as illustrated in Box 1.2.

Conflicting standards of correctness can be viewed as issues of audience. At one point, our school district's administrators had a strict policy that work could not be published unless it was completely free of grammatical, spelling, or punctuation errors. First, second, and third graders are not yet ready to complete all of these steps constructively and independently without a huge investment of time scaffolding them to use correct writing conventions, often at the expense of other concerns. One strategy we devised was for adults to sit with students at the computer at the publishing point, with adults typing on the keyboard, conferring about edits, and holding students increasingly responsible for editing decisions. Although this strategy involved less constructivism and ownership than we liked, it responded to the concerns of an important audience and allowed students to move stories to the level of publication. Other stories were stamped with a label that identified them as "works in progress," and one teacher mounted two versions side by side in portfolios, the final published version next to the student's best independent effort.

Audience concerns from parents and other adults about controversial content in students' stories, such as violence, slang, or dialectal language, can be treated as learning opportunities as well. Our strategy with late elementary to high school students has been to conduct classroom discussions on audience values during which students set limits and standards for their writing that coincide with the boundaries of policies and preferences of their schools, parents, and other important audience members. Students identify who will read their stories and discuss what those groups will expect. Then, they decide on appropriate guidelines. This can present opportunities for class discussions that lead students to engage in higher-order thinking.

For many students, the most important audience—the one that can motivate them as no adult can—is their peers. Many writing lab activities, such as author chair and peer conferencing, are designed to take advantage of students' natural desire to be valued by their peer group. We have been amazed to see the rapt attention that students give to each other when they read their works. Watching a student who is being included for the first time experience the pleasure of reading from the author chair gives the instructional team a strong feeling of satisfaction. With scaffolding, author chair experiences can provide the context for a class of students to express acceptance of a student who heretofore had been unaccepted socially.

Box 1.2. Implementing the Authentic Audience Principle

Zak was a sixth-grade student in the CREW Lab. He had a difficult time starting a task or even staying seated in front of his computer, which seemed to press his instructors toward heavy-handed, authoritarian demands. We responded by establishing consistent expectations for Zak to write, while providing scaffolding to help him select his research topic, take notes, and write about the topic. In the first project, Zak decided to write about Porsches, but when it came time for the publishing party, he had produced only a few sentences. One of them was incomplete, showing a pause in the heavy scaffolding that had been required to keep him writing:

> A Porsche is a very fast sports car and it is made in Germany . The first Porsche was made in 1948 . The first person that made the Porsche was Ferdinand Porsche. He invented and made the Porsche at 25 years old. . THAT THE PORSCHE LOOK DIFFERENT AND MORE HIGH TECH TODAY.
> And it can go from 0 to 60 MPH in 4.4 SECONDS . It can stop from 125 to zero in 5.0 SECONDS. The Porsche top speed is 180 MPH.

Zak loved an audience. He got down to business on the day of the publishing party when he arrived in his dress clothes, prepared to read his first published piece aloud. He was in the midst of his presentation when he realized that he needed help from his instructor to revise the incomplete sentence. He first asked the audience in a mature way to wait a minute. Then, after a quick conference with his clinician, he informed his audience that he would be starting over and reread the piece with the revision.

The next project involved writing expository pieces about space. Zak selected the topic of black holes with minimal scaffolding but soon was back to his pattern of avoidance. Again, as the publishing party date approached, he had written little. This time, however, Zak knew what would happen if he did not finish his piece. We learned from the school librarian that Zak had asked his mother to take him to the city library to gather some additional information about his research topic, and he had arranged to use a computer in the school library to add detail to his article. He also revised one sentence independently and produced capital letter edits in the title and to start a sentence. The published version, with Zak's new information in the second paragraph, follows.

> Black Hole
> Black holes are one of the most phenomenon objects in space. It is so powerful it can suck up light and it could not come out. The reason why black holes are where they are because of the big bang theory. The big bang theory is the reason why everything is here today . It was formed over 20 billion years ago.
> But then later at about 14 billion years ago black holes, white holes, and worm holes where formed. I bet that some of you are thinking what would happen to me if I got stuck in a black hole, well the answer is that you would get over heated or melted why because there is alot of energy trapped inside.

Constructive Learning Principle

Making learning "stick" and making sense of language both require active, reciprocal involvement in the construction of meaning. Constructivist instruction is designed intentionally to mediate experiences so that students can make discoveries on their own with scaffolding. It is important that students learn to use self-regulatory strategies when involved in this process or they may become dependent on their instructors (Graham & Harris, 1997; Harris & Graham, 1996; Hogan & Pressley, 1997; Tharp & Gallimore, 1989).

Constructivist approaches focus on teaching students to use self-questioning strategies to guide themselves through the writing process with systematically reduced scaffolding (see Chapter 5). When the focus is on constructing meanings for appreciative audiences, students learn to organize their thoughts and select words to achieve communicative purposes. In the process, they learn to become more observant of the world and how words can be used to talk about it. In addition, they become more sensitive to the ideas and needs of their fellow authors, as illustrated in Box 1.3.

Keep It Simple Principle

When implementing any new instructional practice, it is important to maintain one's own perspective. It is also important to control the number of competing demands on all of the participants—teachers as well as students. When instructional demands include, for example, an unfamiliar discourse genre, taking notes from challenging texts, incorporating core democratic values from the district's social studies curriculum, editing for all writing conventions, and adding a new student with challenging behaviors, the demands may be overwhelming for everyone.

Together, the team needs to set a reasonable number of new demands to tackle at one time—for both themselves and their students. Teams can adopt the keep it simple principle to remind themselves to control the complexity. They can do this by keeping track of the number of factors that are new (e.g., cognitive, communicative, discourse genre) as they plan a project, as well as the levels of complexity and abstraction inherent in each. Awareness can lead to strategic decisions about how to up the ante systematically for the instructional team and students without overwhelming anybody (Tattershall, 2002).

The team might decide, for example, to spend the first session with a new student with challenging behaviors and emergent literacy abilities at a computer, with scaffolding to help this student learn interesting software features while the rest of the class engages in free writing at computers or at their desks. During this time, an adult whom the student already trusts could introduce key elements of the writing lab routine and construct a story jointly with the student, typing from dictation if needed and assisting the student to select clip art for stimulating ideas or illustrating the brief story. The session could end with students sharing from one of their pieces in the author chair to convey the joyful aspects of writing for an appreciative audience. This gives the new student an opportunity to present his or her work, with reading support from another student if needed. The introduction of the new genre could be allocated to the next scheduled lab session. It might involve a minilesson with a clear outline of key components that the planning team has brainstormed collaboratively, along with supports

Box 1.3. Implementing the Constructive Learning Principle

Marina participated in an after-school homework lab for middle school students. In this lab, the writing lab approach was combined with curriculum-based language intervention using the students' homework assignments as the learning context. Marina was an eighth grader who was a "classroom leader" in math, but who avoided any work that required her to read or write. When asked to produce her first story, Marina scrunched up her face, twirled her hair, and stared at the paper. With encouragement, but with no apparent planning or organizing, she finally produced a story of 71 words about a fight. In it, she repeated the phrase *to fight,* three times and the phrase *I did not want to* four times.

One day, Marina showed the clinician her writing assignment from class, but she said she did not know how to work on the assignment. Her SLP asked her whether directions had been given in class. Marina reported, "I didn't read them, but a guy in my class read them out loud." After further discussion, it was discovered that when someone reads aloud in class, Marina just sits back and relaxes. When Marina pulled out her next assignment, it became clear that she once again had not followed along in the classroom as another student read aloud, and she could not remember what the text was about. The clinician read the passage with Marina and, together, they began to seek the answers to the comprehension questions, but then Marina just looked around the room and rocked back and forth in her chair.

For Marina, goals were established within the writing process for her to take a more active and constructive approach to learning. Marina will:

- Use the first step of the writing process to plan and organize before beginning to write.
- Select varied vocabulary to describe events and situations, using a specific phrase only once within a paragraph.
- Use a read-aloud strategy to
    Make sure the writing makes sense
    Check for appropriate writing conventions and word endings
    Correct errors with minimal scaffolding

The day after Marina's passive listening approach was uncovered, she came in prepared to do her assignments. The clinician reported, "She quickly answered questions 1 through 4 and was able to explain her answers. She even asked me a question (to which she found the answer in reading), and put it on her vocabulary sheet without prompting. She said she could use the vocabulary sheet for tests and homework." Marina was becoming a constructive learner.

Marina also demonstrated her more constructive approach to learning during writing. For example, a few sessions later, in the context of writing paragraphs to enter in her journal, Marina produced the sentence, "I had the same coach from last year."

After using the rereading strategy, Marina said that what she meant to write was "softball coach." She deleted the original sentence. Then, she typed "I had they same softball coach from last year."

Again, Marina used the rereading strategy. This time she moved the cursor and deleted only the additional *y.* Marina was learning to construct meaning both while reading and writing, and she began to use that knowledge to approach other learning tasks.

Box 1.4. Implementing the Keep It Simple Principle

Belvatich (1997) was a middle school teacher who had decided to implement a writers' workshop approach. She had pored over Atwell's (1987) *In the Middle* and had pictured how her own writers' workshop would look. The first few months of real-life experience, however, taught her several lessons about keeping multiple demands in perspective.

In October, Belavitch began to evaluate some of the things she had been doing and decided that "First, keeping a journal for 120 students was completely idealistic. Idealistic is being kind; I was an idiot!" (1997, p. 42). Then, she decided that

> *There needed to be some individual instruction. The size of my classes— 32, 28, 29, and 27—made my task even more challenging. A lot of the assessment tools I was trying to implement, such as journal tracking of the students and meeting with each child every day, proved impossible. I needed much more structure to succeed in creating writers. I didn't want to start assigning topics because it went against the very teaching of process. However, in hindsight, topic assignments would have given me a grasp of students' capabilities and a starting place from which to work. I finally devoted a whole class session to discussing topic searching. (p. 44)*

---

that will help students in their research and planning. In addition, the range of topics could be limited to those for which resource books appropriate to the reading levels of the students could be located. These are just a few of the ideas a team might arrive at with the keep it simple principle as a backdrop.

Box 1.4 describes how educators can keep this principle in mind when setting expectations for themselves as individuals. Belavitch (1997) discovered this in her initial attempts to establish a writing workshop as a middle grades English teacher.

Dynamic Principle

The key elements of the writing lab approach are the components—writing process instruction, computer supports, and collaborative inclusive practices. How the approach is implemented, however, depends on the unique set of circumstances in a particular school and community. It is not a static model that must be implemented according to a rigid script and set of procedures. Rather, it is a dynamic one, which is expected to grow as each team implementing the approach grows in the members' mutual grasp of the principles and components and how to make them work in their unique situation.

In our experiences in developing the approach, we have found that each school-based team brings a unique set of strengths and its own school culture. Each team also grows in its own ways. When empowered to view the approach as dynamic, teams can focus on developing the approach further to achieve maximal outcomes in their own situations rather than feeling constrained by expectations to replicate a static model exactly as originally designed.

In similar ways, our hope is that the users of this book will start with the supports we provide, but go beyond them. We envision interdisciplinary collaborative teams, with parental and student participation, working to build a community of learners in their own schools. The strategies and materials in this book are intended to serve as tools of support for that dynamic process. By focusing on common goals to help all children become literate and successful as students and communicators, teams can create a writing lab learning environment designed to take advantage of their own contextual strengths and to address their particular needs.

Research and Reflective Practice Principle

One way to keep the approach dynamic is to base it on ongoing research conducted by those who are using it. The writing lab approach is grounded in others' research as well as our own (see Chapter 17). The research principle also emphasizes the importance of ongoing *action research* by instructional teams using the writing lab approach.

Action research, as described by Kinnucan-Welsch (2000), is also called teacher or practitioner research. It is based on the notion that teachers can link their practice with evolving theory and that the process can be a valuable source of knowledge about educational practice (Anderson, Herr, & Nihlen, 1994; Branscombe, Goswami, & Schwartz, 1992; Myers, 1985). Action research offers a unique opportunity to view life in classrooms from an insider's perspective (Cochran-Smith & Lytle, 1993, 1999).

Action research involves an ongoing cycle with several steps (Hubbard & Power, 1993):

- Frame a question.

- Gather data designed to answer the question.

- Analyze the data.

- Improve practice based on the analysis.

Like the writing process, these steps are implemented in recursive rather than lock-step, sequential order. Plans and questions can be modified along the way to be more relevant to current needs.

The *R* in BACKDROP also stands for *reflective practice*. When teams begin to implement the writing lab components of writing process instruction, computer supports, and inclusive collaboration, they begin an evolutionary process that extends over time. We have noted three broad phases. The first starts with building a collaborative team and establishing a routine in which all components of the approach are in place. During this phase, probes of students' writing are gathered and analyzed (see Chapter 15). This is also a time when it is helpful for team members to begin to keep reflective journals with dated entries noting what works best and their evolving thoughts about the process. The team often is guided by organizing questions about students' initial levels of functioning and how to make instructional activities run smoothly and yield positive results.

The second phase begins when the team has established a routine, permitting members to focus more on students' individualized objectives and how to accomplish them. This stage might involve a question about which scaffolding techniques and author group pairings help a student who typically avoids talking in the classroom to participate more actively. Another question might be which sound–symbol associations are under a particular student's automatic control. The classroom teacher might assume the lead role in gathering data to answer the first question, and the speech-language pathologist or special educator might assume that role for the second, but the entire team benefits from the answers.

The team begins to enter the third phase when the individualized focus feels more comfortable. At this point, the team can relax enough from meeting the routine demands of everyday practice to reflect on how the approach is working for them. At this point, the questions can be framed in a way that might lead to more generalizable knowledge. An action research question at this level, for example, might address whether more or less structured graphic organizers lead to different results for students with varied incoming abilities.

It is a challenge to frame questions that can be reasonably addressed. Practitioner researchers often start by asking broad questions, such as "How can I improve student writing?" or "How will computers support the writing process?" These are important questions but often too much to tackle. The trick is to frame a question that is broad enough in scope to be important, yet small enough to be manageable. Our colleague in writing this section, Kinnucan-Welsch (2000), advises team members to think of something that has frequently perplexed them or to think of one child who has posed some unique challenges. She suggests focusing on questions you have at the end of the day after working with that child.

Box 1.5. Implementing the Research and Reflective Practice Principle

When we work with classroom teachers to implement the writing lab approach, we gather assessment probes at the beginning, middle, and end of the school year. In one group of third-grade classrooms, after the second probe, our team met to reflect on the results, considering both the writing processes and products we had observed. Most of us had the same concerns: 1) many students had difficulty generating topics in response to the directions to write a story that should include a problem and what happened; 2) too many students seemed to struggle with the task and find little joy in story writing; and 3) the resulting products were less well-developed at the discourse, sentence, and word levels than we had hoped. We hypothesized that the students needed more opportunities for free writing—in which they would generate their own topics and pick their own genre—and more frequent use of the author chair (see Chapter 4).

We introduced a 15-minute free writing period at the beginning of the Tuesday and Thursday classroom writing lab sessions and had author chair activities at least once per week. (Fridays were in the computer lab.) The outcomes of these modifications were measurable as more time on task writing independently, students' explorations of varied genres, excitement at taking the author chair, and better feedback to peers in response to their free writing attempts. Reluctance to write and suppressed efforts were not a problem on the final probes, especially when the students were told they would do author chair on the stories they produced for that probe.

The notion of collecting data may seem daunting until educators realize that they collect data every day in their classrooms. Examining students' writing samples from the beginning of the year to the end is an example of collecting and analyzing data, which routinely occurs in many classrooms. Making tally marks as students volunteer suggestions during author chair or group discussions might be a way of collecting data on spoken language that could help answer questions about supports that help all children participate.

Schleper (1996) described a process for collecting anecdotal data from students who are deaf or hard of hearing. In his classroom, instructors carried clipboards with peel-off sheets of mailing labels. When any team member observed something to record, he or she wrote it on a mailing label with the student's name. Later, team members peeled off comments that related to a single student and placed them on a separate notebook page. What brings such routine observation and data collection into the realm of action research is the intentional connection between data collected and analyzed and the question posed (Kinnucan-Welsch, 2000).

Across time, a team's action research questions may evolve from how to get the process started, to how to make sure individual students are growing in specific targeted areas, to how to modify certain aspects of the process to maximize their effectiveness. By the third stage, we have seen teams begin to share their results and findings with others in their own schools and districts and broader regions. The research and reflective practices principle is illustrated in Box 1.5.

Ownership Principle

The ownership principle operates on two levels. First, all members of an interdisciplinary team need a sense of ownership for implementing the approach and helping students under their joint charge improve their academic and communication skills. Second, students need to feel a sense of ownership for the decisions they make as authors and as members of a writing community social group.

Ownership starts by giving students some control over the selection of their topics. It is important that instructors convey positive expectations that all students will be able to generate appropriate topics and that they will be given sufficient time to do so (Swoger, 1989). Authors also should have a sense of control and responsibility about writing decisions. In the process, students learn to be less dependent on adults for their learning and to communicate directly with their peers about works in progress. As a result, students with special needs begin to acquire ownership for their own decisions and self-confidence about their capacity to construct valuable ideas and contribute to the social climate of the classroom. The ownership principle is illustrated in Box 1.6.

Patience Principle

The patience principle (illustrated in Box 1.7) plays a central role in implementing a student-centered, collaborative writing lab approach. Focus on process means that works in progress may not look as mature as one would like. Granting students true ownership, however, means conveying trust in their ability to make authorship deci-

Box 1.6.   Implementing the Ownership Principle

Isaac was a seventh grader diagnosed with a learning disability, unilateral hearing loss, and speech-language impairment involving rapid speaking rate, imprecise articulation, and phoneme and syllable deletion. Isaac also had difficulty judging his listeners' needs. His instructors often were confused because of partially communicated meanings and unintelligible words. Features of African American Vernacular English appeared in both his spoken and written communication.

It was extremely difficult to get Isaac to write original stories. He was an expert at using avoidance strategies, but he also had a number of topical interests. His writings tended to focus on professional basketball players and recounts of their games, video game players and lists of their "fatality" moves, and instruments of war and battle statistics. Isaac's preferred writing style was a sketchy "play-by-play" genre, which generally started with enumerated lists of any of his favorite elements. The Mortal Kombat people, X-Men characters, or jet fighters and tanks were then removed as the battle proceeded.

Ownership was important to Isaac, but he often brought in books to copy names and statistics. We tried a variety of techniques to scaffold Isaac to produce more mature narratives than the temporal sequences he generally wrote. For example, we would ask him to explain what had caused a particular battle or to imbue his players or fighters with personal motivations. Our most intensive efforts, however, met with small success. Only occasionally would Isaac venture momentarily beyond his safe formula to consider how one of his players might feel or plan, or how effects in a particular battle scene might be influenced by causes. One example is this excerpt from a story called "America's Top Guns" (See Figure 1.1). By this point, Isaac had begun to use his listing strategy to plan, an example of which appears at the beginning of the first page of his story.

When he wrote personal narratives, Isaac was more effective at combining ownership with literary risk taking. (See Chapter 7 for the use of a story grammar scaffold that was effective for Isaac at an early point.) One of Isaac 's later stories, produced one year later, was titled "My Two Dogs." In this narrative, Isaac shows emerging ownership and responsibility for his actions as well as his topics, as well as growing awareness that actions have consequences.

MY TWO DOGS

THE FRIST DAY I WENT IN THE GARAGE AND FEAD MY TWO
DOGS. AFTHER I FEAD THE DOG I WENT BACK TO THE HOUSE.
THEN I LEFT THE HOUSE TO GO TO SCHOOL. AFTHER I CAME HOME
FROM SCHOOL I SAW KIZZY AND HOUND TO GET IN THE GARAGE.
THE NEXT MORNING I FORGET TO FEED MY DOGS. AFTER I CAME
HOME FROM SCHOOL, I SAW TRASH ON THE GROUND. I PICKED IT
UP OFF THE GROUND. AFTER I PICKED THE TRASH OFF THE
GROUND, I WENT IN THE GARAGE. I SAW TRASH ON THE GARAGE
FLOOR. THE GARAGE WAS A MESS. AFTER I CLEANED THE MESS UP,
I WENT TO PUT THE BOARD AGAINST THE GARAGE. THE NEXT DAY
I FORGET TO FEED MY TWO DOGS. AFTER I CAME HOME FROM
SCHOOL, THE DOGS WERE GONE.
THE END

Story #1
AMERICA'S
TOPS
GUNS

AMERICAN AIR POWER
APACHE: WILD
WEST WARRIOR
THE WEST WARRIOR IS THE FASTEST HELICOPER . 989 ROUNDES.
38 MISSILESAND 48 BOMBES
　　the f-15 eagle is a fighter plan
F-15 EAGLE f-15 has 1o missles and 48 rounds of machine guns
LOCKHEAD
BLACK BIRD is fastest -plane the in the world . the blackbird does
not have bombs or guns
F-112 STEALTH FIGHTER
Stealth fighter the fastest fighter plane . The stealth fighter have 4
missiles.

It is summer.. It is a clear weather.Today is monday. all the fighter planes at losan-
geles.They are at the navy station. The fighter go to training . The planes
took off the navy staiton . the ploits check the clouds to make sure if the
sky was clear . the clouds were clear . they saw there fighter planes in
the sky . The three planes fire the three missles .　　🍎 The emeny
planes blew down there planes . The ploits called in more planes .

🍎🍎🍎🍎🍎 One of the planes crashed nto the air froce base. More
planes took of and blew up three planes.

part 2
　　it is about fighters planes. tuesday morning the stealth fighter took
off . when the ploits woke up they saw the black bird taking off . three
emeny planes fire ten misslies at the blackbird . 🍎🍎🍎🍎🍎 . the black
bird blew up three planes . the stealth fighter blew up 12 planes . the
black bird landed on the air force base . the stealth fighter landed on the
air force base.
the f- 15 eagles took off . the f-15 eagles did in the air. 14 emeny planes
flew up the sky . the emeny planes fired 16 missiles , the f-15 eagles
fired 18 missiles . the 14 emeny planes crased into the navy base . the
war over .

part three

Figure 1.1.　Isaac's "America's Top Guns" story. *Note:* the apple logos embedded in the story represent sound effects that could be heard in multimedia playback of the story.

Box 1.7.　Implementing the Patience Principle

Bill was a third grader with a great need for structure and organization. He was the youngest participant in an after-school writing lab experience, which included mostly middle-school students. Bill's mother had referred him for language assessment as a preschooler because of concerns about his communication and social interaction skills. As a third grader, Bill's spoken language sounded like his peers'. His remaining difficulties were in the area of pragmatics. Bill also had low tolerance for frustration. He needed firm closure for each activity before switching and found it difficult to work on the same story for more than one day. Thus, it was difficult for Bill to use writing processes to work on a single piece over several sessions. In fact, in his early days in the writing lab, Bill seemed unable emotionally to leave a story unfinished from one day to the next. One of Bill's early stories about robots, which he wrote at the end of his fourth-grade year, appears in Figure 1.2.

We used the patience principle to accept Bill's need for daily completion in the short term. At the same time, we used the balance principle to target growth in Bill's flexibility and tolerance for change. Just telling him to write for more than one day on the same story was not effective. With his instructors' patient scaffolding, however,

Robots are Back Again

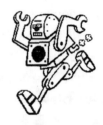

The robots are back again and they are big and bad and they killing people and they are recking down houses and they are livenig on are house and we have to stay in are house and not go outside. If we go outside the robots will kill us and we will never see are mom and dad and they will miss us.

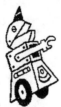

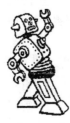

Figure 1.2.　Bill's robot story.

(continued)

Box 1.7. *(continued)*

Bill began to write about his main characters having an adventure, only to return in later chapters written on subsequent days, to have another and another. Bill devised a strategy of writing something like chapters, each of which ended with the phrase "to be continued..." At this stage (during the fall of Bill's fourth-grade year), his favorite topic was killer dogs. Although we were not thrilled with the violent theme, we exerted the patience principle in helping Bill to take difficult next steps. The first chapter of Bill's four-part series on killer dogs read:

> TODAY ON THE NEWS THERE WAS A REPORT ON THE KILLER DOG
> THAT WAS STILL LOOSE ON 24TH STREET. THEY CAUGHT THE
> PEOPLE WHO WERE TRETING THE DOG BAD. ONE OF THE PEOPLE
> WAS ABOUT 36 YEARS OLD. THE OTHER WAS 40 YEARS OLD. THEY
> WERE BOTH MEN AND THEY WERE NOT SMART. THEY SAID THEY
> WERE GOING TO PUT THE DOG ASLEEP. BUT THEY DID NOT KNOW
> THEY DOG NEW WHAT THEY WERE SAYING. SO THAT NIGHT THE
> DOG WENT OUT THE WINDOW AND GOT LOST. BUT THE OTHER
> NIGHT THE DOG CAME BACK AND KILLED THE PEOPLE WHO WERE
> BAD TO HIM! I'M GLAD THAT DID NOT HAPPIN TO ME. WELL ANY-
> WAY THE DOG WHO KILLED THE PEOPLE GOT RANOVER BY A CAR
> THAT WAS A VAN. THE TWO MEN CAME BACK TO LIFE AND THEY
> WENT TO JAIL. THE DOG WAS BURIED IN A GRAVE YARD AND WAS
> TO NEVER BE SEEN AGAIN. BUT ONE DAY THE DOG MAY COME
> BACK TO LIFE. THE DOG GOT RANOVER 24 HOURS AGO. BUT
> WHOEVER KNOWS, WILL THE DOG COME BACK TO LIFE?
> TO BE CONTINUED . . .

With patience, balanced with deliberate scaffolding, Bill was able to move beyond the bridging step. By the beginning of his fifth-grade year, he was willing to work on the same story over an extended period of time without having to finish one per day. He also had matured in his sense of story and had begun to write about much more positive relationships (although not entirely positive; he titled this story "Garfield Kicks the Dog"). By this point, Bill had given up the all-caps strategy and was writing in the voice of his alter-ego, "Dave Arbucle," using a more literary style with multiple episodes, figurative language, direct quotes, and clear character motivations. Missing from this rendition (which is true to the original in punctuation and spelling) is the imported clip art Bill added in the form of a cat, hamburger, and dog, which he used partially to plan his story (see Chapter 7) and partially to illustrate it (see Chapter 10).

> Today when I went in the kitchen for a midnight snack I herd a little
> noise outside, I opened the door and I saw a Dog and a cat in the
> snow. I took them inside my house and I kept them warm and fed
> them. I named them Garfield and Spot, soon they started recking

(continued)

Box 1.7. *(continued)*

my house. Today when I was eating, Garfield took my hamburger and said, "Thanks for the hamburger Dave, I love to eat."

I couldn't belief what came out of his mouth and what he said. The last time I came home, Spot and Garfield toleidly recked my house and I said,

"O.K. who recked my house while I was gone."

"I did," said someone from below.

Yes it was Garfield, that one big lousy cat. I looked in the ice box and there was nothing, just nothing in the ice box not even the ham, the RAW ham. Then I said to Garfield,

"Did you eat the raw ham Garfield."

"Did you say RAW HAM?" said Garfield.

Yes I said raw ham, before I said yes he ran through the hall into the bathroom and barfed in the toilet. Today when i went to my chair I saw Garfield sitting in my chair and playing on the computer. I said to him,

"Garfield I have to do some computer work, so get out of my chair.

"Not in your hole life I will not get out of this chair I won't, he said. "Make me get out of this chair."

So I did make him get out of the chair by using a hamburger to lead him in the kitchen for supper. While I was eating, Garfield was eating like a pig. I said to him

"Garfield you have the manners of a pig, stop hogging around and get out of here."

Then Garfield went to bed and forgot about everything till tomorrow.

Sincerely

Dave Arbucle

---

sions on their own. This requires strategic scaffolding in balance with explicit instruction and high standards while conveying patient expectation that students will make effective decisions as authors.

The patience principle also addresses instructional team challenges of collaborating across discipline boundaries. Collaborative working relationships, with shared responsibility for making decisions and providing instruction, are sometimes frustrating for all partners. At some point, almost everyone thinks, "It would be so much easier to do this alone." Working through the stiff early stages of a new collaborative relationship takes patience and recognition that the long-term benefits are worth the effort. We have found that, as trust builds, team members begin to enjoy moments of synergistic highs during planning and more frequent moments of enjoyed shared experience, both of failures and successes. In our team-building experiences, we have noted that the point at which members can feel safe about gently teasing one another about foibles represents a milestone toward truly becoming a team. It takes patience to reach that point, but it feels great when it arrives.

SUMMARY

The writing lab approach includes three major components—writing process instruction, computer supports, and inclusion of students with disabilities with their typically learning peers. Through writing process instruction, students are engaged in projects that take them recursively through all writing processes—planning, organizing, drafting, revising, editing, publishing, and presenting. The learning contexts of the writing lab include instructional scaffolding by transdisciplinary team members; minilessons; author groups and other forms of peer editing; author notebooks; author chair; and other forms of publication, presentation, and performance. Each of these components is discussed in greater detail in later chapters.

When implementing the writing lab approach, a team makes decisions against a background of values and guiding principles. The values are *respect* for individual students, their diverse cultural experiences, and their strengths and *trust* in collaborative partners and the research behind good instructional practices. The principles that form the BACKDROP for everyday decision making are balance, authentic audience, constructive learning, keep it simple, dynamic, research and reflective practice, ownership, and patience. Balance is achieved by accepting students' ideas and efforts while challenging them systematically to achieve higher levels of competence. Authentic audience opportunities are built into projects so that students learn to adjust their communicative attempts to achieve authentic purposes. Constructive learning opportunities are focused on meaning-making and mediated rule discovery as the pathway to higher-level independent language competence. The keep it simple principle is aimed at controlling the cognitive load on students, as well as on the instructional team. The dynamic principle reminds teams that the approach is flexible, not static. The research and reflective practice principle refers not only to the use of published research but to the conduct of action research and other reflective practices by instructional teams. Ownership is built into projects to help students assume responsibility for their own written language and learning, as well as to be assumed by instructional teams for how the approach is implemented in their own settings. Finally, the patience principle sustains teams through short-term frustrations or challenges to keep ownership in students' hands as they work toward long-term success together.

Language Targets

To understand the nature of language-learning struggles and to know what to target with the writing lab approach, it is necessary first to understand the nature of language. This chapter provides a primer about the five systems of language that characterize what language users need to know: phonology, morphology, syntax, semantics, and pragmatics. It also considers distinctions and similarities between spoken and written language forms and how to draw on reciprocal relationships to support language learning in the writing lab approach. Finally, it introduces the language targets and the structure we suggest for organizing individualized assessment and intervention activities.

FIVE SYSTEMS OF LANGUAGE

Language is complex and abstract, but it is also rule based. Competent language users can generate and understand an infinite variety of sentences that convey all varieties of meanings—literal and figurative, informational and emotional, social and personal. Among its most important interpersonal uses, language allows people to communicate socially with others and to learn about remote ideas and concepts. Among its most important intrapersonal uses, language allows individuals to guide their own thinking and, indeed, to find out what they think. It also allows them to control personal actions and procedures through executive control and self-regulation (Denckla, 1994; Graham & Harris, 1999; Singer & Bashir, 1999a).

Although individual users can be shown to have implicit knowledge of the rules of language, it is difficult to build an explicit catalog of those rules or to figure out what to teach first when children are not learning the systems of language automatically. We do not pretend to provide a complete catalog in this brief discussion, but we do outline some of the major elements of the five basic systems that are often used to describe language. Table 2.1 provides a summary of these interrelated and overlapping systems. In addition to this table, our intention is for instructional teams to refer to their own implicit and explicit knowledge of language systems as they build balanced and dynamic writing lab activities to target language growth objectives for individual students.

Phonology: System of Speech Sounds

The phonological system has come under increasing scrutiny as educators and researchers have gathered consistent evidence that children with weak phonological awareness abilities are at high risk for having difficulty learning to read and write (for summaries, see Blachman, 1994; Catts & Kamhi, 1999; Lyon, 1995). Phonological awareness involves the ability to focus directly on the way words sound. It requires a degree of metalinguistic skill; that is, a conscious focus on language as an object of attention as opposed to the automatic use of language as a tool to communicate a message (Menyuk & Chesnick, 1997). Phonological awareness and other metalinguistic skills generally are present when children reach school age, but even toddlers and preschoolers show budding signs of phonological awareness when they engage in word play and delight in the sounds of language.

The term *phonemic awareness* refers to the conscious awareness and manipulation of individual speech sounds within words. "It involves a more or less explicit understanding that words are composed of segments of sound smaller than a syllable, as well as knowledge, or awareness, of the distinctive features of individual phonemes themselves" (Torgesen, 1999, p. 129). Children who have reached the stage of phonemic awareness can hear a word, detect its separate speech sounds, and pronounce each one in sequence. Or they can listen to a set of isolated speech sounds and blend them into recognizable words.

Phonemic awareness usually is first observed among children in their early school-age years, around first grade. It is required any time a teacher asks students to tell what sound a word begins or ends with, and it plays an important role any time an emergent writer uses invented spelling to construct a word on paper. Although phonemic awareness is a developmental skill, many children, especially children whose homes have limited print-rich materials and children who have language-learning disabilities, do not develop it without special instruction (Catts & Kamhi, 1999; Snow, Burns, & Griffin, 1998; see also Chapter 3). A number of research studies have shown, however, that phonemic awareness can be taught (Ball & Blachman, 1988; Bradley & Bryant, 1983, 1985).

The writing lab approach is designed to help students make connections between how words sound and how they are spelled (see Chapter 6 for scaffolding techniques). It offers opportunities to build phonological concepts and articulation abilities in the interrelated acts of learning to speak, read, and write more clearly for an audience of peers, teachers, and parents. An example of this concept appears in Box 2.1.

Morphology: System of Meaningful Units

A *morpheme* is the smallest meaningful unit of language. Every word is made up of at least one free morpheme (defined as a meaningful unit that can stand alone). In addition,

Table 2.1. The five rule systems of language

Phonology	System of language form rules that governs language sounds	Phonemes are categories of speech production that speakers of a language perceive as being individual "sounds" of the language.
		Changing a phoneme makes a difference in a word's meaning (e.g., in *bat* and *fat*, /b/ and /f/ are distinctive phonemes; in *catch* and *cash*, /ch/ and /sh/ are distinctive phonemes).
		Although the number of letters in *cat* is 3 and *catch* 5, both have only 3 phonemes. The English language has 26 letters, but more than 40 phonemes, so some phonemes are represented by letter combinations (usually digraphs, e.g., *ch, sh, th, wr*).
Morphology	System of language form/content rules that governs meaningful units	Morphemes are the smallest meaningful units of a language.
		A morpheme may be as small as a single phoneme, such as the plural or possessive /s/, or as large as a multisyllabic word.
		Morphemes may be free or bound.
		Bound morphemes may be derivational (prefixes or suffixes that change a word's meaning) or inflectional (suffixes that make a word fit the syntax of a particular sentence).
		Before children enter preschool, language specialists usually compute mean length of utterance (MLU) for 100 utterances by counting all morphemes (words and their inflectional endings) and dividing by the number of utterances.
		Caution should be used in counting bound morphemes for children learning some dialects (e.g., African American Vernacular English) that are less marked by inflectional morphemes than standard English (e.g., *That boy like treat,* has 4 morphemes, whereas the standard English version, *That boy like/s treat/s,* has 6 morphemes). Both are grammatically correct according to their own rule systems.
		During the school-age years, utterance length is generally computed in words rather than morphemes unless a child is having unusual difficulty acquiring the rules for adding inflectional endings.
		Although speech-language pathologists must distinguish dialectal rule use for judging typical versus atypical development, school districts and parents from all dialectal and multilingual groups generally stress the importance of student gaining fluency with standard edited English through schooling.
Syntax	System of language form rules that governs sentence formation and comprehension	Sentences are units of language that represent one or more proposition, which is the linguistic term for "complete thought," including a subject and predicate.
		Sentences are made up of phrases (e.g., noun phrases, verb phrases, prepositional phrases) and clauses.
		Clauses may be independent (stand alone) or dependent (subordinate or embedded).
		A simple sentence has one independent clause.
		A compound sentence has two (or more) independent clauses joined with *and, or, but, so.*
		A complex sentence has an independent clause and at least one embedded clause (a relative clause starting with *who, which,* or *that*), a secondary verb phrase (with a gerund, participle, or infinitive), or a subordinate clause (beginning with conjunctions such as *because, so that, since, when, after,* or *while*).
		When children are school age, language specialists often compute MLU by dividing a student's discourse into T-units. T-units are defined as one independent clause and any embedded or subordinated phrases or clauses (Hunt, 1965, 1970, 1977). The average also includes C-units (Loban, 1976), which are sentence fragments often found in spoken language, but also in written language.
Semantics	System of language content rules that governs symbolic meaning	The essence of semantics is a set of cognitive concepts, or knowledge about the world (Nelson, 1994; Olson, 1970).
		Words are arbitrary symbols (also called signs) that represent concepts. Words are made up of one or more morpheme. Signs are distinct from reference (i.e., the meaning they represent) and referents (i.e., the specific things, events, or ideas to which they refer) (Nelson, 1986).

(continued)

Table 2.1. *(continued)*

		An individual's vocabulary knowledge forms that person's lexicon.

An individual's vocabulary knowledge forms that person's lexicon.

The semantic system can convey an infinite variety of meanings using morphemes, sentences, and discourse structures.

Case grammar is one system for designating the semantic-grammatic roles of words in sentences relative to the verb phrases that govern them. Cases include agent, action, state, object, instrument, locative, temporal, descriptor, patient, and so forth.

Verb tense and aspect choices also convey shades of meaning. Tense describes temporal relations, and aspect indicates notions of current relevance, completion, or duration. For example, *We were wishing we were home* includes both a past progressive and a subjunctive form of the verb *were* to convey that the state of wishing was ongoing in the past and that it had to do with the possibility, rather than the reality, of being home. The perfect tense phrase *I've finished my dinner* indicates both temporal relationships and completion information. It also has a pragmatic component in that it "implies the existence of something in the situation to which the sentence relates, such as a desire to leave the table or a refusal to eat more" (Duchan, 1986, p. 31).

Figurative language includes similes (e.g., *as clean as a whistle*), metaphors (e.g., *She skated through her exams*), idioms (e.g., *He pounded the point home*), and proverbs (e.g., *Absence makes the heart grow fonder*). Proverbs occur in all languages, but are one of the most difficult types of figurative language to process (Nippold, 2000). To learn figurative language one must hear (or read) idiocratic language forms and relate them to the world knowledge being represented at the moment, which is one reason that figurative language is so difficult for people with hearing impairments or limited literacy skills.

Verbal reasoning involves the use of thinking language to plan, organize, predict, speculate, and hypothesize (Paul, 2001). These functions involve the mental manipulation of ideas. Manipulating symbols on paper or computer screens, both integral aspects of the writing lab approach, can facilitate them.

No simple or single system has been designed to measure semantic growth, but language specialists look for numbers of different words (Greenhalgh & Strong, 2001; Klee, 1992; Miller, 1991; Paul & Smith, 1993; Watkins, Kelly, Harbers, & Hollis, 1995) and unusual or specific word choices (rather than such all-purpose words as *thing, stuff, do,* and *make*) as signs of increased language maturity and freedom from word-finding difficulty (e.g., German, 1994).

Pragmatics	System of social communication rules that governs language variation and selection in contextualized language use	Sensitivity to pragmatic rules helps communicators adjust and interpret linguistic and nonlinguistic aspects of communication events according to the sociocultural expectations in particular communicative contexts and groups. Linguistic pragmatic rules include any formulation or comprehension choice that influences social meaning and interpretation. Examples include such cohesive devices as pronominalization, which allows one to replace a previously identified word with a pronoun on subsequent mention (e.g., *The girl noticed her bike had a flat tire*), unless another noun of similar type intervenes (e.g., *Jennifer told her friend that Jennifer's* [*her* would be ambiguous in this context] *bike had a flat tire*).

Pronominalization rules also govern deletion of co-referential words to avoid redundancy of known information (e.g., involving nouns as in *The boy jumped and ran;* or verbs as in *The boy and girl ran*).

Other cohesive devices include conjunctions to convey intention or conditions to a listener (e.g., *If I were you I wouldn't do that*). Some pragmatically driven linguistic choices involve softening requests by using modal verb phrases (e.g., *I want one of those* is less polite than the linguistically more complex *I would like one of those if you have enough*). Socially tuned, appropriate communication requires full, flexible, and integrated use of pragmatic and linguistic rules.

Paralinguistic pragmatic rules involve use of such features as intonation, loudness, or stress to modify the social meaning of a sentence. For example, shifts of intonation can convey that the speaker is being sarcastic, pauses can convey tentativeness, lowered volume can indicate privacy, and shifts of word stress can indicate new or more important information.

Nonlinguistic pragmatic rules involve using nonspoken and nonverbal means to convey such aspects as social closeness or the speaker's feelings about a message. Among these, the term *proxemics* is used to describe the meaning of social distance or positioning while communicating. Gestures and facial cues also provide the body language that augments the meaning of messages. In written language, some of these elements are communicated via verbal description. They also can be communicated with such writing conventions as exclamation points, question marks, commas, quotation marks, ellipsis points.

Knowledge of pragmatics allows individuals to formulate utterances to serve different communicative functions. The two major classifications are assertive functions (e.g., requesting action or information, greeting a friend, commenting on observable phenomena, making statements of opinions or rules) and responsive functions (e.g., providing verbal acknowledgements or responding to requests for information).

Knowledge of pragmatics allows individuals to act appropriately with partners in various discourse events, such as conversations, joke telling, story telling, or giving information.

Knowledge of pragmatics allows partners to structure discourse, introduce or change topics, take turns appropriately, and convey just the right amount of information for an audience.

Metapragmatics is the child's conscious awareness of expectations for using language appropriately in context (Wilkinson & Milosky, 1987). Classroom success depends on metapragmatic skills for reflecting on communicative behaviors, detecting and judging inconsistencies, recognizing inadequacies, understanding communicative failures, and changing communicative behaviors in varying situations (Kaufman, Prelock, Weiler, Creaghead, & Donnelly, 1994).

The social essence of pragmatic rules makes them particularly sensitive to social-cultural variation.

Instructors need to be aware that their communicative style may be perceived differently depending on students' backgrounds and cultural knowledge, and conversely need to seek to understand possible diverse cultural influences on their students' communicative styles when they seem odd or inappropriate (Patterson, 1994).

---

there are two groups of bound morphemes. Derivational morphemes make up a large class of meaningful units that are used to derive different forms of words. The class includes prefixes (e.g., *non-*, *dis-*, *re-*, *un-*) and suffixes (e.g., *-less*, *-tion*, *-able*, *-ness*). Ehri (2000) reported that the suffixes *-ed*, *-ing*, *-y*, *-ate*, *-er*, *-ion*, and *-ly* are the most common morphographs (i.e., morphemes spelled a certain way).

Inflectional or grammatical morphemes make up a smaller class that appears only as suffixes in English. Grammatical morphemes inflect words to fit the syntax of a particular sentence. As noted in Table 2.1, rules for inflectional morphemes vary across dialects. Thus, measures that treat morphemic variations as errors are particularly prone to cultural-linguistic bias. The importance of recognizing this factor during diagnosis of language disorder, however, does not preclude an educational team from setting educational goals for all students to gain facility with Standard American English (SAE) morphology. The inflectional morphemes that appear on nouns in SAE are

- Plural *-s*, usually spelled as "s" or "es," but pronounced as /s/, /z/, or /ez/, depending on whether the phonemes that precede it in a word are voiceless (e.g., *hats*, *books*), voiced (e.g., *bugs*, *names*), or sibilant (e.g., *houses*, *witches*)

Box 2.1.   Interfaces Among Phonology Problems and Spelling

Aaron was a fourth-grade student diagnosed with a specific language impairment and learning disabilities. Aaron's speech was influenced by persistent difficulty differentiating the liquid and glide phoneme categories of /l/, /r/, and /w/. Despite several years of speech therapy, Aaron continued to confuse the sounds, not only in his speech but also in his reading and writing. For example, Aaron tended to spell the word *was* as "ros." Examples appear in the following story he wrote using a software program (*My Words*) that allowed him to insert sound effects, shown in square brackets:

the family

I saw a cow that said [moo] the cow was a big cow and the cow did marry a hors the horse he made thes moos [neighhh]. Thay lovd ech Other efery day the other day thay got a babey the babey is a bird he made this nooes [chirp] the nex day thay had another babey the babey wos a dog he said [woof]. Then the babya dide I ros sad I said this nose [wahhh] .

The unstable spelling of *noise* as "moos" and "nooes," with possible interference from the word *moo* on the first occasion is typical of some students with combined speech-language and learning disabilities. Intervention for Aaron focused on feedback that helped him connect phonemic awareness across contexts involving speech production, auditory discrimination, spelling, and reading. He had several personal minilessons and an author book page that highlighted the word *was*. The result was that approximately 2 months later, he was able to spell *was* consistently and demonstrate spelling in the transitional stage by beginning to use -*er* and -*ed* morphemes in the following story. The high degree of violence in this and similar stories by peers was addressed subsequently in minilessons and lab activities, using the authentic audience principle, by discussing the story's negative effects on some readers, particularly parents.

Aaron has a batl with a monster

I was hafing a batl with a moster it was 9'000 feet long. It was red, its nails were poisin . I had a sword and a flashliet. I cut his head off head it was still alive. I used the flashliet, the monster got stroger . I cut his arm, its blod was black. The arm grew back. It was mad . It terned green. It shot poisin at me. It missed me and hit a tractor. It melted. I was mad . I chopped it in haf . It was dead , I thot the monster was dead . The monster tried to cut my head off . I stabbed the monsters hart . The monster was dead . I was happy .

- Possessive *-'s*, usually spelled as "s" but pronounced differently, like plurals, depending on preceding phonemes (e.g., *cat's* /s/, *boy's* /z/, *Chris's* /ez/)

The inflectional morphemes that appear on verbs in SAE are

- Present progressive *-ing*

- Third-person singular *-s* or *-ez* (e.g., he *bats*, she *reaches*)

- Past tense *-ed* (painted), usually spelled as *ed* but pronounced as /t/ after voiceless consonants (e.g., *walked*)

- Past participle endings on verbs, spelled as *ed* or *en* (e.g., he *has walked*, we *have taken*), but pronounced differently depending on preceding phonemes

Writing lab activities are designed to help children acquire deeper understandings of the morphemic makeup of words and to use that information for spelling, reading, and talking. For older students, this may include teaching them directly about the Anglo-Saxon, Latin, or Greek origins of most English words. In fact, Latin and Greek origins are responsible for approximately 60% of English words (Adams & Henry, 1997). Adams and Henry noted that students who learn to recognize such patterns have an important tool for recognizing the hidden regularities in English spelling, notorious for its unpredictability.

Anglo-Saxon morphemes provide most of the short, everyday words common in elementary school texts. These words are prone to compounding (e.g., *pigtail, flashlight*), and to the addition of common prefixes and suffixes (e.g., *like, unlike, likely*). Adams and Henry (1997) suggested second grade as a time to start teaching the most common prefixes *un-, in-, mis-, re-, be-,* and *de-* and suffixes *-ing, -er, -ed, -less, -ful,* and *-ly.* Anglo-Saxon morphology also influences three common spelling patterns: 1) the one-syllable doubling rule before suffixes beginning with a vowel (e.g., *hot* becomes *hotter*); 2) the silent *e* dropping rule before suffixes beginning with a vowel (e.g., *blame* becomes *blaming*) but not a consonant (e.g., *blame* becomes *blameless*), and 3) the final *y* rule for changing the *y* to *i* when a consonant precedes it unless the suffix begins with *i* (e.g., *try* becomes *tried* or *trying*).

Latin morphemes often function as bound roots (e.g., *-rupt-*), which are combined with other bound morphemes in such words as *interrupt* and *disruption.* Understanding the Latin influences on morphology helps students see constancy in spelling patterns that otherwise seem inconsistent, such as shifting pronunciations of vowels in unaccented syllables (e.g., *divide* versus *division, serene* versus *serenity, confide* versus *confidential, local* versus *locality, compete* versus *competition*).

Greek morphemes compound two roots or derivational forms rather than affixes (e.g., *tele + phone, phon + ology, ortho + graph*). Words of Greek origin generate several peculiar sound–spelling correspondences (e.g., the *ch, ph,* and *y* representing the /k/, /f/, and /I/ sounds in words such as *chlorophyll*). Many words in the language of science are generated from Greek origins.

From the beginnings of literacy development, students must be able to pick out individual words as separate entities within the slippery stream of speech in order to learn to read and write. Those who can recognize the patterns of morpheme chunks have a powerful tool for decoding and spelling unfamiliar or multisyllabic words, regardless of whether they can label them as Anglo-Saxon, Latin, or Greek. For example, a student who knows the words, *can* and *racer* might figure out how to spell or pronounce the word *cancer* by morphographemic (or orthographic) analogy. An example of how scaffolding was used to increase a third-grade student's metalinguistic attention to the morphemic structure of words (but without requiring him to memorize the rules) appears in Box 2.2.

Syntax: System of Sentence Structures

Syntactic structures serve as the basic unit of communication, both for spoken and written language. Complete ideas (sometimes called *propositions*) lead to complete sentences. When communicators use language to convey ideas, they use sentences.

The structure of sentences can be explained in a variety of ways. Universal grammar theorists use more abstract terms from the work of Chomsky (1980, 1981) to describe syntactic elements, but we recommend using terminology that most teachers recognize. Sentences are constructed around predicate phrases as the central core of meaning to indicate action or state of being. The action may or may not involve an object. The verb is called *transitive* if it can take an object and *intransitive* if it cannot. The subject of the sentence does or is what the predicate specifies. To be judged complete, a sentence must have at least a subject and predicate. The only exception is an imperative sentence or command; however, it is not really an exception because the subject (*you*) is understood, as in *Shut the door*. A complete subject-plus-predicate structure is also considered to be an independent clause because it can stand alone.

Students with underdeveloped spoken syntax are at a disadvantage for using this important language system to generate and evaluate sentences as they formulate language across modalities, including figuring out unfamiliar words while reading and checking word choice and syntactic appropriateness while writing (Gillam & Carlile, 1997). They lack the inner language skills to judge if a sentence sounds right.

Students with language needs at the level of syntax include students learning English as a second language, as well as students with disabilities. Both groups may handle syntax adequately for use in spoken social interactions but run into difficulty with the more decontextualized structures of academic language, whether spoken or written (Cummins, 1984; Tattershall, 2002).

SLPs measure advancing syntactic ability in the preschool years by counting morphemes (i.e., any base word + its inflected or contracted morphemes) in a spoken language sample, then dividing by the number of utterances to compute *mean length of utterance* (MLU). This measure captures advancing maturity because as young children learn language, they use more morphemes in each utterance to communicate more information. Even toddlers can combine more than one idea in a sentence, but they probably use listing rather than syntactic deletion strategies, and their utterances still are limited in length (e.g., *Mommy Daddy go/ing bye-bye*, five morphemes, with compound subject; *Puppy jump scratch me*, four morphemes, with compound verb).

Tables of normative data are available for comparing children's MLU in the early language-learning years with expected means and standard deviations for children of that level (e.g., Miller, 1981). For example, the predicted MLU for 18-month-olds is 1.31 (with a range within one standard deviation of 0.99–1.64 morphemes per utterance); the predicted MLU for 60-month-olds is 5.63 (with a range of 4.44–6.82 morphemes per ut-

---

Box 2.2.　Personal Minilesson Focused on Derivational Morphology

Garrick wrote a touching poem about how much he cared for his mother. One line, in which he spelled *knowing* as "noing" provided a teachable moment for morpheme-level scaffolding. The instructor first listened to the creative use of words and commented on the feelings that came through so nicely in the poem, then asked Garrick to pull out his author notebook and turn to his personal dictionary. The scaffolding language was as follows:

Adult:　Let me show you some interesting things about that word *no*. There are actually two ways to spell that word—N-O, as you have here, and . . .

Garrick:　K-N-O-W [he volunteered, clearly having experienced the other spelling before, but not having connected it with the meaningful use in the current context]

Adult:　Great, let's write that word in your dictionary. Where should we put it?

Garrick:　Under *K*

Adult:　Good, let's do it. Here's another word that goes along with *know*. Have you ever heard of the word *knowledge*?

Garrick:　[Shakes head no]

Adult:　When you "know" something, you have "knowledge" in your head. You might hear, "Garrick has a lot of *knowledge* about dinosaurs."

Garrick:　Oh yeah!

Adult:　Let's add it in your dictionary next to *know*. Here, I'll write *know*, but this time I'll add *-ledge*. So what does this word say?

Garrick:　Knowledge.

Adult:　Great!

---

terance). After age 5 years, sentence length explodes, and the MLU measure no longer works. The main problem at this point regards how to segment utterances as children master conjoining strategies, stringing many simple sentences together in compound sentences with the conjunction *and*. Especially in students' writing, *and then* . . . sentence-combining strategies have the potential to yield sentences that go on and on.

Researchers studying the typical language development of school-age children have suggested methods for solving this problem by segmenting utterances at main clause boundaries instead of at the end of sentences. Such a method divides utterances into separate independent clauses, including any embedded or subordinated elements that make a unit more complex. Hunt (1965, 1970, 1977) named these *T-units*, for minimal "terminal" unit. Loban (1976) added fragments common in spoken communication and called them *C-units*, for "communication" unit. Data from Loban's study of low- and high-achieving students appear in Table 2.2. Scott (1988a) compiled data from various research studies and summarized systematic increments in *mean length of T-unit (MLTU)* (computed in words rather than morphemes) in both spoken and written syntax from third through twelfth grade. We have added data from our research. These data appear in Chapter 15 (see Table 15.7).

As noted, a T-unit is defined as an independent clause (i.e., with a subject and predicate) along with any phrases or clauses embedded in it (e.g., *Reading books is my favorite thing to do; I like to read books; The book, which I forgot to bring, was my favorite*) or subordinated to it (e.g., *She thanked me when I gave her the book*). When clauses are elaborated, more information is packed into each T-unit. As a result, MLTU rises. Younger children and children with language difficulties tend to string together independent clauses with the coordinating conjunctions *and, but, or,* and *so.* Their T-units are generally shorter than T-units in which more information is embedded. For example, the string *I forgot the book/but I can bring it tomorrow/and I will give it back/so I hope that is okay* is made up of 4 separate T-units, with 22 total words, and an MLTU of 5.5 words. In comparison, the utterance *I forgot the book that I need to give back, although I am coming tomorrow and can bring it then* conveys the same information in 1 T-unit with an MLTU of 20 words. Even mature language users tend to formulate less elaborate sentences in their spoken than in their written discourse because of distinctions in language processes and uses within the two modalities (discussed later in this chapter).

Studies of spoken and written grammar that have tracked syntactic changes in spoken and written language through the school-age years have shown a consistent picture of increasing later developing forms in the period from mid-elementary through high school (summarized by Perera, 1986; Scott, 1988a, 1999; Silliman, Jimerson, & Wilkinson, 2000). In particular, older children's written language samples show more relative clauses (*It was the boy who probably did it*), expanded noun phrases (*The large, green, hairy monster . . .*), nonfinite clauses (*Keeping the room clean was her responsibility*), and adverbial fronting (*There sat the big king elephant*). As students learn to write stories and reports with clearer details and more information, they naturally need more complex sentences with structures like these to express their meanings. This, in turn, prepares them to understand the increasingly complex sentence structures in the language of others, which they read and hear.

Although sentence length could be expanded ad infinitum through embedding and subordination, at some point an upper limit in desirability is reached. Overly complex sentences are too difficult to process. Stylistic differences also come into play, as in the literary contrasts often drawn between Hemingway and Faulkner (Wells, 1986). More mature writers try to detect overly complex sentences during the revision process and break them down into simpler ones. The writing lab approach is designed to encourage students to develop syntactic abilities to produce sentences that are increasingly complex and correct but that reflect audience-sensitive communication decisions. Improved outcomes are measured as advancing proportions of sentences scoring in the higher-level categories along the continuum, simple incorrect [si], simple correct [sc], complex incorrect [ci], and complex correct [cc] (see Chapter 15).

In this coding system, the number of verbs in the sentence determines simple or complex. If there is only one verb, a sentence is rated as simple; if there is more than one, the sentence is complex. Additional verbs might appear as main verbs (i.e., finite verbs) in compound verb phrases (e.g., *She hid and forgot about it*) or subordinated clauses (e.g., *After she hid it, she forgot where*). They might also appear as secondary verbs (nonfinite verbs), which are infinitives (e.g., *She decided to look for it*), gerunds (verbs used as noun phrases; e.g., *Looking for it proved difficult*), and participles (verbs

Table 2.2.　Mean length of C-unit (MLCU) data from Loban's (1963) studies of spoken school-age language

Grade	Lowest group Mean	SD	Highest group Mean	SD	Total group Mean	SD
Kindergarten	4.18 (N = 22)	1.29	5.76 (N = 30)	1.53	4.81 (N = 338)	1.33
1st	4.89 (N = 22)	1.36	6.89 (N = 30)	1.39	6.05 (N = 260)	1.37
2nd	5.49 (N = 22)	1.18	7.04 (N = 30)	1.18	6.57 (N = 261)	1.18
3rd	6.08 (N = 22)	1.82	7.73 (N = 30)	1.33	6.65 (N = 259)	1.81
4th	6.42 (N = 24)	1.20	8.77 (N = 25)	1.08	7.70 (N = 246)	1.26
5th	6.90 (N = 24)	0.93	8.85 (N = 25)	0.95	7.89 (N = 243)	1.10
6th	7.19 (N = 24)	0.88	9.48 (N = 25)	1.12	8.37 (N = 236)	1.25

From Loban, W.D. (1963). *The language of elementary school children.* (NCTE Research Report No. 1). Urbana, IL: National Council of Teachers of English. Copyright 1963 by the National Council of Teachers of English. Reprinted by permission.

used as adjectives; e.g., *Looking for it, she forgot about the time; She found the toy broken*).

The writing lab approach's analysis system is designed to capture evidence of children's advancing syntactic maturity by giving some credit for main clause coordination without overcrediting it. Students' sentences are coded as complex when they use a coordinating conjunction to combine two independent clauses into a compound sentence. For example, *He saw her/and then he turned around* is scored as 2 T-units and 1 complex correct [cc] sentence. If more independent clauses are compounded, they are segmented and coded separately, following the rule to credit a maximum of two conjoined T-units as complex. For example, *She putted the dog's collar on/but he shook it off/so she ran after him/but she did not catch him/and he got away* is scored as 5 T-units. The first two are scored together as 1 complex incorrect [ci] sentence; the second two are scored as 1 complex correct [cc] sentence, and the last is scored as 1 simple correct [sc] sentence.

Targeting more mature syntax contributes to the writing lab mission to help students develop knowledge of all the systems of language sufficient to support them in their communicative interactions, whether listening, speaking, reading, or writing, in both academic and social contexts. Box 2.3 illustrates how this happened for a sixth-grade girl.

Semantics: System of Meaning

The semantic components of language include "knowledge of vocabulary and knowledge about objects and events" (Paul, 2001, p. 5). The study of semantics by semanticists tends to become hugely philosophical and abstract. Writing lab teams need to focus on how to encourage authors to *need* specific words and phrases to convey particular meanings when they write in order to help students elaborate their semantic systems.

As indicated in Table 2.1, an individual's internal vocabulary, which is available for language comprehension and production, is called the person's *lexicon.* A rich and varied lexicon provides advantages for both reading and writing. Numerous studies have established word knowledge to be a major correlate of reading comprehension, and others have established that comprehension scores can be improved by providing training aimed at word/concept development (Snow et al., 1998). When assessing written language samples (see Chapter 15), we look for evidence that a child is using mature and interesting word choices, as opposed to overreliance on particular words, inexact word selection, or usage errors.

Linguistic meanings are acquired in meaningful contexts (Nelson, 1974). Traditional pull-out therapy activities designed to teach new vocabulary by using flash cards to help students with the complex meanings of literate language have limited effectiveness. Similarly, general education activities that require students to memorize dictionary meanings from textbooks rarely transfer to real communicative interactions. Figurative meanings also are best learned in meaningful contexts, and the school-age years are filled with expectations for students to understand and apply figurative meanings, particularly as they move into adolescence (Nippold, 1988a, 1988b, 2000). The writing lab approach helps students connect reading and writing with meaningful communicative purposes. As they experience authentic audience responses to their own more elaborate meanings, students begin to tune into the expressions and vocabulary of other speakers and authors (Swoger, 1989).

Incorporating more complex meanings into writing may be easier than obtaining them from reading for students struggling with literacy. Composing language to convey intended meanings may increase expectations for written texts to make sense. Each bit of writing success can help students intensify their focus on words in other oral and literate language contexts. Box 2.4 illustrates how this worked for Swoger's (1989) high school student with disabilities.

Pragmatics: System for Using Language Appropriately in Social Contexts

The pragmatic system is unlike any of the others because it relates more closely to communication than to language per se (Gallagher, 1991). Pragmatic elements are conveyed through nonlinguistic as well as linguistic means. For example, judging how close to stand or how to respond to a listener's facial expressions are pragmatic social-communicative behaviors but not linguistic ones. Pragmatic skills also are called on when speakers and writers make linguistic judgments about how to tailor their language to fit specific social contexts. Listeners and readers use pragmatic skills to interpret underlying meanings and intentions of communicative partners.

The development of social competence is dependent on cognitive, motor, and receptive and expressive language skills (Guralnick, 1992). The opportunity to practice those skills, in turn, is dependent on social competence (Odom, McConnell, & McEvoy,

Box 2.3.   Revising Sentence Structure

Eboni was a fifth-grade student with learning risks (including frequent absences from school to care for younger siblings) and failing grades. She had been referred for special education assessment but had no diagnosed disability. Eboni prepared the following report on the Milky Way galaxy.

> But what I really think the milky way is it's a galaxy in which it can be discovered in it's own way. And sometimes it can be seen but not with a telescope you can cut off all the lights in your neighborhood and stand on top of your roof and it for the last 40 years if you are careful of what you cut off in your neighborhood.

Although she read the report aloud a number of times while drafting, she could hear nothing wrong with how the sentences sounded and declined to revise the anomalous ones. The instructors concluded that Eboni had processed the language of her research sources enough to grasp their meaning. This was evident in her use of the dialectal features of her African American Vernacular English home language when she described the need "to cut off" lights in order to be able to view the Milky Way. Apparently, Eboni was able to apply her spoken language abilities to paraphrase the material but not to identify the anomalous syntax.

True to the ownership principle, the instructors left Eboni, as author, in control of decisions to revise. The instructors did use scaffolding techniques to frame the anomalous syntax and focus Eboni on cues indicating problems with the syntax. The scaffolds were gentle and noncorrective, however, because Eboni was emerging from being a reluctant writer. The team did not want to jeopardize her newfound willingness to take risks.

It was in the process of rehearsing on videotape to read the report aloud at a publishing party that Eboni finally was able to hear the anomalies in her sentences and to know where the language did not sound right. At this point, she decided to revise the sentences so that they would make sense. Reading sentences aloud during daily author group sessions did not provide sufficient feedback for Eboni to recognize the anomalous syntax. By contrast, reading sentences aloud in high-stakes anticipation of a real audience added enough salience to make the problems apparent so that she could revise the sentences that did not make sense.

1992). Spoken and written language both are forms of social communication. Writing lab contexts provide numerous opportunities for supporting enhanced social competence and using enhanced social competence to support learning.

Appreciating reading and writing as communicative acts involves pragmatic skills of social interaction. Students with special language and learning needs may require extra help to consider authors' intentions and discourse organization cues when they read and to think about audience needs and organizational strategies when they write.

Box 2.4.   Using Writing Processes to Stimulate New Attention to Word Meanings

Swoger (1989) was a high-school English teacher who described how her student, Scott's, language system started to bloom in the context of a writing workshop. After many years of special education, Scott was enrolled in Swoger's general education "basic writers" class. Perhaps for the first time, Scott was encouraged to write about his own ideas.

With a great deal of patience and encouragement, after 3 weeks Scott finished his first story about his dog, Hambone, who became sick and died. Scott and his friends found the dog and buried him but not before some time had passed. Scott's story was three paragraphs. The last one read:

> So then we got a shvle and dig a good hole for him very deep. Then we buiried him. It was a little sad. We knew he would die sometime. So we buirded him in that hole and we covered it up, Tom and me. We were pretty sad. (p. 62)

After the first story, Scott was off and running. His next topic came easier. Equally important, his sensitivity to new vocabulary began to exude the language development phenomenon in which children's brains are capable of soaking up dozens of new words per day. At the school-age level when this happens, students consciously select words to achieve unique communicative purposes. Swoger (1989) wrote:

> It is interesting to me that although Scott seldom used language, he had language. It's like those millions of seeds and deep roots lying dormant until the rains come. Scott's desert began to bloom. I first noticed changes in his choice of words. He wrote "obnoxious," his first three-syllable word, when describing his two new puppies. No doubt he had picked up some of his mother's vocabulary in relation to those dogs.
>   One day, later in the year, he came to my desk and asked if there were two meanings of the word, "hospital." He wrote: "The friend's sister had a lot of people over to celebrate Mardi Gras. I met a lot of them and they were very hospitable." Scott seemed to be noticing words. He needed words; he was a writer. (p. 62)

Two activities of the writing lab approach that can make a difference for such students are peer conferencing and the author chair. Both activities, when supported by instructional scaffolding, make the audience immediate and explicit. As students revise their stories, feedback from peers can help them to think about how well their ideas are communicated by their language choices. As they contemplate their own written discourse, students develop new strategies for judging the clarity of their language and whether it is likely to have intended effects on their audience (McAlister, Nelson, & Bahr, 1999). Although peer interactions may require heavy scaffolding by educators at

---

Box 2.5.   Writing Lab Contexts Can Help Students Develop Social Empathy

Shawnda was a third-grade student in an inclusive writing lab. She had frequent flare-ups of anger in both academic and social situations. Although Shawnda was not identified as having learning disabilities, her learning problems ultimately resulted in a recommendation to repeat third grade. In a poetry unit, Shawnda wrote about her anger:

Feelings About People

By

Shawnda

i am mad at my grama

i haer whin peopol toke abowut me

i smake my brathr cus I am mad

i beat sum bute because I am mad

Shawnda shared her poem in peer and teacher conferences. She received positive feedback about the clarity with which she conveyed her feelings, but her instructors indicated that it must be hard to feel so angry all the time. We asked Shawnda if she knew anything she could do when she found herself feeling so angry. She thought a minute, then returned to her desk and independently added a final line to her poem:

i am sorry every body.

---

first, an important outcome of the writing lab approach may be greater independence and social awareness on the part of all students. Box 2.5 provides an example.

Summary of Language Systems and Implications

Throughout this book, readers are encouraged to think about how to facilitate growth in all five systems of language using the activities of the writing lab. For example, the balance principle of Chapter 1 and the assessment activities of Chapter 15 are designed to encourage attention to all of these language systems for individuals as well as the whole class. Chapters 4, 5, and 6 show how to use minilessons, author group interactions, and scaffolding to focus on multiple aspects of language learning.

Knowledge of any of the systems of language can be affected in children with disorders of communication, either specifically or in conjunction with other problems (Nelson, 1998; Paul, 2001). In such cases, a student's own written language, displayed on paper or computer screen, can provide the therapeutic material for fostering the development of any language system with signs of impairment. Growth in language knowledge and use are legitimate targets of the general education curriculum as well.

SPOKEN AND WRITTEN LANGUAGE: DISTINCTIVE BUT RECIPROCAL

Language expectations and opportunities vary when language is used for listening, speaking, reading, writing, or thinking. The key to successful intervention is to capitalize on intermodality distinctions, similarities, and reciprocal relationships to support improvements in both spoken and written language forms. Receptive and expressive systems do not develop in exact parallel, however, and at times, one may develop before the other (Paul, 2000).

Distinctions Between Spoken and Written Language

One distinction between spoken and written language relates to universality. Spoken language is universal, whereas literacy is not (Perera, 1984). That is, all cultures have spoken languages that are equally complex, that evolved naturally over thousands of years, and that people learn without being formally taught. On the contrary, all cultures do not have written language systems. Systems for representing a language in writing must be invented. Literate language skills are generally taught and learned through formal schooling. Although not universal, literacy is a mandatory ticket to power and independence in literate cultures, and every effort should be made to help all learners become literate.

Some distinctions between spoken and written language are physical (Berninger, 2000; Kamhi & Catts, 1999a; Perera, 1984; Scott, 1994). Physical differences exist, for example, between primary sensory modalities of input (i.e., audition for listening versus vision for reading) and motor modalities of output (i.e., oral motor for speaking versus fine motor for writing). Similarities exist between reception and expression as well. This is especially true for higher levels of formulation and comprehension whether language is spoken or written. With scaffolding, students can make connections across language modalities they may not make on their own, and they also can learn to connect language more directly to thinking and self-regulation.

Most people think of receptive language as easier than expressive. This conclusion is supported by observations that 1) most receptive vocabularies are larger than expressive ones; 2) understanding someone else's message, whether spoken or written, makes fewer demands on word retrieval and sentence formulation than expressing one's own; and 3) responding to multiple-choice test questions is easier than composing essays. There is another side to this coin, however. Speaking or writing in one's own words may be easier than listening to a teacher's complex explanations that are filled with unfamiliar words. In formulating language for spoken or written expression, students start with their own ideas and vocabulary, which reduces the demands to make sense of unfamiliar ideas expressed with higher-level words and complex syntax. Switching expressive for receptive pathways can be effective in helping students overcome learning blocks and fear of failure. The result is enhanced access to the tools of language learning, including increased opportunities to interact. For example, as described in Box 2.6, a child who worked with his teacher to construct rules for learning basketball became a more constructive listener for learning from the teacher in other instructional contexts.

Other differences between spoken and written language can be found in the degree of nonlinguistic context for supporting the linguistic message. Contextual supports are generally greater in spoken communication because of the immediate presence of a communicative partner. Partners lessen the message load on senders by providing support for topic selection, cues about breakdowns indicating need for repair, and support for word finding and sentence generation. Several writing lab activities are designed to take advantage of this distinction. For example, persuading a reluctant writer first to tell a story orally may provide a necessary bridge for getting the student's own words on paper, either via dictation or scaffolded spelling. At other points, the instructional team uses author groups and teacher and peer conferences to provide spoken communication support for helping authors recognize the need to clarify and revise some element of written language.

Distinctions between spoken and written language also can yield advantages in favor of written language. One place this occurs is in the availability of time (Kamhi & Catts, 1999a; Perera, 1984). The temporal difference has the following effects:

- Spoken language choices must be instantaneous, whereas written language choices can be reflected on and revised.

- Speakers construct and convey language with the pressure of an immediate audience, whereas authors decide when language is ready for others to read.

- Once produced and heard, spoken elements remain only briefly in working memory, whereas written elements remain available for readers and writers to ponder.

This relative permanence of written language makes it available for instructors to scaffold and for authors to revise. SLPs traditionally have used tape recordings to encourage clients to listen to their spoken language for the purpose of correcting it. The writing lab approach allows SLPs and other team members to work with students, contemplating their relatively more permanent language jointly on the page or computer screen for the purpose of making it clear and interesting as an authentic act of communication.

Distinctions and similarities in spoken and written language can be found at the level of discourse as well as in the ways they are transmitted. Some discourse genres are more common in spoken communication (e.g., conversation) and some in writing (e.g., expository essays). Most, however, find at least some expression in both spoken and written forms (Gillam, Pena, & Miller, 1999; Kaderavek & Sulzby, 2000). Examples include oral storytelling and written narratives, spoken expository lectures and written reports, oral conversation and e-mail. Chapter 4 discusses ways in which discourse genre choices can be used to support enhanced communication growth across spoken–written language boundaries.

Box 2.6.   Interplay Between Learning to Write Instructions and Listen to Them

Birch was a third-grade special education student who had a seizure disorder (controlled by medication) and cognitive and emotional difficulties. He spent part of the day in a special education classroom, but during writing lab activities Birch was included in a third-grade general education classroom. Birch was having difficulty participating in that classroom. He struggled with group instructions and showed language comprehension difficulties. Both he and his third-grade teacher had questions about how he would fit into the general education classroom. Birch was inattentive in group discussions, and his teachers seemed uncertain about which behaviorial standards to apply. The SLP encouraged the teacher to hold Birch to class standards of behavior and conveyed that there was no "special" knowledge the teacher lacked for teaching Birch. Birch needed heavy scaffolding, at first, to find topics to write about and to get his words on paper. Things began to turn around when Birch's teacher worked closely with him to construct the rules for learning to play basketball, in a story Birch called "Mario":

MARIO

by Birch

Mario is the best basketball player.

he palays basketball   all   of the time. He plays at the Oakwood
gym.

David is on my team

the rest   of   the   team   naes

buddy   chris   Birch Joanna   David, Robert, Michael, Latonya, and
Devon. My team plays about 19 games a year. My team pays attention to the bal and works together. I will bounce the ball before I
shoot. I will pass the ball when I don't have a shot. The name of my
team is the warriors

In Birch's case, the individual interaction between general education teacher and special education student led to better understanding and closer matches of teacher talk and child listening. The teacher learned to check Birch's comprehension and to expect Birch to pay attention in group discussions. This, in turn, yielded more successful communication experiences across the school year. These experiences enhanced participation for Birch in his third-grade general education classroom. By the end of the school year, he was participating actively in group discussions and producing stories independently.

Reciprocal Relationships Between Spoken and Written Language

The writing lab approach is designed to take advantage of the reciprocal relationships between spoken and written language so that development in one area may contribute to the other. In research, it is easier to demonstrate association than causality between spoken and written language (Catts, 1993; Ehri, 2000; Kaderavek & Sulzby, 2000; Kamhi & Catts, 1999a). Studies designed to show that growth in one area can cause improvement in another have been concentrated in the area of phonemic awareness and word decoding (Ball & Blachman, 1988; Bradley & Bryant, 1983, 1985) or in spelling and word decoding (Ehri, 2000).

Reciprocal Relationships at the Word Level

Berninger (2000) suggested a two-pronged structure for conceptualizing the relationship between spoken language development and spelling. She differentiated problems at the phonetic level of perceiving the features of speech production from problems at the phonemic level of representing the abstract sound categories of language in long-term memory. Symptoms of speech perception difficulty can be detected in students' invented spellings, when they add or delete syllables or make other changes that may reflect speech perception difficulties (Moats, 1983, 1995). Students who are experiencing problems at the phonemic level are likely to have difficulty learning phoneme–spelling correspondences. Such associations are needed to spell in an alphabetic writing system in which phonemes map onto spelling units, represented sometimes by a single letter but often by two. These students may require experiences that help them conceptualize phonemic categories and the ability to manipulate them mentally. Berninger concluded from her research that "learning to spell is a matter of the mind's ear learning to communicate with the mind's eye and that this communication can occur at multiple levels between corresponding units of speech and writing" (2000, p. 75).

The writing lab presents many opportunities to help students connect their speech production and speech perception processes to spelling patterns. Scaffolding techniques focus on pronouncing words slowly, syllable by syllable, feeling the sounds, and thinking about letters that make those sounds. For example, we have worked with a number of students who viewed *in* and *and* as the same word (both spelled *in*) until they were scaffolded to hear the difference and to pronounce each word distinctly. Other students have learned to disentangle phoneme sequencings in pronouncing multiple syllabic words. For example, one student learned to say "position" rather than /po zhi sun/ when reading the directions for an assignment; another, to change pronunciation of /am i nal/ to "animal."

The best results in intervention studies with at-risk spellers have involved a focus on speech and language units as the underpinnings of spelling (Berninger, 2000; Scott, 2000). In early intervention, this involves helping students first learn the alphabetic principle (connections between phonemes and one- or two-unit letter spellings), then whole word and onset–rime feedback, traditionally known as *word families.* In later intervention, this involves work at the morphological level (free and bound morphemes, inflectional and derivational affixes, roots, and compounds), helping students detect morphemic and orthographic patterns that repeat across words with a degree of regularity despite being often dubbed as "irregular" spellings. Each of these levels can be targeted within the writing lab approach, as discussed more fully in Chapters 6 and 16.

Reciprocal Relationships at the Discourse Level

Phonology, spelling, and word-level studies are important, but studies that cast a wider net are needed to yield more comprehensive pictures of spoken–written language relationships. For example, Catts (1993) found that, although phonological awareness and rapid automatized naming predicted reading decoding well at the word level, standardized measures of language ability in kindergarten were better predictors of reading outcomes at higher levels, especially of reading comprehension.

By the time children enter school, they can produce simple stories with well-developed plot structures in which the story elements are logically connected to one another, are linked to a central theme or character, and demonstrate understanding of cause–effect relationships (Gillam, McFadden, & van Kleeck, 1995; Roth, 2000). Composing written stories builds on this background knowledge but adds several layers of cognitive-linguistic activity:

> Composing written stories is a complex process that requires the coordination of several highly complex cognitive and metacognitive skills including the generation of ideas, organization of those ideas, development of a plan, translation of the plan into action, review and revision of what has been written, and the monitoring of one's performance during the composing process. (Roth, 2000, p. 16)

Some evidence supports reciprocal relationships between narrative writing skill and reading ability. For example, Barnhart (1990) found that stories written by less than average readers with lower levels of reading comprehension were less complex, less clear, and less cohesive than those produced by average and higher than average readers. The suggestion is that students who learn to produce more complex stories when writing have a more complex framework for understanding more complex stories when reading (Roth, 2000).

Reciprocal growth, however, is not likely to occur without focused scaffolding. In one study, students from 9 to 12 years of age with language disorders made greater growth in narrative structure when intervention emphasized language content and greater growth in language form when the instructional focus was on language skills (Gillam et al., 1995). Other authors have described shifts in a spoken–written continuum over time (Scott, 1999; Silliman et al., 2000). For example, students in the early elementary years are more likely to write the way that they talk and to use their thoughts as the landscape of consciousness for the characters they write about, whereas later elementary students gain facility at shifting perspective and using syntactic and lexical devices to convey meanings from diverse perspectives. Box 2.7 shows how Hewitt (1994) took advantage of narrative discourse elements to encourage this shift in perspective taking for a student with autism spectrum disorder.

The relationships between spoken and written language development and higher levels of thinking and social interaction have been studied less frequently, but clinical reports suggest that such abilities can benefit from integrated spoken and written experiences as well (Sturm & Koppenhaver, 2000; Ylvisaker & DeBonis, 2000). As Yoshinaga-

---

Box 2.7. Using Narrative Discourse Structure to Scaffold Perspective Taking

Lynne Hewitt (1994) described how she used narrative discourse to scaffold perspective taking for Barry, an adolescent student with an autism spectrum disorder. She indicated that she used constant feedback on his answers to questions about the texts he read in order to make him aware of monitoring characters' psychological states, as in this sample of instructional scaffolding discourse from a typical session:

Lynne: Do you have any idea why she might have cried when her son said those bad things about himself?
Barry: Uh uh.
Lynne: Why would that make a mother feel sad?
Barry: Itsa . . . It makes them afraid.
Lynne: It makes him afraid? Umm, what about her feelings, what is she feeling?
Barry: Her feelings were hurt.
Lynne: Um hm. I agree. How could her feelings have been hurt by him saying those things about himself?
Barry: I don't know. [almost inaudible]
Lynne: Okay, let's think about mothers. Today's Mother's Day, right? That's one reason I picked this story. How do mothers usually feel about their kids?
Barry: Sad.
Lynne: All the time?
Barry: They feel happy.
Lynne: Do they love them or hate them or they don't care?
Barry: They love them.

Hewitt noted that when Barry was challenged, he tended to look for an automatic surface-level response. An example, was his response "sad," which seemed to relate to Hewitt's earlier question about what might make a mother feel sad; however, when she gave him three choices,

> *He was able to come up with a more conventional response with some confidence, showing an awareness of social norms in mothers' feelings for their children ("they love them"). Although this was a forced-choice task, the fact that Barry did not follow his usual tactic of repeating the last-offered choice suggests that he was consciously selecting his answer. Replies such as these provided evidence that Barry was able to reason about people's psychological states. (1994, p. 99)*

Itano and Downey expressed, "The more knowledge children acquire, the more elaborate schematas become, and more knowledge helps students organize information into accessible pathways" (1996, p. 64).

Language specialists can apply their training to help students make reading, writing, speaking, and thinking connections that go beyond narrow tasks to authentic, integrated, communicative use (Butler, 1999). The writing lab is especially suited to pursuing those aims.

Summary of Spoken and Written Language Distinctions and Possibilities

The reciprocal relationships between spoken and written language, as well as their distinctions, present possibilities for using varied abilities to assist each other. Students who have difficulty writing a story can experience success by telling a story first to an interested listener, or if necessary, by dictating it to an adult or peer. Reluctant writers can learn to compose expository discourse when scaffolded to produce organizing questions orally and in writing before seeking information in books. Students who have difficulty comprehending a teacher's rapid speech may develop advanced syntactic abilities in the context of formulating more complex structures in writing. Reciprocal relationships between spoken and written forms of words may make their patterns more apparent, which, in turn, facilitates pronunciation, spelling, and word decoding skills.

In Chapters 4, 6, and 9, we show how word processing computer software speech-synthesis feedback can help students gain independent access to information about spoken–written language relationships. Conversations in author groups and with peer conferencing partners can assist students to internalize audience expectations, helping them judge whether they are meeting audience needs while writing at their computers. These are just a few of the bridging relationships the writing lab approach can support.

LANGUAGE TARGETS

Language intervention is a deliberate process by which instructors with explicit intentions design activities and use scaffolding to take students from a level where they are currently functioning to the next higher level. A distinction between the writing lab approach and traditional forms of language intervention is that the next higher level in decontextualized language therapy is often a baby step away from where the student was previously. Meanwhile, the student's general education peers are taking larger and larger steps toward adult competence. Students with disabilities who are receiving services in remote sites and isolated settings get further and further behind.

It was largely in response to this growing discrepancy that parents and professionals who could see the bigger picture advocated for updated language in IDEA 1997. At that point, as noted in Chapter 1, the stipulation was added that a student's IEP should include "a statement of measurable annual goals, including benchmarks or short-term objectives, related to—meeting the child's needs that result from the child's disability to enable the child *to be involved in and progress in the general curriculum*" (Sec. 614 [a][1][A]; italics added).

The goal to keep students in the general education curriculum influences how intervention teams now describe the more specific targets of language intervention. Working in relative isolation, language specialists, such as SLPs, may be accustomed to thinking and planning using the terms *phonology, morphology, syntax, semantics,* and *pragmatics*. Such terminology sounds a lot like jargon, however, to the teachers and parents who are important collaborative partners in the enterprise of helping all students become competent language users. It is not enough to just plan to work on language in general. Teams need to know which specific elements of spoken and written language require attention for individual students.

As a better way, therefore, we recommend thinking about language targets as occurring at language levels: starting at the discourse level, proceeding to the sentence level and word level (which includes the sound level), and then addressing such surface level elements as writing conventions. In addition, our outline of language targets, as illustrated in the writing lab approach (see Figure 1.1), includes elements of spoken communication, particularly as they appear in writing lab contexts. We introduce these elements here and discuss them more thoroughly with suggestions for scaffolding in Chapter 6. Chapter 15 provides techniques for describing current levels of performance for students as an outcome of individualized assessment using written language sampling.

Discourse Level Language Targets

The writing lab is particularly suited to targeting language at the highest level of communication units—connected discourse. When communicating at the discourse level, language users draw on and integrate their knowledge of the five systems of language. This allows them to select and combine words in structures that reflect their knowledge of syntax, semantics, and pragmatics and to produce physical representations of words using their knowledge of phonology and morphology.

Authentic writing projects are the key discourse structures of the writing lab approach. Writing projects are authentic if they communicate to a real audience for a specific purpose. Varied communicative purposes are associated with different language genres. In addition to targeting narrative and expository discourse, the writing lab approach provides opportunities to target language use in poetry, letter writing, conversation, and many other possibilities. Table 2.3 summarizes some of these opportunities.

Britton (1979) described both narrative and expository genres as *spectator discourse* in which a speaker or writer assumes a dominant role, organizing a series of sentences into a preplanned whole, using a structure designed to make the beginning, middle, and end apparent to listeners or readers. In spectator discourse, the speaker or author establishes the theme, and others typically follow along. Conversation, on the contrary, is organized as *participant discourse,* in which communicative partners act as equal participants, negotiating topics and following conversational themes established jointly.

Narrative and expository discourse forms generally are considered to represent literate forms, whether they occur in spoken or written language. When used in spoken communication, either may be embedded in a conversation. For example, in the midst of conversation, one of the partners might launch into a personal narrative, perhaps preceding it with an introduction such as, "Did I tell you about the time . . . ?" Most fictional literature also is structured as some variation of a narrative, often involving a protagonist who comes up against multiple barriers and must plan strategies to get around them on the way to achieving a goal. Spoken expository discourse is encountered when one partner starts an information-giving segment by saying, for example, "I read the other day that . . . " Science and social studies textbooks, which generally are

Table 2.3.   Discourse genres

Conversational	Narrative	Poetry	Expository
Social conversation structure	*Story grammar structures*	*Poetic structures*	*Expository structures*
Initiation	Setting	Acrostic	Beginning/ introduction
Topic introduction	Episode structure	Haiku	Middle
Topic maintenance	Problem or conflict	Ballad	Consistent with subgenre structure
Contingent queries	Internal response		Supporting points
Clarification requests	Goal/intention	*Poetic qualities*	Transitions
Contingent statements	Plan	Imagery	Ending/conclusion
Topic shading	Action	Nonliteral word meanings	
New topics	Ending	Rhythm and rhyme	*Expository qualities*
Termination		Focus on the sound of language	Informative
	Story grammar qualities	Humor	Factual
Social conversation qualities	Structural elements	Romance	Based on research
Partners negotiate topics	Title		
Partners share turns	Once upon a time		*Expository subgenres*
Partners presuppose about each others' knowledge	The end		Description
	Theme/motto		Definition
	Stylistic elements		Classification
Academic "teacher talk" conversation structure	Flashback		Comparison
Initiate (teacher)	Dialogue		Illustration
Respond (student)	Foreshadowing		Analogy
Evaluate (teacher)	Point of view		Example
	Landscape of:		Sequence
	Action		Process
Academic "teacher talk" qualities	Consciousness		Cause and effect
Known-answer questions			Temporal order
	Subgenres		Argument
Partners unequal	Personal narrative		Persuasion
Teachers take longer turns and control	Biography		Deductive reasoning
Student take shorter turns	Fairy tale		Inductive reasoning
	Fable		Time lines
	Mystery		Historical events
Student-centered academic discussions	Western		
Brain storming and divergent answers encouraged	Humor		
	Science fiction		
Many students participate	Drama		
Ideas are appreciated for their contribution to the discussion but not evaluated specifically			

From Nelson, N.W. (1992). Performance is the prize: Language competence and performance among AAC users. *Augmentative and Alternative Communication, 8,* 3–18; adapted by permission of Taylor & Francis (http://www.tandf.co.uk).

organized as expository texts, assume increasing importance with advancing grade level. Direction giving is another commonly encountered spoken expository discourse event.

Both narrative and expository discourse offer rich language learning and cognitive development opportunities. They differ, however, in their demands and opportunities. Narrative discourse often is targeted before expository discourse in school curricula, but even early elementary students are capable of reading and writing informative texts as well as narrative ones (Calkins, 1983). Both genres are essential for school success. Story writing provides opportunities to reflect on important life themes for the purpose of enlightening or entertaining. Report writing provides opportunities to extract and re-organize content from multiple sources for the purpose of conveying information. Other differences are discussed relative to each genre in the following sections. They are summarized in Table 2.4.

Narrative Discourse Learning Opportunities

Part of the task facing children in school is to learn about the classic genre forms and purposes. For example, classic Western story grammar structures include setting, problem, internal response, plan, action, outcome, and ending (Stein & Glenn, 1982). Most children are natural storytellers: budding with toddlers' accounts of events in their young lives (Westby, 1994), blossoming in the dramatic play of preschoolers (Paley, 1981, 1990, 1994), and coming into full bloom in the school-age years (Applebee, 1978; Westby, 1994).

Narrative structures vary by culture and context, but storytelling is universal (Heath, 1983; Hester, 1996; Hyter & Westby, 1996; Scott, 1994; Westby, 1994). Every culture has a way of telling stories. From the earliest toddler accounts of hurt fingers to the most eloquent works of playwrights, storytellers capture the subjective human experience and interpret its emotional, moral, and cultural meanings. Narratives serve as a primary mode of making sense of the world and help children develop a theory of how other people's minds work (Astington, 1990; Bruner, 1986, 1990).

Storytelling also is thoroughly intertwined with social interaction values and universal themes, such as "villainy, lack, loss, and trickery" (Westby, 1994, p. 193). Bruner (1986) noted that stories could have what he called a landscape of consciousness or "subjectivity," as well as a landscape of action (essentially, the plot). Most stories told by children older than 9 years "devote considerable attention to the landscape of consciousness, that is, how the world is perceived and felt by the characters in the story" (Westby, 1994, p. 198). In advocating the use of narrative in interventions with adolescents with autism, Hewitt described stories as

> Essentially a means for exploring the nature of people's lived experiences . . . Talking about the thoughts and feelings of characters leads naturally to a holistic approach to the text, that is, an approach in which plot elements, cohesive devices, and other elements of structure can naturally be seen to relate directly to the underlying purpose of representing individual experience. (1994, p. 91)

Establishing causal connections, explaining character motivations, and exploring consequences of actions all require complex and abstract thinking. Chapter 15 discusses methods for judging the maturity of narrative development. Chapter 6 suggests scaf-

Table 2.4. Narrative and expository discourse comparisons and contrasts

		Narrative discourse	Expository discourse
Use	Purpose	To entertain To gain control of life's fears and frustrations To illuminate how people deal with the problems of life	To inform, describe, or persuade To organize information or oneself To develop theories about logical-scientific and historical relationships
	Subgenres	Personal narratives • Accounts—telling to a new audience • Recounts—shared retelling • Eventcasts—commenting on plans • Imaginative stories—*once upon a time . . .* Fables/myths/historical tales/trickster tales/tall tales Mysteries/westerns/romances Novels (chapter books)	Descriptive/elaborative Sequence/procedure "how to" Comparison/contrast Cause–effect explanation Problem/solution
	Personal/cultural style	Voice Sense of audience	Unique and enlightening questions Perspectives from domains of knowledge Sense of audience/authorship
Structure	Macrostructures—story grammar	*Beginning—middle—end* Story setting (characters, time, place, initiating event) Action and follow-up (temporally, causally, goal oriented, planful, or not) Conclusion	*Beginning—middle—end* Introduction of topic Elaborating statements Conclusion
	Sentence-level structures	Temporal connectors (*and, then, next, after, while*) Causal sequence (*so, because, since*) Elaborated descriptions (relative clauses with *that* or *who*) Adverbial conjuncts/disjuncts (*really, probably, actually, however, although, nevertheless, yet*)	Temporal connectors (*and, then, next, after, while*) Causal sequence (*so, because, since*) Logical relations (*if…then, therefore*) Adverbial conjuncts/disjuncts (*really, probably, actually, however, although, nevertheless, yet*)
	Word-level structures	Selecting words to serve communicative purposes	Selecting words to serve communicative purposes

folding questions and author group strategies for helping students develop their narratives into increasingly mature structures. Selecting words and constructing sentences for the purpose of telling a story and engaging an audience gives importance to language choices that cannot be matched by many sessions of language drill and practice.

Beyond changing the stories that students tell others, the writing lab approach attempts to change the stories of personal failure that many students have learned to tell themselves. These are the "I'm so stupid," "I can't learn this," and "Everybody else understands it, but I don't" stories. Most of us have felt momentary doubts about our abilities, but some children live stories of failure and decide that there is not much use trying to be the hero when the outcome is predetermined. Students who internalize such stories are the ones who repeatedly say, "I hate writing," "I can't," or "I don't know." We have seen a number of them who, through the writing lab approach, begin to experience the joys of successful writing and publishing and to start to rewrite negative stories of themselves (see stories of change in Chapters 5, 13, 16, and 17).

Expository Discourse Learning Opportunities

Whereas narratives address the human challenges of life, its emotions, and relationships, expository texts offer structures for organizing factual information about the world in forms that make broader meanings and patterns more clear. Expository texts can be presented in a variety of relatively distinctive structures. Some are sequences, organized around a timeline of events or a structured series of steps or procedures. Others have a more hierarchical structure, organized as an outline with a series of superordinate and subordinate topics and their relevant details. Yet others are structured to persuade, compare and contrast, or explain cause-and-effect relationships. Any of these expository organizations is intended primarily to convey information.

Narrative and expository discourse are not always crisply separate. Box 2.8 illustrates how one student was stimulated by a direct quotation in a CD-ROM encyclopedia to write a report on astronauts. The direct quotation from this personal narrative seemed to allow the student to consider how another person might take a different perspective and to move the student toward higher-level thinking. It helped the student get into a report-writing framework.

Some students resonate more with expository than narrative discourse. Even those who resist expository writing at first may light up when they select their own topics. Research in an area of passion can help students learn how to read for authentic purposes. For example, Ellen, a typically developing third-grade student, loved penguins. She announced to her mother at the beginning of the school year that she planned to write about penguins every Friday during free writing. When her mother asked her if she thought she might get bored writing about the same topic all year, Ellen replied, "Oh no, you can write facts about penguins, stories about penguins, poetry about penguins . . . " (and her list went on).

By their nature, expository texts require research. A person must know something about a topic in order to write about it. The search for information often requires reading, discussing, interviewing, and even arguing. When a whole class pursues aspects of an issue, students may support one another in these discussions and group efforts. For example, Calkins (1990) described how students studying topics of homelessness and

Box 2.8. Direct Quotations Can Stimulate Perspective Taking

In the writing lab, an SLP worked with Cody, a fifth-grade student with special needs, to help him learn to use the computer with increasing independence. When the group began to research topics related to space, Cody found a CD-ROM encyclopedia item with a quotation from a Russian astronaut. Beginning his article with the quotation allowed him to get started and to write the piece, but it also helped him to consider another person's point of view. This report, which appears in Figure 2.1, includes an expression of personal goals, as well as a report on the astronaut. With Cody's selection of this quotation, he seemed to be reflecting on the power and possibilities of using language for literary effect.

Astronauts

"It was a great silence, unlike any I have encountered on Earth, so vast and deep that I began to hear my own body: my heart beating, my blood vessels pulsing, even the rustle of my muscles moving over each other seemed audible."–Aleksei Leonov.

Here are some facts about astronauts. I have to fly with astronauts. I have to float in the air when I'm in space. I'm playing music. I will put on my coat and gloves. I have to turn on my music, and air so we have oxygen. I have to put on my helmet for safety.

I can make my own goal. I can run. I can Join the astronauts and I could be a engineer. I can learn a different things about astronauts.

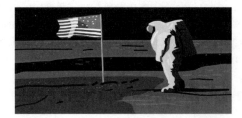

Figure 2.1. Cody's astronaut story.

immigration used interviews and other research techniques to address important societal problems in the context of joint expository writing projects. These are, in fact, primary advantages of using expository texts to create needs and opportunities for more complex language use. A question-guided information-gathering process can bring topics to life for children and create natural bridges from what students know already to what they want to learn (e.g., Atwell, 1990; Calkins, 1990).

Other Variations Across Genres

Authors can also use discourse forms such as journal entries, poems, plays, letters, editorials, or persuasive discourse while developing their language and thinking abilities. Any genre targeted by the general education curriculum can be a target of writing lab activities.

Persuasive writing is loaded with cognitive and communicative challenges and opportunities. To persuade someone of something sets up direct communicative links from author to audience. To persuade an audience (parents, principal, friends), students must first think about who the audience is and then take the audience's perspective. In the early stages, it helps to draw the topics from immediate, personal experiences. This process can be scaffolded with some strategic questioning by teachers; for example, "What might persuade your parents to let you stay up later?" or, "What might persuade the school district to repaint our classroom?"

Poetry writing is particularly rich with opportunities to focus on the effect word choices can have on listeners or readers. This benefit not only applies to composing poetry that rhymes but also to the semantic aspects of language, which are often the focus of free verse or haiku. Students can be encouraged to shut their eyes and think of how something looks, sounds, feels, or tastes, and then find words and phrases to help others experience something similar when they read the students' words or hear them read aloud.

Many other genre possibilities exist. We have worked with middle school students to write, produce, act, videotape, and do live performances of skits or televised news interviews. Another SLP worked with students in a special education classroom to help them write scripts for product and movie reviews. Her students also prepared cue cards to use when filming their presentations. A third-grade teacher taught her students to review library books and write persuasive pieces for other students. The school librarian displayed the reviews with the books just inside the library door where other students would see them as they prepared to leave the classroom, taking full advantage of the authentic audience principle.

The possibilities are endless. Our hope is that readers will be stimulated to experiment with a variety of learning contexts, finding the rewards of each and exploring new ways to expand their learning opportunities.

Sentence-Level Language Targets

Sentence-level language targets of the writing lab approach include 1) grammatical sentence formulation, in which noun–verb agreement is observed; 2) inclusion of articles, auxiliary verbs, and other grammatical function words; and 3) communication of ideas in structures that make sense. These targets require the application of semantic as well as syntactic knowledge about meaning making. Other sentence-level targets include cohesive language devices that link sentences; make pronoun references clear; and provide smooth, logical transitions from one sentence to the next.

In addition, students need to be able to produce a variety of syntactic structures and to use more complex structures to convey more complex ideas. For example, more detailed descriptions can be conveyed with expanded noun phrases and relative clauses. Cause–effect relationships can be expressed with subordination using *because* and *if . . . then* clauses. Written language contexts make it possible to work with students on many sentence structures that give them difficulty in speaking, listening, reading, and writing. The writing lab approach makes it possible to target reciprocal processes for producing more complex sentences to achieve communicative purposes and for comprehending them in the discourse of other speakers and writers.

Word-Level Language Targets

Word-level language targets can be divided broadly into vocabulary and spelling targets. The writing lab approach also makes it possible to target the word-retrieval problems experienced by many students with language impairments.

Vocabulary Targets

Students with larger vocabularies consistently perform better on almost any measure of literacy and school success (Catts & Kamhi, 1999; Snow et al., 1998). By focusing on word choice elements for improving written products, students can be taught to pay attention to vocabulary in the world around them, including attention to new words in spoken conversations and written texts (Swoger, 1989).

The acquisition of new vocabulary and the development of literacy are known to occur in tandem. This is the phenomenon Stanovich (1986, 1988a) dubbed as "the Matthew effect," with biblical reference to the phenomenon in which the rich get richer. That is, as students learn new words, they increase their capacity for learning even more.

Acquiring new vocabulary involves learning fine distinctions in meaning and association, including figurative meanings, in which words and phrases are used in non-literal ways. It also involves learning how to pronounce words clearly as well as to spell them. This is why we categorize spelling targets at the word level rather than as a writing convention.

Spelling Targets

Within writing lab contexts, spelling is targeted and scaffolded as a developmental skill. In the early grades, this means helping students grasp the alphabetic principle that written spellings represent spoken words (Snow et al., 1998). In alphabetic systems like English, spelling requires students to learn sound–symbol association rules (Kamhi & Hinton, 2000) and to use their phonetic speech production capabilities to "hear" and "feel" the sequences of sounds in words so that they can produce invented spellings. Research indicates that learning to decode words supports learning to spell them and vice versa (Ehri, 2000).

Beyond phonemes, words are made up of morphemes. As students begin to grasp the orthographic principle, they can relate word spellings more directly to word meaning without reference to how the words sound when spoken (Kamhi & Catts, 1999b). At this point, they begin to spell more words conventionally and find it easier to learn to spell new words by analogy as well as by sounding them out. Although orthographic word knowledge may appear to be largely visual, actually it represents deepening understandings of word roots, derivational morphology, and the histories and language origins of groups of words (as discussed previously in this chapter). Within the writing lab approach, students develop sound–symbol associations while learning about morphemic-orthographic patterns to spell and read the words in their own written products. In the process, they learn to tune-in more completely to the spellings of words when reading materials written by others.

Word-Retrieval Targets

Word-retrieval problems probably are more common among students with all kinds of language disorders than is generally recognized (German, 1993, 1994). Word-finding impairments are diagnosed when individuals struggle (with abnormal frequency) to retrieve and produce words that are clearly part of their vocabulary (Denckla & Rudel, 1976; German, 1979). All language users have experienced this phenomenon at one time or another as an annoyance, but in severe forms, word-retrieval difficulties are disabling. They can lead to such secondary symptoms as

1. Talking around a word (circumlocution) or telling a referent's function rather than its name (e.g., *thing you cut with* instead of *knife*)

2. Using long pauses or pause fillers (e.g., *ah, um, well*)

3. Overusing all-purpose words (e.g., *stuff, thing, make, do*)

4. Using indefinite or personal pronouns with unclear referents (e.g., *something, someone, he, she, it*)

5. Substituting gestures for words

6. Attempting to self-correct, with negative effects on fluency

7. Producing extra verbalizations (e.g., *What's that word? Oh, I know it.*)

Alternatives for explaining word-finding impairment have ranged from information processing deficits, to impaired phonological representation of words in a person's inner lexicon, to limited semantic elaboration within the lexicon. German (1993) observed at least three patterns. Some individuals have retrieval difficulties in combination with intact receptive language. Others, such as those described by Kail and Leonard (1986), have receptive language problems associated with unstable word meanings. A third group has complicated problems involving all systems of language.

The writing lab approach can target the abilities and skills implicated by any of these explanations. It helps students develop stronger vocabulary with richer and deeper semantic associations. It also helps them increase the clarity and automaticity of multi-modality skills for representing words accurately in spoken and written forms. Scaffolding techniques include teaching students to use both meaning and sound/letter cues to retrieve just the right word to express their meaning and have the desired effect on their audience. In addition, the temporal advantages of written language permit reflection and revision, thus making it easier for students with word-finding impairments to compensate for them while strengthening their skills.

Writing Conventions as Language Targets

Most instructors have no difficulty thinking of writing conventions as targets of instruction in learning to write, but many do not necessarily conceive of them as targets of language intervention. Treating writing conventions as elements of communication can help students learn why they should use punctuation and other writing conventions, which can increase the likelihood that they will produce mature, well-written products.

Writing conventions include such apparently surface-level features as punctuation, capitalization, and paragraph indentation. These features often are the focus of final editing when a piece of written work is nearing publication. They influence how people evaluate the work and, more important, how easy it is to read. Although writing conventions have the appearance of being surface-level features, their presence or absence can provide rich information about the deeper state of a student's language knowledge.

Consider some of the first writing conventions to be learned—periods at the end of sentences and capital letters at the beginning. Knowing how to use these devices requires first that students have a metalinguistic awareness of what a sentence is. Interacting with students around their use of periods and capitals can serve as a form of dynamic assessment (see Chapter 6) in which instructors are able to learn about a student's knowledge of sentences so they can scaffold strategically to advance that knowledge. As students learn other forms of final punctuation, such as question marks and exclamation points, instructors can scaffold them to acquire concepts of syntactic structures that can be used for varied pragmatic purposes, all stimulated by discussions of writing conventions.

Learning to capitalize words in addition to those at the beginning of sentences can lead to increased metalinguistic understanding at the word level. Metalinguistic ability is widely recognized as an accompaniment (and possibly a prerequisite) to literacy learning (van Kleeck, 1994). Knowing which words to capitalize in the title of a written work, for example, requires implicit understanding of the differences between content words and grammatical function words. Although it probably is not wise to teach such abstract terminology to young students, they can learn to apply implicit knowledge about distinctions between categories of words and, in the process, extend that knowledge. Special educators and SLPs collaborating with general education teachers can help students learn appropriate meta-language, such as "main words" and "linking words," or whatever terminology is introduced in the school's curriculum. Similar issues arise as students learn to capitalize proper nouns but not common nouns. The exact terminology is less important than the opportunity to reflect on, and become aware of, language and to learn the same terminology as general education peers for referring to important concepts of formal schooling and literacy learning.

Quotation marks are another writing convention with richer implications than apparent on the surface. When students begin to introduce dialogue into their stories, they need to use quotation marks. This signals an important transition in students' awareness that written language is more than just spoken language written down. Before they make this transition, students often incorporate oral language features in their writing. Examples include direct address to the audience (e.g., *Hi, my name is Josh.*), associative sentence linking strategies (e.g., *And then the guy got on his horse.*), other oral transition devices (e.g., *Well, I think I will tell you about last weekend.*), and apparent dialogue but without identifying the speakers (e.g., *Let's get them. No, I don't want to.*). When dialogue does begin to appear, as in the last example, instructors can indicate delight and help students find examples of how dialogue is punctuated in books.

The introduction of dialogue also presents opportunities to scaffold students about cohesion in communication to make sure that readers can understand clearly who said what and how they said it. Such discussions can help link students to sentence-level understandings of comments, questions, and explanations and to word-level understandings of the value of replacing everyday words, such as *said*, with interesting words, such as *shouted* or *whispered*.

The point is to help students recognize the communicative value of writing conventions rather than treating them as rules to be learned. Chapter 6 offers additional suggestions about how to scaffold such understandings.

Spoken Communication Targets

Writing lab contexts offer many opportunities to assist students to work on their spoken as well as written communication. SLPs generally categorize spoken communication components as articulation, language, voice, and fluency. Traditional speech goals are potential targets within the writing lab approach as well. In the writing lab approach, SLPs can find multiple opportunities to scaffold students' speech production skills as they interact with peers and adults in formal and informal settings.

Articulation Targets

Articulation refers to the production of phonemes in words and connected speech. As discussed in Chapter 3, most American children can articulate all of the sounds of English by the time they enter school. Some children, however, have difficulty developing linguistic concepts for the phonemes of English and understanding how they fit together in words within their spoken communication. Such children persist in using immature phonological processes to simplify the phonological structures of words, reducing consonant clusters (e.g., saying "scape" for *scrape* or "keam" for *scream*), or leaving off final consonants (e.g., saying "beer" for *beard* or "claw" for *clock*).

A few students need help to differentiate later-acquired phonemes, such as the liquids, /l/ and /r/. They round their lips, as for /w/, rather than shaping their tongues to produce the sounds accurately. Other children confuse the similar sounding phonemes, /f/ and /th/. This articulation problem should be differentiated from dialectal variations in production of /f/ and /th/ by speakers of African American Vernacular English. Additional sounds likely to cause difficulty for children with impaired articulation are the sibilants, /s/ and /sh/. If students have not learned to produce these sounds by second or third grade, they may need therapeutic interventions to learn to do so without a protruding tongue (the interdental /s/ or "lisp") or without forcing air out the sides of their tongue rather than down the center (a lateral /s/).

Students with severe articulation impairments involving many phonemes and sequencing and transition problems may be diagnosed with developmental apraxia of speech (DAS; Hall, Jordan, & Robin, 1993). DAS is presumed to have neurogenic origins. Children with DAS have extreme difficulty learning the smooth, automatic movements of connected speech.

The writing lab offers opportunities to target both speech articulation and phonemic awareness for all of these children by emphasizing the reciprocal nature of spoken–written relationships. As discussed previously in this chapter, when children learn standard sound–symbol correspondences, they have a concrete referent for sounds that may have been too fleeting and ephemeral for them previously to conceptualize. For assessment purposes, invented spellings also give instructors a window into how a student is hearing speech sounds, and they present opportunities to scaffold the student to higher levels of spoken language skill.

It may be necessary to teach isolated productions of sounds a student cannot produce correctly in a pull-out setting. Then, by working in the classroom in writing lab contexts, SLPs can greatly speed up the time-consuming process that is traditionally called *carryover*. The presence of an authentic audience of peers is as powerful a motivation to improve one's spoken communication as it is to improve one's written communication. Reading one's work aloud in the author chair presents opportunities for students to learn that if others cannot understand them, they need to work on their articulation accuracy, phrasing, and speaking rate.

Spoken Language Targets

Spoken language targets are similar to written language targets. As described previously in this chapter, language involves five interactive systems. Our dissatisfaction with traditional language intervention for school-age children, which often targeted only speech production, initially stimulated our focus on written language and its potential for supporting spoken language reciprocally.

Spoken–written language connections are many and deep. Some distinctions do exist, however, and writing lab activities are designed to take advantage of those. The social-communication demands of conversation can be targeted within the small group activities of peer conferencing or author groups. Instructors can scaffold students to understand the pragmatic expectations of their peers, with resulting increases in their social acceptance (see the story of Spencer in Chapter 13). Peers can be scaffolded to indicate their discomfort in ways that are helpful rather than hurtful to students who have inappropriate turn taking or other pragmatic skills. Students with language needs can be scaffolded to use their growing semantic and syntactic abilities to formulate comments or questions that make sense and fit logically in the conversational context. In many cases, by taking advantage of teachable moments in classroom communication contexts, SLPs can achieve with one trial what might take hundreds of trials in isolated settings of traditional therapy rooms. When teachers take over this role, the learning opportunities multiply throughout the week and are not limited to two times per week with the SLP.

Voice and Fluency Targets

Voice problems are another traditional target of speech therapy. Hypertensive voice production or vocal abuse, usually from too much yelling, can lead to the development of vocal nodules, which are callus-like growths on the vocal folds. Once students acquire a set of new voice production skills in the therapy room, the major challenge is to get them to use (carryover) those new skills in the classroom, on the playground, and at home. Other students who do not have voice disorders nevertheless need to learn to speak at appropriate levels of loudness to be heard by others in formal communication settings. We call this using a "public voice."

Similarly, students who stutter or who have other rate and fluency problems need to learn basic production skills in a small group or one-to-one setting. Skill development may take a few weeks in isolated one-on-one settings, and reminder sessions may be needed occasionally, but the main challenge to get students to use the new speech production approach all of the time and automatically can be addressed readily in writing lab contexts.

In writing lab activities, SLPs can signal privately to students with voice and fluency targets that they are expected to use their newly learned skills. In addition, SLPs working in classrooms can model for classroom teachers and peers how to support the student to independent, automatic use of the new voice or fluency skills as well.

Summary of Language Targets

Assessment and intervention activities of the writing lab approach are organized to target language growth at the levels of discourse, sentences, words, writing conventions, and spoken communication. Using this leveled structure for language targets helps teams decide how to focus their instruction and moves the questions of instruction beyond "What will we do tomorrow?" to "How can we help each student acquire the skills he or she needs to achieve success in school and life?"

SUMMARY

Language and learning are thoroughly intertwined during both the preschool and school-age years. This chapter provides an overview of the five rule systems of language—phonology, morphology, syntax, semantics, and pragmatics. Differences and similarities between language in its spoken and written forms are noted for their potential in supporting intervention efforts. Language targets are discussed at levels of discourse, sentences, words, writing conventions, and spoken communication. The message is that children need higher-level language skills to participate fully in school, and that writing in different genres and communicating orally about writing can help them acquire those skills.

3

Students with Language-Learning Needs

Language learning is a complex, integrated, indeed *miraculous,* process. Nevertheless, it proceeds without fanfare for most children. This fact may be partially because language is so firmly intertwined with all other aspects of human interaction and partially because language learning is usually so commonplace that no one pays much attention to it. Even when academic or social difficulties occur, they are not always attributed when they should be to problems with learning language.

For some children, language-learning barriers, such as hearing loss, Down syndrome, or general developmental delay, are recognized early. Children with disabilities such as these may enter intervention programs by 3 years old or even earlier. For others, parental concerns are minimized at first, but they grow and become acknowledged as children fail to meet developmental milestones.

For children who struggle with language and literacy learning, the early elementary years often are filled with anxiety and withdrawal, and the later school-age years are characterized by the cycle of failure (Fujiki, Brinton, Morgan, & Hart, 1999; Gerber, 1993). Reading and language problems generally do not disappear but continue into adolescence and early adulthood (Apel & Swank, 1999; Aram, Ekelman, & Nation, 1984; Bashir, Conte, & Heerde, 1998; Records, Tomblin, & Freese, 1992). In a decade of clinical experiences across the age span of schooling and in multiple settings, we have found benefits of the writing lab approach for students with all kinds of disabilities, needs, and abilities.

All students—not just those with disabilities—have language-learning needs and strengths. The writing lab approach, with its collaborative, inclusive, individualized instruction is appropriate for all students. Students who are academically talented can be challenged at appropriate levels with the same activities that are designed to meet the IEP goals of students receiving special education and speech-language intervention.

The discussion of students with language-learning needs in this chapter starts with a description of students identified as needing special education. In the writing lab approach, however, labels diminish in importance. Although IEP goals are addressed in writing lab activities, all students have individualized goals. In addition, specialists assist teachers to meet the needs of all students.

This chapter also touches on the needs of students whose language is different rather than disordered, including both second-language learners and dialectal speakers. The importance of valuing other cultural influences is emphasized, along with responsibility for helping all children acquire standard literate language forms. This brief overview of students' special needs is far from exhaustive, but it sets the stage for the rest of the book (especially Section III), which emphasizes techniques for addressing students' individualized needs.

STUDENTS WITH IDENTIFIED SPECIAL EDUCATION NEEDS

The phrase "special language and learning needs" applies to students with a range of disabilities and with a diverse set of language-learning issues. Students with identified special education needs include those with specific language and learning disabilities as well as those whose language-learning problems are related to other disabilities.

Types of Disabilities

Children with speech-language impairments usually are identified during their toddler or preschool years because of delays in learning to talk (Friel-Patti, 1999; Rescorla, 1989; Thal & Bates, 1988). Some children who demonstrate early expressive delays do not, however, end up demonstrating disabilities, especially if their comprehension and gestural communication systems are unaffected (Paul, 1991, 1996, 1997; Thal, Tobias, & Morrison, 1991). Paul (1996) recommended a watch-and-see approach for such children to avoid over-identifying them, but some researchers worry that underidentification may result if a watch-and-see approach is used—especially for children with multiple risks including poverty; they believe that earlier treatment, including a focus on emergent literacy, is important to prevent later difficulties (van Kleeck, Gillam, & Davis, 1997).

When problems in spoken-language acquisition persist and are observed among children with typical cognitive development and no other disabilities, the problems are termed *specific language impairments* (SLIs) (Tomblin et al., 1997; Watkins & Rice, 1994). SLI often involves core challenges acquiring skill with morpho-syntactic features of language, although difficulties with the linguistic details of language may be relative to the particular language a student with SLIs is attempting to learn (Bedore & Leonard, 2001; Leonard, 1998; Leonard & Bartolini, 1998; Rice & Oetting, 1993; Rice & Wexler, 1996; Windsor, Scott, & Street, 2000). Short-term memory deficits, auditory processing problems, and slow naming speed also are associated with SLI, as are difficulties with phonological awareness and learning to read and write (Butler, 1999; Catts, 1991, 1993; Catts, Fey, Zhang, & Tomblin, 2001; Catts & Kamhi, 1999; Friel-Patti, 1999; Torgesen, 1999).

As noted in Chapter 2, problems of phonological or phonemic awareness should not be confused with single phoneme articulation difficulties. Speech and language problems overlap, but they also may occur separately (e.g., Catts et al., 2001; Zhang &

Tomblin, 2000). Parallel treatment of phonological feature awareness and production does not necessarily result in parallel improvement in each area (Harbers, Paden, & Halle, 1999). Although some children need intervention to produce such speech sounds as /l/, /r/, and /s/, many of these children have no difficulty discriminating these sounds in the speech of others.

Lewis and colleagues (2000) followed students with phonological disorders (with and without other language problems) from the time they were 4–6 years old until they were in third or fourth grade. Articulation measures did not differentiate the students in follow-up investigations. The children who began the study with combined phonology and language problems performed worse than the phonology-alone group on measures of phoneme awareness, language, reading decoding, reading comprehension, and spelling. The phonology-alone group demonstrated poor spelling abilities relative to their reading and language abilities.

When children with language-learning difficulties are not identified until they reach school age, it is usually because their spoken language and cognitive abilities approximate those of typical development. Many students with no history of parental concern or special education diagnosis, however, first come to their teachers' attention when they struggle in learning to read and write. Some have difficulty from the earliest stages of formal literacy instruction. Although preschoolers may be identified as having learning disabilities, problems with reading and writing and other language skills are more likely to become apparent in kindergarten and first grade. When language problems are primary, SLPs in particular may diagnose students as having language-learning disabilities (LLDs; Butler, 1999; Wallach & Butler, 1984, 1994).

Other students reach second or third grade before their difficulties are formally diagnosed as learning disabilities, and some pass through the early stages of literacy learning with relative ease but struggle with advancing cognitive-linguistic demands in the upper grades. These students may wait even longer to be identified with LLDs (Butler, 1999; Keogh, 1993). The category of learning disability per se is unique in that it is defined in federal law:

> "Specific learning disability" means a disorder in one or more of the basic psychological processes involved in understanding or in using language, spoken or written, which may manifest itself in an imperfect ability to listen, speak, read, write, spell, or to do mathematical calculations. (U.S. Office of Education, 1977, p. 65083)

Although the category of students with learning disabilities consistently is the largest in U.S. reports of disability demographics, not all students with learning disabilities are adequately diagnosed. Some are misidentified. Others are not identified at all, even though they struggle with school (Zigmond, 1993). Concerns have been expressed about the policy of waiting until students experience academic failure before diagnosing learning disabilities and about the numerous flaws in learning disability definitions that use cognitive referencing to compare "achievement" with "ability" (Francis, Fletcher, Shaywitz, Shaywitz, & Rourke, 1996; Lyon, Gray, Kavanagh, & Krasnegor, 1993).

Most students with LLDs have problems in the use of language for listening, speaking, reading, or writing (Wallach & Butler, 1994). Numerous other similarities appear between students with spoken and written language problems. Even children with learning disabilities in the area of mathematics may have difficulty manipulating abstract symbols.

Students with SLIs and/or LLDs often have difficulties with limited phonology and syntax use into the school-age years, accompanied by heightened difficulty learning the sound–symbol associations so critical to word decoding and spelling (Blachman, 1997; Catts et al., 1994; Catts & Kamhi, 1999; Stanovich, 1988a, 1988b). Five variables among kindergartners—letter identification, sentence imitation, phonological awareness, rapid naming, and mother's education—have been found to predict reading outcomes best in second grade (Catts et al., 2001). Students with reading difficulties concentrated in the area of word decoding (often related to phonemic awareness difficulties) but who demonstrate intact comprehension skills may be labeled as having dyslexia (Catts, 1991; Catts & Kamhi, 1999). As noted in Chapter 2, the evidence is mounting that reading, spelling, and phonological awareness abilities and problems are reciprocal (Clarke, 1988; Menyuk & Chesnick, 1997; Torgesen, 1999). The good news is that the reciprocal relationship means that progress in one area can stimulate progress in others (Ehri, 2000).

Students with SLIs commonly have difficulty with language expression beyond the production of single words. Some have relatively fewer problems comprehending or interacting socially with peers. This does not mean, however, that pragmatic issues are nonexistent for students with SLIs, especially when comprehension and pragmatic problems are part of the profile (Donahue, Szymanski, & Flores, 1999; Fujiki & Brinton, 1994). Table 3.1 summarizes difficulties faced by children with a history of LLDs when they reach school age. It highlights distinctions between language abilities needed for less formal, spoken language contexts of nonacademic interactions with those needed for more formal, written language contexts of schooling.

Some students with borderline language and/or learning disabilities experience difficulties that do not reach thresholds for special education identification until the middle elementary school years, at which point their marginal language systems become overtaxed by the increased complexity of school language and processing demands (Keogh, 1993; Nelson, 1998). Students included in this group include those who are out of step with peers because of difficulty organizing discourse, judging audience needs, and grasping deeper meanings of narratives heard and read (Roth, 2000).

Students with other special education diagnoses (see e.g., Batshaw, 2002) often have language-learning problems that accompany them. Some students, particularly those with higher-functioning autism spectrum disorders (see e.g., Wetherby & Prizant, 2000), have relatively greater difficulty with semantic content and pragmatic use than with phonological, morphological, and syntactic form. Literacy skills still are rare targets for language intervention programs of students with autism and other developmental disabilities. For example, reading, writing, and literacy do not even appear as entries in the indexes of some classic textbooks on autism (e.g., Koegel & Koegel, 1995), although they do appear in more recent ones (e.g., Quill, 2000; Wetherby & Prizant, 2000).

Yet some students with autism spectrum disorders, in fact, have unusual abilities for processing the surface aspects of talking and reading that can serve them positively in reciprocal written–spoken language-learning interventions. For example, some students can repeat what they hear or read aloud at remarkably early ages but still have limited ability to integrate literal, figurative, and social meanings. When students develop early word recognition skills in reading, along with limited language comprehension abilities, they may be diagnosed as having hyperlexia (Catts & Kamhi, 1999). When they experience social interaction difficulties along with sense-making problems, they may be diagnosed as having semantic-pragmatic disorder or autism spec-

Table 3.1.   Characteristics associated with specific language-learning disabilities in school-age years

Language system	Spoken language needs (Listening and speaking)	Written language needs (Reading and writing)
Phonology	Few problems remain in speech production after early grades. Phonological awareness weaknesses may show up in rhyming, word segmenting and blending, and other metalinguistic tasks throughout school.	Persistent phonological confusions affect reading decoding and spelling abilities.
Morphology	Residual regular/irregular confusions may persist after typically developing children cease regularizing (e.g., *feets* and *finded* are still considered normal in the early elementary years).	Problems relating patterns to morphemes and orthographic patterns affect reading and spelling: Free: *tan, man, fan; low, bow, show* Bound: derivational: *dis-, -tion;* inflectional: *-ing, -ed*
Syntax	Few problems are obvious in simple expressive syntax but problems may go undetected in complex syntax, both for understanding and formulating complex messages.	Problems in basic comprehension affect reading for some students. Some students have adequate simple syntax skills but cannot handle complex syntax while reading or writing.
Semantics	Inadequate and inaccurate basic/foundation vocabulary may be an undetected cause of failure to respond appropriately to oral directions. Students may not recognize or "fast map" academic/curricular/sophisticated vocabulary.	Ability to recognize unfamiliar words as "new" may be affected by both semantic difficulties and low reading-decoding skill. Students with adequate semantic systems may not use them strategically while reading or writing.
Pragmatics	Some students have no particular pragmatic difficulties in social conversation, but have difficulty producing organized, clear narrative and expository spoken discourse. Others have marked problems in social conversation and interaction as well as in narrative and expository production and comprehension.	Most students with language-learning disabilities have difficulty drawing on all systems needed to understand and produce complex written texts— whether narrative or expository.

Sources: Johnson and Grant (1989); Lewis, Freebairn, and Taylor (2000); MacArthur (2000); Nelson, (1998); Roth (2000); Scott (1999, 2000); Silliman, Jimerson, and Wilkinson (2000).

trum disorders (Rapin & Allen, 1983; Tiegerman-Farber, 1997; Twachtman-Cullen, 2000). In an investigation comparing social conversation conducted orally and in writing (by passing a notebook back and forth), we found that some students with autism were measurably better at staying on topic and interacting appropriately in writing (Schairer & Nelson, 1996).

Paley (1994) described several children with exaggerated communication needs in her kindergarten classes, in which story dictation and dramatization were features of every session. One of the students Paley described was Serena. Although Paley avoided labeling any of her students when describing them, others might recognize elements of hyperlexia and possible autism spectrum disorder in Paley's description of Serena as a child who spoke perfectly but stored "memories in verbal rituals and compulsive behaviors" (p. 12). Box 3.1 describes how Paley responded to Serena's needs by showing her classmates—including Dylan, a child with symptoms of SLI—how to be sensitive to Serena's more compulsive needs. The example also shows how, in a classroom focused on storytelling, Serena was able to use storytelling to process some of her own fears about losing control by being granted ownership and patience.

Box 3.1. Storytelling for Students with Diverse Language-Learning Needs

Serena had amazed her parents with her early interest and ability in literacy, but they had become concerned about her strange uses of those talents. For example, as Paley (1994) read to the class, Serena neatly printed the names of her classmates alphabetically on cards, which she then passed out to them: "NOT-LIBBY," "NOT-ARIANNE," "NOT-PETER," and so on. Paley commented, "We have all been alphabetized and organized by color into nonpersons" (p. 12).

Another student with special needs in Paley's class that year was Dylan. Dylan's profile is consistent with specific language impairment. At 5 years old, Dylan had mastered neither language nor appropriate social behavior. "'Me'en a tiger,' he growled, pouncing on a child who sat quietly listening" (p. 11) while Paley read aloud to the group.

In the community of storytellers, Dylan had opportunities to improve his social skills in the context of responding to Serena's perfectionism. One of her compulsive needs was that every story must have more than one character. Paley described what happened one day during story dictation:

> Before Dylan tells his story, he warns Serena that no one else will be in it. "Only me. Just fox is me only that." He is preparing her for what he knows she will do: run away from the table. Serena panics when a story has only one character. She has made a number of compromises for the sake of storytelling but she cannot accept a single-character story any more than an empty space on a line, or an unfinished sentence at the bottom of a page.
>
> Dylan's story is brief, so Serena doesn't have to stay away long. "Once upon a time come a fox. That me. Growl! Jumping on the hill. And I make my teeth like this. And then running around. Look how strong the fox."
>
> He shows me his muscles and then puts a finger on an "and," while whispering Serena's name.
>
> "Speaking of Serena," I whisper back, "do you want to add another character? So when we act out your story, Serena won't cry and run away."
>
> He considers the option for a moment but then shakes his head. Later in the year, he and all others will methodically avoid one-character stories. (p. 15)

In Paley's class, it was okay to be different. Serena was able to participate because the other students learned to accept her idiosyncrasies, but she also used her stories to create a bridge that helped others understand her. One day, the day after she had refused to help others clean up, Serena told this story:

> Once upon a time there was a school of kids but there was only five kids in the school. Number 1 liked to jump, number 2 liked to play, number 3 liked to build things, number 4 liked to draw, and number 5 liked to be the leader. One day number 5 was the leader but the teacher said number 1 couldn't jump. And then number 5 told number 2 not to play. And then when he was getting the milk, he told number 3 not to build, and when number 5 was going to music, the teacher told number 4 not to draw. And number 5 was the only lucky one that day. (p. 16)

Paley observed that this story helped her "understand, in a less emotional context, [Serena's] great need to control everything in a world in which she controls very little. She spells out—in exaggerated form—feelings the children recognize" (p. 17).

Excerpts from Judith Felson Duchan, Lynne E. Hewitt, & Rae M. Sonnenmeier (Eds.). *Pragmatics: From Theory to Practice.* Published by Allyn and Bacon, Boston, MA. Copyright © by Pearson Education. Adapted by permission of the publisher.

A broader group of students without clear special education needs might have difficulty with the abstract meanings of language and its pragmatic-social uses. One possible reason for this may be the difficulty of diagnosing pragmatic difficulties with standardized tests (Westby, 1999b). It has been estimated that approximately 10% of preschool-age children fail to demonstrate adequate social competence (Elksnin & Elksnin, 1995). Children with disabilities are particularly at risk. Students with developmental disabilities involving cognition and students with emotional and behavioral issues face particular challenges with the pragmatics of language use (Cole, Coggins, & Vanderstoep, 1999; Donahue, Hartas, & Cole, 1999; Rogers-Adkinson & Griffith, 1999; Sturm & Koppenhaver, 2000).

Many students with SLIs primarily in the area of syntax have comparatively few difficulties with pragmatic aspects of social communication (Craig & Washington, 1993; Rapin & Allen, 1983). Nevertheless, students with language impairments are at greater risk than typically developing peers of demonstrating problems with social skills (Fujiki & Brinton, 1994), particularly social withdrawal (Fujiki et al., 1999; Fujiki, Brinton, Isaacson, & Summers, 2001). They also experience greater social disvalue by their peers (Gertner, Rice, & Hadley, 1994; Redmond & Rice, 1998), particularly if their language problems extend into the areas of language comprehension, semantics, and pragmatics (Craig & Washington, 1993). Yet students with even mild disabilities traditionally have been given fewer opportunities to express themselves, particularly in writing (Christenson, Thurlow, Ysseldyke, & McVicar, 1989).

Adolescence is a challenging time for any individual's concept of self, but the risks skyrocket when those years are compounded by the presence of a language impairment associated with hearing loss, traumatic brain injury, or developmental disabilities (Stinson & Whitmire, 2000; Sturm & Koppenhaver, 2000; Tattershall, 2002; Whitmire, 2000; Ylvisaker & DeBonis, 2000). Some students find a sense of accomplishment in their written language activities that can support them in developing new social relationships, either through co-authoring activities, peer conferencing, or author group experiences. Box 3.2 shows how this occurred for one student described by Donahue, Szymanski, and Flores (1999). Chapter 4 describes how author groups and other peer conferencing can contribute to social-interaction learning, and Chapter 8 describes the use of co-authoring software features to provide unique opportunities for peer interactions.

Students with hearing impairments or who are deaf find it particularly difficult to gain access to spoken and written language even though their cognitive-linguistic and emotional systems may be basically intact (Musselman, 2000; Stinson & Whitmire, 2000). Yoshinaga-Itano and Downey (1992) reviewed literature on the written language problems of children with hearing impairments or deafness and noted that earlier studies had emphasized difficulties at word or within-sentence levels. Yoshinaga-Itano and her colleagues added evidence about semantic, discourse-level problems. They pointed out that children who lack earlier developing language competencies face extra challenges when attempting to acquire literate discourse abilities during their school-age years; they produce stories that have fewer words, use fewer syntactic and semantic tools for conveying information, and include fewer high-level story grammar elements, such as those conveying psychological causality (Yoshinaga-Itano & Downey, 1996; Yoshinaga-Itano, Snyder, & Mayberry, 1996b).

Luckner highlighted that "Unlike their hearing peers, who learn to read and write in a language they already know, many students who are deaf or hard of hearing learn

---

Box 3.2.   Written Language Supports for Social Interaction Learning

"Emily Dickenson" was a 16-year-old girl whose LLDs had been identified in kinder-garten. Donahue, Szymanski, and Flores described her as a student with "a long his-tory of oral language problems and social isolation" (1999, p. 275). By the time she reached high school, Emily could understand basic semantic and syntactic structures, and, with some scaffolding, could respond to basic instructions and simple literal and inferential information. She also could use story grammar frameworks to aid her comprehension of stories. Her language production was characterized by short state-ments and questions, appropriate answers to *wh-* questions, correct verb tenses, and subject–verb agreement. Despite such strengths in basic communication skills, Emily's language impairment was characterized by "significant difficulties in comprehending and participating effectively in social-communication interactions, processing rapidly presented auditory information, comprehending complex literal and inferential in-fromation, and formulating fluent, concise messages" (p. 275).

At this point, Emily's social and emotional difficulties were more salient than her per-sisting oral language deficits. Her hesitancies in oral language communication were characterized, for example, by an incident in which she grabbed a marking pen she needed from a peer, rather than requesting it verbally. Not surprisingly, Emily was socially isolated. She did, however, possess significant strengths in reading, spelling, and writing. In fact, her self-identity seemed "to revolve around her literacy talents and interests" (p. 175), which she used to support her peers with disabilties in read-ing and spelling tasks.

Donahue, Szymanski, and Flores (1999) reported that a turning point came for Emily in her development of social skills around a co-authoring event with another student who had a similar passion for screenplays and watching movies. At one point, this was the description of their interaction:

> *Sitting together at one computer, continuing their Sailor Moon screen-play, Emily and Steven are engaged in an animated conversation about their writing. The computer teacher comes in and scolds them for forget-ting to turn their computer off the day before. Each is embarrassed, but jokingly blames the other, engaging in typical teenage bantering. After the computer teacher leaves the room, they laugh and whisper together, clearly pleased to be caught in collusion. (p. 281)*

---

to read and write while simultaneously learning their first language" (1996, p. v), or in the case of students whose first language is American Sign Language (ASL), learning a different language. The method of instruction or communication used by students who are deaf or hard of hearing (i.e., oral–aural versus simultaneous/total communication) appears to be less influential, however, on their written language development than more basic lexical/semantic issues. Yoshinaga-Itano, Snyder, and Mayberry (1996a) drew this conclusion when they compared written language samples produced by students around the age of 12 years who were communicating primarily via oral–aural versus simultaneous/total communication. The researchers found no significant differences between compositions of the two groups. Although literacy expectations for deaf and hard of hearing students are generally grades below their hearing peers, research has provided success stories for all kinds of educational possibilities and environments, and these stories indicate that "given the appropriate student and environmental variables, deaf and hard-of-hearing students can achieve at levels commensurate with normally hearing peers" (Yoshinaga-Itano et al., 1996a, p. 54).

Mode of communication does not influence the nature of scaffolds students require. Although the basic experience of communicating ideas through print is common to all literate language users, scaffolds should be matched to students' prior experiences with language. Schleper (1996) described how early adolescent students who were deaf developed spelling strategies for remembering how to spell difficult words based more on analogical morphology than phonology. For example, one student whose first language was ASL signed MONDAY + KEY after asking for the spelling of *monkey*. Schleper also described the strategies of a deaf early childhood educator who introduced her students to three little words in the word *snow*: *no, now, ow*. He indicated that "the students were thrilled with the word play, just like my middle-school students, and they all quickly learned to fingerspell and write this new word" (p. 203).

Students who have severe physical and/or multiple disabilities also may experience challenges at all levels of language and literacy acquisition. As discussed in Chapter 11, students with physical disabilities or sensory impairments, such as blindness, may benefit from specialized access methods, including alternative keyboards, word prediction, or other computer supports to enable them to get their words on the page independently (Beukelman & Mirenda [with J. Sturm], 1998; Hunt-Berg, Rankin, & Beukelman, 1994; Koppenhaver & Yoder, 1993; Pebly & Koppenhaver, 2001; Sturm et al., 1997; Zorfass, Corley, & Remz, 1994). For students with severe physical and speech impairments, literacy skills can make the difference between dependence on rote messages prepared by others and the ability to communicate unique messages they have constructed themselves. Formal instruction historically has been provided rarely for such students (Beukelman & Mirenda, 1998; Koppenhaver & Yoder, 1992; Light & McNaughton, 1993; Mirenda, 1999). Although this pattern has begun to change, instructional teams have much to learn about how to help these students develop full access to literacy learning.

Written Language Problems of Students with Disabilities

Written language acquisition for all students is a primary target of the writing lab approach. This approach provides interdisciplinary opportunities to target reciprocal spoken and written language growth for all students. Essentially any of the goals on the IEPs of students with disabilities can be targeted through writing lab activities. Similarly, any general curriculum written language goal can be addressed through the writing lab approach (see Chapter 16). Nevertheless, it is helpful to consider special challenges facing students with LLDs and various related conditions when approaching writing tasks. Problems have been observed at all stages of the writing process, including planning, drafting, revising, and editing (Roth, 2000).

Planning Problems

Students with LLDs engage in relatively little planning and, even when prompted, have relatively few planning strategies on which to draw (MacArthur, 2000). They often start impulsively with little reflection about audience or situation, write linearly on a topic using only a "what next" or "knowledge telling" strategy, and stop when they have written all their easily retrievable knowledge on that topic (Graham, Harris, MacArthur, & Schwartz, 1991; Roth, 2000; Scardamalia & Bereiter, 1986; Troia, Graham, & Harris, 1999).

Students with LLDs also have less knowledge about the characteristics of good writing and the writing process. They tend to emphasize mechanical issues over substantive ones (Graham, Schwartz, & MacArthur, 1993), and they may be less sensitive than peers to the requirements of different genres or text structures (Englert, Raphael, Anderson, Gregg, & Anthony, 1989; Roth, 2000).

Some typically developing students can produce stories with adult structures by age 6 years. The majority are expected to do so by age 9 or 10 (Applebee, 1978; Peterson & McCabe, 1983; Stein & Glenn, 1979). After that point, students tend to elaborate their stories through increased numbers of episodes and complex embedding strategies (Roth & Spekman, 1986). In contrast, students with LLDs produce stories that are shorter, less detailed, less cohesive, and less syntactically complex (Barenbaum, Newcomer, & Nodine, 1987; MacArthur & Graham, 1987; Montague, Maddux, & Dereschiwsky, 1990). Students who are deaf and hard of hearing may still be developing basic story elements until they are 18 years old (Yoshinaga-Itano & Downey, 1996).

The narratives of students with LLDs also include fewer internal responses, plan statements, and complete episodes. Roth (2000) summarized explanations for lower quality written narratives as involving reduced language processing abilities, less interest in and understanding of the writing process, lower levels of written language automaticity, trade-offs of attention on the mechanics of writing at the expense of higher-level discourse abilities, and reduced self-regulation and self-monitoring strategies. Graham and Harris (1989) showed that strategy instruction had a positive effect on story grammar elements for students with LLDs but that these students' stories remained shorter and received ratings of lower quality than typically developing peers.

When writing expository texts, students with LLDs may: 1) take longer and write less, 2) apply limited concepts of what makes a good product (e.g., equating a good essay as one with no spelling errors), 3) substitute inexact vocabulary for desired choices when word-retrieval or spelling problems interfere, 4) make quantitatively more errors in spelling, punctuation, and grammar, and 5) require more practice to achieve mastery of a writing strategy (Wong, 2000).

When Englert, Raphael, Fear, and Anderson (1988) questioned students about their knowledge of expository text construction, students with LLDs showed less knowledge than either their high- or low-achieving peers about how to control and regulate the writing process, use organizational strategies or text structures to generate or group ideas, and monitor the quality of texts. Their expository compositions also tended to be less well developed than those of their peers.

Although students with LLDs start out with difficulties in planning, organizing, discourse knowledge, and self-regulation strategies, research indicates that specialized interventions can make a difference (Englert et al., 1991; Graham & Harris, 1989; Graham, Harris, & Troia, 2000; Montague & Graves, 1993; Wong, 2000). Chapter 5 suggests scaffolding techniques for targeting problems involving planning, organizing, and self-regulation.

Drafting Problems

The ability to draft written discourse requires a complex set of cognitive-linguistic and motor acts. Berninger described these abilities as *transcription;* the young child:

> First discovers that scribbling with a crayon or pencil leaves a visible trace; following this discovery, handwriting follows a predictable developmental course, beginning with random scribbling, and proceeding in order to zigzag lines, letter-like marks, true letters, single words, clauses, and sentences. (2000, p. 68)

Transcription is more than a motor act; it is a language act as well. To be able to draft, students must be able to spell, at least well enough that they and others can read back the words they have written. Both handwriting and spelling are problematic for students with learning disabilities, and these skill areas seem to be related (Johnson & Grant, 1989). Students with limited motor abilities still can compose written language using keyboards and specialized key access if necessary, but they must be able to spell if they are to move beyond a stage of symbol writing to use an alphabetic system like English.

The definition of conventional writing, as suggested by Sulzby, is "connected discourse that another conventionally literate person can read without too much difficulty and that the child can read conventionally" (1996, p. 27). Most students can demonstrate enough understanding of Sulzby's key traits to be considered capable of conventional writing by the end of first grade (Scott, 1999). Critical traits include knowledge of 1) sound–symbol relationships, 2) words as memorable and stable units, and 3) text as an object. Scott added that emergent writers are expected to have a belief that they can write and that many who at first profess to be unable to write can be scaffolded to write when given sufficient encouragement and support (see Chapter 5).

Part of the recursive nature of the writing process is that drafting involves the ability to keep in mind and further develop planned discourse structures to guide the organization of text (Hayes & Flower, 1980). While writing, expert writers carry on an active internal conversation with themselves, deciding what they know and think about a topic, along with how best to organize and communicate the information (Bereiter & Scardamalia, 1987). Simultaneously, drafting involves constructing sentences and selecting words for the purpose of conveying intended meanings and relationships, keeping audience needs in mind all the while. Novice writers, in contrast, are more likely to engage in a "knowledge telling" approach, which seems to be guided by a strategy to "say what you think and then give reasons" (Bryson & Scardamalia, 1991, p. 45).

The multiple and integrated discourse-, sentence-, and word-level demands of skilled authorship are challenging for all students, but without intervention, they are beyond the reach of students with weak language abilities. Even in their spoken narratives, children with language impairments use fewer conjunctions and less elaborate noun phrases (Greenhalgh & Strong, 2001). At about age 9 or 10, typically developing students demonstrate "differentiation" in their written (compared with oral) grammatical constructions, including 1) elimination of such oral language devices as *well* and *you know;* 2) fewer clauses coordinated with *and* and more subordinate clauses; and 3) increases in such written language structures as passives and nonfinite forms (e.g., infinitives, gerunds, participles). These abilities present challenges to most students with language problems.

Wong (2000) summarized research that students with LLDs make quantitatively more errors in grammar than their typically developing peers. Johnson and Grant (1989) noted particular problems in the area of syntactic morphology. In addition, Wong noted that problems beget problems. For example, word-retrieval and spelling problems can lead students to substitute inexact vocabulary for desired choices. A general outcome of all of these difficulties, as shown by numerous studies, is the production of shorter texts, measured both in total numbers of words and total numbers of sentences (Scott, 1999). Scott also noted that "when researchers have looked at lexical and syntactic variety, poor writers have been shown to have a more limited repertoire of complex sentence structures" (p. 250).

Spelling problems are treated as word-level language problems in the written language analysis system we propose (see Chapter 15). Spelling issues for students with LLDs often are severe and long term. Many such individuals struggle with spelling across their lifespan (Blalock & Johnson, 1987; Juel, 1988). In general, however, "poor spellers follow the same general developmental stages as better spellers," and, "best practices for good spellers will likely benefit poor spellers" (Scott, 2000, p. 67). Chapter 6 describes these strategies.

Drafting is the core language-production act of writing. Its complexities should not be underestimated. Students with LLDs, as well as those with other disabilities, can face challenges at the sound, syllable, word, sentence, or discourse levels. Such difficulties can be detected through individualized assessment (see Chapter 15). The writing lab approach offers multiple opportunities to scaffold all students, including those with disabilities, to develop more mature language skills and competencies (see Chapter 6).

Revising Problems

Revising and editing sometimes are treated as part of the same process, but they really address two different kinds of internal questions. In order to revise, students have to be able to ask themselves such questions as, Is this organized the best way? Will my readers understand it? Is there enough detail? Is the sequence logical? In other words, revising requires metacognitive reflection and making changes that involve substantive issues, mostly at the discourse and sentence levels. In contrast, editing addresses questions such as, Is this correct? Is my punctuation okay? Are the words spelled correctly? Editing also requires careful rereading, and it may lead to revisions of content as well as correction of spelling and writing conventions, but editing is focused more on surface issues and mechanics than discourse structure. Both revising and editing require linguistic abilities as well as proofreading and self-reflective skills.

Revising is challenging to all students, but Tully (1996) questioned if the concept was too difficult for early elementary students to tackle:

> I believe that children in grades two and above can handle revision if they are taught the skills that enable them to do it and if revision is presented to them as process of developing—rather than correcting—writing. Kids have to know that it's not about fixing errors but about making their meaning clear . . . . Revision means "to look at again." Children grow as writers when they experience themselves as active revisers and shapers of their writing. (1996, p. 8)

If revising is challenging for all students, it is even more so for students with LLDs. Research shows that they are less likely to spend time revising than skilled writers (MacArthur, 2000). In one study, MacArthur, Graham, and Schwartz (1991) investigated the metacognitive awareness of seventh- and eighth-grade students with LLDs by asking them what changes should be made to improve a paper they wrote. Most of them suggested revisions that would address surface elements only, such as spelling and neatness. Only one fourth of the students made any recommendations for revising their own papers based on content. When evaluating other students' papers, however, the students suggested revisions to improve discourse content, including suggestions to add information and to change the beginnings of papers. These findings support the use of peer conferencing and peer "editing" (including revision) activities, which are key instructional components of the writing lab approach (see Chapter 4).

Editing Problems

Editing problems stem from basic language problems, as well as from metalinguistic and metacognitive difficulties. Students with LLDs tend to have difficulty with capitalization, often omitting it. They also have difficulty with punctuation—producing sentences without end punctuation, leaving large segments of text unpunctuated, or using end punctuation at points other than sentence boundaries, which creates sentence fragments (Scott, 1999). They also lack the metalinguistic abilities to know clearly what a sentence is, and they lack the metacognitive and self-regulatory abilities to reread their work and notice when problems are present. Within the writing lab approach, we scaffold students to notice how punctuation problems interfere with communication of their intended meanings (see Chapters 5 and 6). Students are taught directly when basic skills are found lacking. They also are taught directly to reread their works carefully and to identify problems within them using the procedures of the writing lab approach.

STUDENTS WITHOUT DISABILITIES WHO NEED INSTRUCTIONAL SUPPORT

In some cases, students' language-based learning problems are attributed to behavioral issues such as not paying attention, not trying, being "slow," or many other labels that relate to observable behaviors but provide little insight into underlying problems. Some of these children may indeed qualify for services when they are referred and evaluated for the presence of specific LLDs or other disability-related language disorders.

In many cases, however, a teacher who is convinced that language-learning problems are at the root of a student's academic difficulties is disappointed to find that formal testing does not qualify the student for special services. Many such students do indeed score low on formal language tests compared with their classmates, but they do not qualify for services because of "cognitive referencing" or "discrepancy model" policies (see Nelson, 1998, for a review). Such policies require students to score low compared with younger students with similar mental ages or intelligence quotient (IQ) scores, rather than to same-age peers. Meanwhile, these students are expected to compete with same-age peers to be successful in classrooms.

Particularly when language problems involve comprehension, language factors may depress IQ scores, making it difficult for children who are slower learners to qualify. Such children then may find themselves in a gray area in which their teachers know they need special attention, but no one is available to provide it. Students like these do not necessarily need to be labeled, but they do need attention from professionals knowledgeable about how to foster language development. Being held back is not the answer. For example, one 7-year-old girl, who had repeated first grade but had not been diagnosed as having a language disorder, observed a peer's jeans with holes and asked, "How come your pants are all in a hole?" Without assistance, and without understanding the language basis for many aspects of her learning difficulties, this child and others like her fall further and further behind their classmates. Eventually, many drop out before completing secondary school.

Most gray-area students continue to struggle without special help except from dedicated classroom teachers, who already may be dividing their attention among 20–30 other students and who often have no special training in how to foster language development that does not proceed typically. Although formal testing makes it clear that students with combined cognitive and language delays do not have the skills to progress academically with their same-age classmates, professionals with specialized skills to help them acquire those skills may be prohibited by policy from working with such students.

Underlying such maladaptive policies is the assumption that children with commensurate cognitive and language abilities cannot benefit from intervention. A growing body of evidence suggests, however, that this assumption simply is not true (Cole, Coggins, & Vanderstoep, 1999; Cole & Harris, 1992; Fey, Long, & Cleave, 1994). Evidence also is growing that the language abilities of children with specific and nonspecific language impairments are similar and that students with nonspecific language impairments are particularly at risk for continuing difficulties with spoken and written language (Catts & Fey, 2001).

Collaborative, classroom-based interventions can make it possible for all children to develop the language skills to be successful in school, and policies should promote this. The answer is not to label more children and pull them out of their general education classrooms but to bring teams of professionals together who can address all special needs in general curricular contexts. The inclusive contexts of the writing lab approach, which combine language intervention methods with general education experiences, can do just that (see Chapter 17).

STUDENTS WHOSE LANGUAGE IS DIFFERENT

Students whose first language is different from SAE have specific language-learning needs despite the fact that they may not have any disabilities. These students include bilingual children, second language learners, and children who speak a dialect of English other than SAE.

Bilingual and Second Language Learners

School-age bilingual children and second language learners have to learn a new language at the same time they are learning to cope with the demands of schooling (Gutierrez-Clellen, 1999). Cummins (1984) recommended distinguishing basic interactional conversational skills (BICS), which might serve English language learners well in informal social settings, from the cognitive academic language proficiency skills (CALPS) of schooling that present greater challenges to English language learners. In other words, academic concepts often are expressed in unfamiliar language, have fewer contextual supports, and require world knowledge that may not be in students' realms of experience. This explains why some second language learners can communicate adequately in most social conversations but still experience language-related difficulties when attempting to meet the academic literate language expectations of classrooms. The writing lab approach offers opportunities to help such students strengthen both their spoken and written English skills in supportive but challenging and integrated events.

Students Who Speak a Different Dialect

Everyone who speaks a language speaks a dialect of it, and the rules of dialectal grammars are just as regular and complex as those of SAE (Pinker, 1994). Problems arise, though, when written forms of the language dialect differ significantly from SAE. Examples of dialects with this characteristic include African American Vernacular English (Ebonics), Appalachian English, European-influenced nonstandard English, and Spanish-influenced English of many varieties.

Societal judgments of whether a person is literate and educated are strongly influenced by language use and communicative style. Although most educators agree that all students should learn to use correct SAE grammar, there is little agreement about how best to teach it. Exhortation and correction do not work. If a student's natural oral language is corrected when the student attempts to communicate, he or she may feel confused, inadequate, and detached from the rewards of schooling. The writing process approach can bridge this student's spoken language skills to the expectations of written language and SAE proficiency without such social penalties.

Using an "anything goes" approach (i.e., being overly accepting of students' efforts) is also not the answer. Delpit (1995) was particularly critical of "liberal" educational practices that do not assist all students to develop fluency in literate language forms. She quoted a fellow black educator talking about the notion that African American children had to learn to be fluent in writing before they could be expected to conform to SAE standards:

> I've got a kid right now—brilliant. But he can't get a score on the SAT that will even get him considered by any halfway decent college. He needs *skills,* not *fluency.* . . . White kids learn how to write a decent sentence. Even if they don't teach them in school, their parents make sure they get what they need. But what about our kids? They don't get it at home and they spend all their time in school learning to be *fluent.* (p. 16)

Delpit (1995) used this quote to make the point that dialect speakers need explicit instruction in SAE grammar. She explained her concerns:

> Although the problem is not necessarily inherent in the method, in some instances adherents of process approaches to writing create situations in which students ultimately find themselves held accountable for knowing a set of rules about which no one has ever directly informed them. . . . If such explicitness is not provided to students, what it feels like to people who are old enough to judge is that there are secrets being kept, that time is being wasted, that the teacher is abdicating his or her duty to teach. (1995, p. 31)

Smitherman (1994) expressed a slightly different perspective. She cautioned against equating language differences with "problems" or "mismatches." In a piece called, "The Blacker the Berry, the Sweeter the Juice," she demonstrated that stories written with more elements of African American discourse styles (for the National Assessment of Educational Progress) received higher ratings than those with fewer elements, regardless of the inclusion of African American grammatical features. The issues are not simple, however, and opinions are not necessarily aligned with racial and ethnic identities.

As we noted when discussing the balance principle in Chapter 1, some school districts have policies that mandate published works to be written in standard edited English. Although this mandate presents challenges to the ownership principle, instructional teams can use a variety of strategies to help students bring written products to publication standards within curricular deadlines (see also Chapter 6 regarding revising and editing). This can be accomplished while working toward increasing independence and teaching the features of SAE grammar.

Figures 3.1 and 3.2 show how the revision process provided opportunities for students to revise their home dialects to literate SAE conventions. In Figure 3.1, a fifth-grader named Ray made a number of changes during the revision process with minimal scaffolding. It was particularly interesting that when rereading, Ray stopped when he read, "My sister she likes to play basketball and tea kwon toe." He spontaneously crossed out the redundant *she* in apposition, which is a common feature of spoken African American Vernacular English. While doing so, he noted that the revised sentence sounded more like language used in books. Ray was developing literate language skills.

Figure 3.2 shows an About the Author piece for a fifth-grader named Lidia. Lidia's family had immigrated from Mexico, and her first language was Spanish. When scaffolding this piece, it was important to consider the Spanish rule for pronominalization, which indicates that a pronoun is not needed when a second clause clearly has the same subject and pronominalization is coded on the verb. During revision, the SLP had Lidia reread the sentence, "All the teachers I have are helpful and nice, made me go on and begane a new grade level that I should begane and start a new life that is ahead of me." When Lidia indicated that she thought it sounded all right, the instructor, recognizing the Spanish-language influence, made explicit the need for the pronoun. She pointed out that, although it was acceptable in Spanish to omit the subject for the second sentence because it was clear, in English it was important to say that it was "they" (the teachers) who made Lidia go on and start a new grade level. Without criticizing Lidia's home language, the distinction was clarified, and her English literacy skills were advanced.

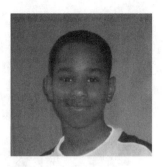

ABOUT RAY I LIVE IN PLAINWELL NOW. I EAT CHICKEN BLUE AND

PIZZZA TOO I AM 10 YEARS OLD. MY FAVORITE MOVIE IS DEEP SEA MY

FAVORITE T.V. SHOW IS WRESTLING.   I HAVE 1 BROTHER AND SISTER

MOM DAD. I'm the oldest. My sister is 9 end
my brother is 3 he talks too
much and likes to play my games.
he loves to eat sausage and eat
chicken. It is his favorite food
My sister she likes to
play basketball and tea kwon toe
I have been going to Spring valley for
5 years. Oh yeah I was born on
April 8,

Figure 3.1.   Ray's About the Author piece.

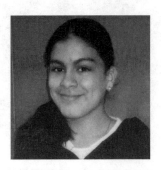

About the author

Lidia

My favorite state is   California (that's where I was born.)

I like to play (sports) .but my favorite sport is soccer and

hockey. I like my familiy who lives with me now. I like

studing about the weather.I want to be someone special like

my teachers. All the teachers I have are helpful and nice, they

made me go on and begane a new grade level that I should

begane and start a new life that is ahead of me and you

know what, I thank them. my favorite food is pizza,

macoroni, spageti. This helps me.I love writing and hope you

enjioed my writing. My mom or dad help me
when I need help.

Figure 3.2. Lidia's About the Author piece.

STUDENTS WITH DIFFERENT
CULTURES OR ECONOMIC DISADVANTAGES

Beyond grammatical linguistic and dialectal differences, a number of other cultural factors influence how children are socialized to learn discourse and the knowledge they have when they come to school. Children in all ethnic groups hear narratives in the family gatherings of their early childhood long before coming to school, but not all children are socialized to organize their spoken and written narratives in the same ways (Gee, 1990; Heath, 1983; Westby, 1994). Understanding this fact helps educators to use assessment and instructional practices that accommodate cultural differences, meanwhile helping students to acquire strategies that are valued by mainstream society.

This appreciation has particularly strong implications for individualized assessment. All children do not experience language-sampling tasks in the same way. Students from Native American cultures, for example, might find it hard to share a piece of work before they consider it finished (Robinson-Zanartu, 1996). Such cultural factors must be taken into account when conducting informal assessments (Gutierrez-Clellen & Quinn, 1993; Gutierrez-Clellen, Restrepo, Bedore, Pena, & Anderson, 2000; Lidz & Pena, 1996). A danger also exists that teachers might lower their evaluations of students' stories because of unrecognized signs of cultural diversity (Michaels, 1991).

Mainstream children from a variety of ethnic groups come to school already having been socialized to tell stories with European-tradition discourse structures (Roth, 2000). Children in other cultural groups may be socialized differently, but all tell stories (Gutierrez-Clellen, 1995; Heath, 1983, 1986; Hester, 1996; Westby, 1994). Some African American children, for example, have been socialized to tell stories that are more topic-associative in that they are constructed by linking each topic associatively with whatever precedes it (Michaels, 1981). Topic-associative narratives contrast with topic-centered narratives, in which a central topic is developed through a series of related events. To be nonbiased, assessments of personal narratives must account for such variations.

Variations in elicitation tasks also result in changes in discourse structures. Personal narratives, which discuss one's own experiences, are more likely to be topic associative than other types (Hester, 1996). Differences also occur when children from diverse cultures produce spoken versus written narratives (Hyter & Westby, 1996; Michaels, 1981; Scott, 1994). Children from Hispanic cultures may expect to relate their personal experience stories through dialogic conversations rather than monologic narratives (Gutierrez-Clellen & Quinn, 1993). Westby's (1994) literature review also showed that children from white working class families are more likely to have extensive experience in giving tightly scaffolded narrative recounts of shared daily events, (e.g., "Tell me about what you did today."). Although these children are exposed to children's books, parental scaffolding in such families is often focused more on rote learning (e.g., colors or numbers) than comprehension. Children from African American working class families may have less experience with children's books and more expectations to produce expressive accounts of events, often involving teasing, exaggeration, and cooperative telling. Young Mexican American children may have more exposure to stories about historical events and less to children's literature. Children in Chinese American families often are exposed more frequently to informational books and stories designed to teach values and convey historical events, than to fictional stories.

Different analysis schemes also yield diverse results for students from different cultures. Labov (1972) used "high point analysis" to describe narratives in inner-city communities in which the narrator 1) orients the listener to who, what, and where something happened; 2) relates a series of events that build to some sort of climax or high point; and 3) then resolves the story by telling how things turned out. The high point is the "emotional heart of the narrative or the climax." It contains a "high concentration of evaluative statements or words" (Rollins, McCabe, & Bliss, 2000, p. 228). To elicit high-point narratives from a child, examiners may tell their own personal event narratives first (e.g., about being stung by a bee or scared by an animal). Using this technique, McCabe and Peterson (1984) found that European North American children could be expected to produce a "classic high point narrative" by 6 years of age.

Rollins and her colleagues (2000) reviewed other research that yielded evidence of cultural differences.

- African American children produced more classical narratives in structured interviews with adults than European North American children.

- Algonquin and Chinese children used high-point narrative structures, but ended them at the high point.

- Japanese- and Spanish-speaking children elaborated less on actions.

- Spanish-speaking children emphasized evaluations over events.

- Hawaiian children sometimes told "talk-stories," weaving teasing and fantasy into repetitive routines for groups of listeners.

As this review suggests, assessments are less likely to be biased when they are considered from multiple perspectives and when they are based on samples gathered across multiple contexts (Hyter & Westby, 1996). When evaluating the narratives of children from varied ethnic backgrounds, professionals may consult cultural informants, who can help them rate the narratives (Rollins et al., 2000). Dynamic assessment techniques also have been recommended. These focus on measuring children's abilities to employ new discourse organizational strategies after they have been given systematic, guided exposure to primary characteristics of targeted discourse structures (Gillam, Peña, & Miller, 1999; Gutierrez-Clellen, 2000; Gutierrez-Clellen & Quinn, 1993; Lidz & Peña, 1996; Miller, Gillam, & Peña, in press) (see Chapter 5 for a discussion of dynamic assessment).

Cultural diversity presents challenges to instructors but opportunities for enhanced richness as well. Classrooms with diverse students create opportunities for students to tell their stories in different voices and to help others learn about cultural experiences beyond their own. Paley (1979) wrote about bringing parents and grandparents in from their ethnically diverse neighborhood to share stories and special foods in one of her kindergarten classes. Tabors (1997) reviewed evidence that there are a variety of cognitive, emotional, and cultural benefits to first-language maintenance as children learn a second language.

Ethnic diversity is one thing. Poverty is quite another (Payne, 2001). Many children who are raised in poverty, regardless of ethnic identity, come to school less prepared to meet its academic demands. When children have had few experiences with lit-

---

Box 3.3.   Sociolinguistic Differences in How Girls and Boys Tell Stories

A third-grade girl version (with original spelling, capitalization, and punctuation) of a peer conflict story was:

> My friends Trishe and Julie and me all got in a hugh fight. When we
> want on the Playground me and Julie mad up. But me and Trishe
> didn't so me and Juli playd and then Trishe came ofer and sed do
> you wont to be frands agen. So I said yes and we when frands agen.
> the end

A boy version was:

> Me and My Friends
> Me and my Friend John and Mark and Dave and Dionte and Richy.
> Mark and Dave had a Fight and Richy and me and John stot
> [stopped] the Fight. I sad shake hand and they wer Friends agin.
> the end

---

erate language in their homes, they need opportunity to fill those gaps. Educators must seek ways to provide experiences that will bring them to the level of their peers in the area of emergent literacy skills. It is important to remember that every child has stories to tell and the potential to develop and express ideas at higher levels. The writing lab approach is designed to bring those stories to life in literate language that is respectful of the student's home culture.

Sociolinguistic variation allows language users to select from a variety of syntactic and vocabulary choices and stylistic elements to achieve desired effects in particular situations. Within the writing lab, we find that children differ in their personal and cultural choices about how to express that knowledge. Some of the choices are gender related. Westby (1994) reviewed research about gender differences in which young girls (preschool to early elementary) were found to structure their stories around the landscape of consciousness, with themes of deprivation, human relationships, and domestic animals, whereas boys centered their stories around the landscape of action, with themes of unrelated violent actions and endings in which heroes overcome their villains. Even when they start with a similar theme, the narrative styles of girls and boys can be distinguished. For example, Box 3.3 includes two stories written by third graders as assessment probes at the beginning of a school year—one by a girl and one by a boy.

We base this writing lab instructional approach on the values of respect and trust. Every student deserves them. Professionals who accept and appreciate the diverse experiences of the students in their classrooms can establish a classroom culture in which diversity is valued. Diversity includes variations in language production at grammatical and discourse levels, as well as in the broader dimensions in which culture influences world views and common practices.

Author chair, peer conferencing, computers, and joint reflection on written language are some of the contexts that can enhance language learning in the school-age years for any in this diverse group of learners. Most of our own writing lab experiences, which have crossed the grade-span from first through eighth grade, have been conducted in collaboration with the Kalamazoo Public Schools, in which more than 50% of students are African American and as many as 80% of students qualify for free or reduced price lunch in some schools. Many of the illustrations in this book come from those students. Others come from Mexican American children of migrant farm-working families who participated in our summer programs. Still others come from children adopted from war-torn countries who participated in our after-school homework labs. The mother of one of those girls said of her adopted daughter, "It's not that she knew 10 languages in Pakistan; it's that she didn't really know any well." In all of these experiences, the shared focus of our instructional teams, which have incorporated diverse groups of professionals, as well, has been on helping all students become effective written language communicators.

SUMMARY

In this chapter, we have introduced the diverse group of children who can benefit from the writing lab approach. Our interest in this approach has grown from our efforts to find effective means of assisting children with disabilities to become effective communicators and literate language users who can make progress in the general education curriculum.

In the process of our various research, personnel preparation, and outreach projects, we have worked in collaboration with a school district that includes a high proportion of culturally and linguistically diverse learners. We have worked in schools in neighborhoods in which children of all races and ethnic groups face everyday challenges of poverty, familial disruptions, and other pressures that no child should have to face.

In our decade of working together to develop this approach, our experience has been that all students can be challenged at an appropriate level to work on language and literacy. Our experience also has been that every student with whom we have worked could teach us something about the joyful expression of meanings and feelings of accomplishment.

Designing Instruction

4

This chapter describes learning components of the writing lab approach and how to use these components to set up writing lab experiences. It begins with the logistics of setting up a lab. These include scheduling, establishing a routine, and providing environmental supports. Other learning components discussed in this chapter are authentic writing projects, computer lab experiences, minilessons, author notebooks, and teacher and peer conferencing. The chapter concludes with a discussion of author chair and other presentation and publication experiences as contexts for addressing students' spoken and written communication needs.

SETTING UP A WRITING LAB

Setting up a writing lab involves starting with values and BACKDROP principles. This sets the stage for scheduling and other logistic decisions that lead to establishing a daily routine.

Starting with Values and BACKDROP Principles

Although aspects of the writing lab can be implemented in pull-out settings, the approach works best when special service providers collaborate with general educators in the inclusive contexts of classrooms and computer labs. In such environments, students with special education needs and speech-language impairments can be scaffolded to communicate and to participate with their general education peers. Peers without disabilities, in turn, can be scaffolded to respond supportively and to develop more mature language and communication skills themselves. When working as teams, general educators acquire strategies they can use throughout the week to support students with special needs or other learning risks. In this way, students benefit from specialized attention that extends beyond the brief periods of intervention they would otherwise receive in isolated settings.

Establishing a fully inclusive writing lab requires the development of a transdisciplinary collaborative team based on the values of respect and trust. Some groups have team relationships before they start working together in a writing lab approach. Others come together as a team and begin to develop respect and trust coincidentally with developing their lab. In either case, teams require nurturing to bring satisfaction to all participants and to achieve mutual goals. As team members learn what to expect of one another and how to work together, they begin to feel safer in revealing their uncertainties. A sign that a team has begun to jell is when members can share humor in conducting the serious enterprise of addressing students' needs. These critical relationship-building aspects are discussed in Chapter 13.

To be considered transdisciplinary—rather than multidisciplinary or even interdisciplinary—professionals must be willing to learn from each other and to release aspects of their roles to one another. In inclusive writing lab contexts, general educators, special educators, and SLPs work together to establish and address mutual goals, plan activities, and provide instruction. At the same time, they maintain their identities as experts in general curriculum and classroom management or in meeting the needs of students with language, learning, and social-communication issues. Successful teams guide their decision making by basing their planning on the BACKDROP principles described in Chapter 1.

Respecting all students as learners and raising expectations for students with disabilities and other learning risks is a key aspect of the writing lab approach. Early in a new school year, many general education teachers pinpoint those students whom they can count on to be attentive, quick to learn, and responsible in carrying out the teacher's directions. These students are given special privileges, such as passing out papers and carrying messages to the principal's office. The trust and respect of a student's classroom teacher carries special power. In healthy collaborative relationships, special service providers can work with students and teachers to extend the "responsible student" role to those who otherwise rarely experience the magical messages of their teacher's special trust.

Scheduling and Other Logistics

When setting up a writing lab, teams need first to address general planning issues that create a structure and routine. Included in early discussions should be:

- Finding a time to plan

- Scheduling regular times for holding writing lab sessions

- Gaining access to the school's computer lab

- Clarifying classroom rules and teachers' philosophies of discipline, behavioral expectations, and consequences

- Setting up the physical structure of the classroom and using early sessions to establish routines that create a community of authors

Before they can begin planning, team members must decide that it is worthwhile to work together. Without this critical step, it is unlikely that they will be able to carve out the time to meet. Decisions to collaborate often occur because general and special educators and SLPs have students in common, share an instructional philosophy, or even a friendship. Early discussions about establishing a writing lab approach revolve around the possibilities for helping students achieve higher-level language and thinking skills within curricular activities that the teachers deem important. Teachers who may be reluctant to collaborate at first may become more enthusiastic when they hear about successful collaborations from their teacher peers.

Once teams decide to work together, they begin to address basic logistics, starting with a time to plan. Time is mentioned consistently as the major challenge of collaborative service delivery. Collaborative service delivery does indeed take time, but more time is needed for planning in the early stages of setting up writing lab routines than later. School principals should be brought in at all stages—planning, implementing, and celebrating. Administrative support is perhaps the most essential element in finding planning time slots and spaces for planning. Administrative support also can lead to occasional release time to permit team members to engage in more in-depth planning and evaluation. Our teams and others have met over lunch, at teachers' scheduled planning times, and after school. In these meetings, basic plans are outlined by the team. If the division of responsibilities for lesson components is negotiated jointly, then individual team members may do any additional planning for components they are leading outside of the meetings.

Time devoted initially to setting up writing lab routines pays off when predictable structures are established and a classroom culture is in place that supports all students to be productive and successful. After a writing lab routine is established, planning time can shift to a greater focus on meeting the specific needs of individual students. At all points, however, it is worthy to try to raise the level of the discussion beyond, "What are we doing tomorrow?" to "What are the needs of these students?"

Collaboration in general becomes easier and more efficient over time. This is part of the message of the patience principle. After basic routines and relationships have been established, it is easier for collaborative decisions to be made in hallways and in classroom doorways or through messages exchanged in mailboxes, e-mail, and late night or early morning phone calls. As noted previously, school principals may assist by occasionally arranging half-day substitute teachers to allow a team to meet for an extended period to analyze written samples, for example, or to discuss issues facing the team.

One strategy we have used for extending inadequate planning time is to focus on developing relationships with a particular group of teachers one year and to switch the developmental focus to a different group the next. We continue to interact with the first group of teachers but with less intensity. Of course, IEPs must be implemented consistently, but the developmental costs in terms of time in a particular classroom or grade diminish with experience. After a routine is established and roles and responsibilities are apportioned, the intensive focus of new development can shift to building capacity in a different grade level or with a new group of teachers.

Scheduling joint times for writing lab sessions is almost as difficult as finding times for planning. Although it is not necessary for writing labs to take place at the same time each day, predictable schedules are essential. We have found three sessions or more per week to provide the continuity needed to support the process and to maintain interest in and motivation to complete projects. If SLPs and special educators are unable to schedule more than two sessions per week in a particular general education classroom, general educators may need to continue working on writing lab projects at times when the special service providers cannot be with them. The writing lab approach is intended to be part of the curriculum, not an add-on to the curriculum. Although it involves practicing language arts, it is more than just language arts. Therefore, if writing lab time fits best when science or social studies is scheduled, the writing lab projects are designed to meet the goals of the science or social studies curriculum.

Whenever class time is devoted to writing lab projects, students with disabilities should be present. In fact, a sign of inclusive thinking is when general educators are sensitive to providing instruction critical to writing lab projects only when all students are present. Examples include reading a story as a model for fable writing or introducing background concepts for scientific writing. IEP teams (including parents) can decide whether it is acceptable to send a classmate to fetch a student from the special education room for such activities. When it is impossible for the student to be present in the general education classroom, special educators or SLPs can use the same materials to introduce the concepts in other settings. An alternative is to assign learning buddies to orient students who must be out of the room when critical instruction takes place. Dramatic boosts to self-esteem are possible when students with disabilities are assigned to be learning buddies for peers without disabilities who must be out of the room for band practice or other special activities.

The time set aside for each writing lab session varies according to the attention abilities of students at particular grade levels, the routines of a particular school, and the schedules of special service providers. We sometimes start with shorter sessions (45 minutes) for first- and second-grade students, but even young students can build endurance for extended writing over the school year. Each writing lab session also incorporates at least two activities. When constructive learning and ownership principles are implemented, it is easier for students to stay on task. Students at all grade levels can be kept actively engaged in learning during 60-minute sessions. In a computer lab, regardless of grade level, at least 45 minutes are needed to have a productive session that includes a minilesson, writing time, saving, and printing.

Establishing a Daily Routine

A daily routine of the writing lab approach involves nurturing a community of authors, employing classroom discipline as a route to self-regulation, introducing learning components, including free writing, and structuring the physical environment.

Nurturing a Community of Authors

Early writing lab sessions are designed to help students conceptualize themselves as a community of authors who are working productively. Sometimes, students consult with peers or instructors, and sometimes they share their work with the whole class in the author chair, but essentially they work toward goals for which they have ownership. Students learn to call on all members of the instructional team for assistance, including special service providers and classroom volunteers as well as general education teachers. In writing lab contexts, students begin to experience the motivating rewards of having adults and peers as members of an authentic audience interested in their ideas. They also begin to experience the magical power of writing as a way of knowing (Bridges, 1997).

Establishing the surface aspects of such a culture generally takes at least a month, during which the keep it simple principle is used to introduce one new learning component per session. It is important for special service providers to know that they can work toward IEP goals for students with disabilities during these sessions as well as during other phases of writing lab interventions. Establishing the deeper value system of students' trust and respect for themselves and peers generally takes longer than 1 month, often extending across an entire school year and sometimes more. The important point is that it can be accomplished and that major gains can sometimes be made in a single session (see Chapter 13 for illustrations).

Employing Classroom Discipline as a Route to Self-Regulation

When teams begin to collaborate, they need to establish and communicate a joint discipline policy. Communicating clear lines of authority for all team members and following consistent routines can help avoid student confusion and head off any manipulative tendencies to pit one teacher against another. Expectations usually start with existing rules of the classroom teacher and include such things as spoken or unspoken rules for moving around the classroom, using the bathroom, or finding a place to write other than one's assigned seat.

Many students easily infer the rules of the "school culture curriculum" (Nelson, 1998). Others, especially students with disabilities who are removed from the classroom throughout the day, may have difficulty inferring the generally unspoken rules for classroom behavior (Creaghead & Tattershall, 1985; Sturm & Nelson, 1997). They may need a minilesson to make such rules explicit. A minilesson on classroom rules might start with a student brainstorm. The constructive nature of this activity is important for building responsibility for self-regulatory behaviors. The list then can be refined and posted prominently in the classroom or in author notebooks. The appendix to this chapter shows a list of rules brainstormed by students in an after-school writing lab for fourth through sixth graders known as the CREW Lab.

Just stating the rules, however, does not mean that all students understand them or can comply with them physiologically and emotionally. It may take individualized scaffolding to help some students acquire self-regulation abilities (see Chapter 5) and to be full participants in group discussions (see Box 4.1). The goal is to build self-regulatory skills based on feelings of ownership and success so that students begin to discipline themselves from the inside (showing "inner control") with lasting effects, rather than requiring firm "outer contol" on behavior, which often has only temporary effects.

Introducing Learning Components

When initiating the writing lab approach in a new classroom, we use the first session to collect baseline written language samples using procedures described in Chapter 14 and 15. Then, we plan a relatively low demand first project to serve as a vehicle for introducing writing lab components. This makes it possible for students to concentrate on learning routines, to begin to understand writing processes, and to develop a common vocabulary for talking about them. Stories make good first projects. Another good first project is to have the students write About the Author pieces, modeled after those often found on book dust jackets (see examples in Figures 3.1 and 3.2). Digital photographs of the students can be inserted in the documents, and the resulting products can be shared with parents at school open houses and conferences. The About the Author pieces or stories should be dated and included in students' writing portfolios.

A daily writing lab routine might include a minilesson; extended time for students to plan, draft, or revise their written work; and opportunities for peer conferencing or group sharing. Table 4.1 illustrates a sequence of minilessons and session goals using About the Author projects to establish writing lab routines. This example comes from a situation in which students had access to a computer lab every third session because they had to share an hour block with two other classrooms.

Box 4.1.   Story of Thai and Group Discussions

Thai was a fifth-grade student in a fully inclusive writing lab that took place in his general education classroom twice a week. Every third session was held in the school's computer lab. Thai was an outgoing, friendly student, but he had difficulty taking part in group discussions. In fact, during whole-group instruction, Thai had a pattern of avoidance behaviors that included positioning himself physically at the periphery of the group and staring out the window or talking to his peers instead of participating in the group instruction.

Watching this pattern, one member of the team attempted to scaffold Thai to attend to the discussion by moving him to a more central position in the group and encouraging him to listen so he could share his interesting ideas, too. Thai's response was, "Oh, I never talk in class," whereupon he continued his noisy conversation with classmates, distracting them as well as himself. At that point, Thai's teacher asked him to leave the room. The SLP followed a few minutes later, indicating to Thai that this was not about punishment. Rather, it was about helping him to set some goals about making contributions to the group discussion. The instructor emphasized that Thai had good ideas that his fellow students and teacher would be interested in hearing. Together they wrote three goals in Thai's author's notebook:

- Listen to the group discussion so I will know what to say.
- Raise my hand at least once in a discussion.
- Make an appropriate comment every time I am called on.

During the next session, Thai paid attention during the minilesson, raised his hand, and made an appropriate comment. After the session, he approached the SLP and asked, "Did I do better today?" with a smile on his face. His instructors responded, "Did you meet your goals? Let's take a look." Following this personal minilesson, the team looked for opportunities to encourage and comment on Thai's increased participation, and the pattern of improved involvement continued.

Table 4.1.   Planning for About the Author project to establish writing lab routines

Session topic	Group objectives	Individual objectives
Tuesday in classroom • Idea generation • Planning/organizing	List stages of the writing process. Listen to several examples of About the Author discourse and brainstorm categories of information to be included Use a graphic organizer to generate ideas for self. • Include three categories • Include two subcategories with each	Roselani—Work independently for 5 minutes. Shoshannah—Generate words and spell them phonetically. Kwan—Ask for assistance using pragmatic skills. Nailah and Chris—Raise hand and contribute to group discussion.
Thursday in classroom • Organizing paragraphs • Drafting • Taking digital photos	Use ideas from graphic organizer to generate sentences and add details. Use invented spelling to produce descriptive words and phrases. Indent paragraph, and use appropriate capitalization and punctuation.	Continue working on Tuesday's objectives.
Friday in computer lab • Drafting on the computer • Using writing software features	Enter text independently using the computer (tab to indent, shift to capitalize). Reflect on organization and add details. Use spelling checker and other features to monitor text generation.	Roselani—Work independently for 15 minutes. Produce a four-sentence paragraph. Shoshannah—Type words and use spelling checker for highlighted words. Kwan and Nailah—Consider audience needs for adequate information.
Tuesday in classroom • Revising and editing • Peer conferencing • Proofreading symbols	Use revising sheet to evaluate the presence of all important features. Meet with peers to fill the author and editor roles. Use proofreading symbols on peer's paper.	Roselani—Use peer conferencing sheet to guide self through process. Shoshannah—Reread work independently. Kwan—Use pragmatic skills for interacting with a peer. Nailah and Chris—Raise hand and contribute to group discussion.
Thursday in classroom • Publishing and presenting • Author chair	Take turns reading in the author chair. Make a suggestion and ask a question about peer discourse.	Roselani and Shoshannah—Read work independently from author chair. Kwan and Nailah—Raise hand and make appropriate author chair comments.
Friday in computer lab • Revising and editing on the computer • Adding borders and changing fonts	Use cut and paste and insert features to make revisions from draft notes on previous printout. Add borders and change fonts.	

Including Free Writing in the Routine

Adding a free writing component to writing lab sessions contributes to a positive classroom culture and conveys to students the encouraging aspects of constructive learning and ownership. To qualify as free writing, no external demands are placed on topics, spelling, or punctuation. Story starters are not compatible with free writing. To help students develop strategies for generating their own ideas, an early minilesson might introduce them to strategies for brainstorming and making an idea web for topic selection. The appendix to this chapter provides a handout for a minilesson on brainstorming.

Encouraging free writing may require a heavy dose of the patience principle, which Swoger (1989) used with her high school student Scott (described in Box 2.4). Swoger reported the strategy she adopted from her accelerated writers' class for use with "basic writers" like Scott, who had been in special education classes all his academic life. "If they did not perform," Swoger wrote, "I waited, but I revisited each desk every day. 'Tell me about your story,' I would say while looking with interest into their eyes" (p. 61). As Swoger (1989) illustrated, it was important to convey to Scott her trust that he did have ideas worth writing about. The goal of fluency coming from within depended on Scott gaining confidence that his ideas were worthwhile.

During free writing, the only directions are to put pencil to paper and write. For students with physical or visual disabilities, access to a computer with special supports (described in Chapter 11) can serve as their pencil and paper. Students who are very young or who have extremely limited literacy skills might be allowed to draw in combination with writing, but as soon as possible they should be scaffolded toward writing their ideas in words. As students gain experience, they may be encouraged to use free writing time to experiment with different writing styles or genres, but the choice as to what to write remains theirs. Chapter 5 provides suggestions for scaffolding students who are reluctant writers or avoiders. Chapter 7 describes computer software tools designed to support idea generation. Instructors can convey to students that all authors use strategies to generate ideas. Most important, instructors should convey trust that all students have worthwhile ideas that will be interesting to others.

To establish a culture for free writing as one of quiet industry, instructional teams might provide soft background music and a comfortable structure that includes guidelines for what kind of movement is allowed around the room and where students might sit. Although lounging on a couch or beanbag chairs and chatting with friends is not generally conducive to writing, students differ in their needs to move around. Such issues should not be treated as behavioral concerns but as matters of logistics. That is, instructors can point out that authors need a solid surface to write and a quiet place to think. In initial free writing times and periodically thereafter, adults should sit and write as well. Special service providers can use this time to observe the writing processes of their students while engaging in their own writing. When adults share their writing from the author chair, along with personal goals for improving it, the concept that goals are for everyone is modeled, and the values of respect and trust are enhanced.

In the session in which free writing is introduced, students might write for most of a session then participate in author chair. All students are encouraged to take the author's chair, but no one is forced. Chapter 13 provides an illustration of how one student gained the confidence to sit in the author chair.

In later writing lab sessions, 10–15 minutes of free writing might be used to set the tone for in-class writing lab sessions. Starting writing lab sessions with free writing also can give special service providers time to join the group when they are coming from other settings. Once everyone is writing, adults can begin to move quietly about the room, showing interest in students' choices and scaffolding them toward goals, but also writing themselves. The emphasis remains on the fluent expression of ideas. If students start to get distracted vying for adult attention, adults should return to writing themselves.

Students with limited literacy abilities might draw pictures independently until an adult is available to take their dictation and to help them read the words representing their ideas from the page. As students become more proficient, instructors can use a shared pencil technique (taking turns writing words or sentences with scaffolding) to support transition to independent writing. Other scaffolding techniques to get students started are discussed in Chapter 5. Scaffolding techniques to help students gain skill with sound–symbol representation, word choice, sentence construction, discourse organization, or any other language target are discussed in Chapter 6. Although we strongly encourage invented spelling during free writing as an aid to fluency, we do not believe that teachers or students should be bound by any "always" or "never" rules. For example, one student's free writing journal was full of long lists of "I like . . . " phrases, except that *like* was spelled "lak" dozens of times. This misspelling provided a teachable moment for a short personal minilesson on vowel awareness and spelling patterns. In the following session, the instructor again showed appreciation for the student's ideas and commented on how her good spelling made it easier to read those ideas. Then, the instructor expressed interest in knowing more about the student's "I like" topics. This addressed an objective for the student to elaborate her ideas beyond lists.

Many of our teacher colleagues have extended free writing opportunities into other parts of the school day. Students who spend a portion of their day in special education classrooms can take their author notebooks, which include a free writing section, back and forth with them. This allows them to work on ongoing writing projects in both settings. Transporting author notebooks also increases communication between the general and special education teachers about the student's work.

Structuring the Physical Environment

Physical aspects of the environment, as well as social interaction aspects, require organization (Areglado & Dill, 1997; Fiderer, 1993). Teams decide where to store materials such as paper, pencils, drawing tools, staplers, staple pullers, hole punches, resource books, dictionaries, author notebooks, and computer disks. A date stamp is particularly helpful for keeping a portfolio of student works in order. Following the classroom teacher's lead, the physical work environment of desks and tables can be arranged to support both individual writing time and small-group interactions. Space in the classroom can be designated for initiating minilessons, perhaps with the support of an overhead projector or computer monitor to model writing processes for students. Other environmental classroom supports include posters with reminders of such components as stages of the writing process, daily schedules, and classroom rules. Word walls can be established with high-frequency grade-level words laminated and posted around the classroom alphabetically as spelling supports for the students to refer to while writing.

Many classrooms include a station with two or three computers with a shared printer. This arrangement allows teachers and assistants to help students complete projects and print copies that could not be completed during computer lab sessions. Rules need to be established for how and when students can gain access to such computers. For example, a sign-up schedule might help students develop inner goal direction and self-regulatory skills for using time wisely during moments of free choice.

PLANNING PROJECTS

Authentic writing projects give students reasons to improve their written language and to make sure it communicates their meanings. Writing labs are designed to permit a balance of curriculum-driven projects and student-centered projects, such as free writing. Curriculum-driven projects provide opportunities to work on language and communication goals while also working toward goals of the general education curriculum. Free writing and other student-choice projects provide opportunities to work on language and communication goals while emphasizing ownership.

Several decisions related to project planning are listed in Table 4.2 starting with choice of a genre and topic. Prelock, Miller, and Reed (1995) recommended that teams allot 5–10 minutes for brainstorming a lesson activity before making decisions about how to implement it so that they can consider the goals for curriculum and the needs of the identified students as an integral part of the planning. Some school curricula specify which writing genres and competencies should be targeted at each grade level and even the academic semesters in which they should be taught. Other curricula are less tightly prescriptive. In either case, writing projects can support a variety of curricular areas including language arts, social studies, and science. In addition, within each writing project, opportunities exist to address all of the language learning targets introduced in Chapter 2 using techniques discussed in Chapter 5.

We often recommend narratives as early projects because narratives are a valued academic, social, and self-regulatory discourse style. Story-writing projects provide opportunities to teach story grammar components explicitly with goals of more sophisticated storytelling and story comprehension. As students learn to construct both a landscape of action and a landscape of consciousness, they engage in higher order thinking about causal relationships and human motivations and interactions (Bruner, 1986; Westby, 1994). When writing narratives, students have opportunities to engage in writing processes recursively and purposefully. The personal nature of narratives engages listeners, too. Narratives easily capture the interest of peers in author chair activities. In this way, they contribute to the development of a class culture that respects different histories and imaginations.

The first step of planning for any project involves reflection on its cognitive and linguistic demands and opportunities. A form for guiding team-planning brainstorms appears in Figure 4.1. Note that the first two questions encourage brainstorming about the nature of the genre being targeted. The latter three address the three main components of the writing lab approach: writing process instruction, computer supports, and inclusive practices.

Table 4.2.   Project planning decisions

1. Choose a genre for the project, and discuss how students will select their topics.

2. Discuss language-learning possibilities that can be targeted in each of the writing lab components for the whole class and for individual students.

3. Identify expected student outcomes and how individual student needs will be addressed and documented.

4. Consider computer software features that can support writing processes.

5. Decide what minilessons and other supports will be needed.

6. Schedule writing-lab components for each day.

7. Assign instructor roles for each writing lab activity, including minilessons, scaffolding individual students, data collection, and managing time and routines.

8. Decide what the final publication will look like and how it will be celebrated.

1. What is the nature of the genre _____ ?

   What sub-genres should we consider?

   What key elements would we like to see as student outcomes?

2. What are the learning demands of the genre?

   Language demands? (discourse, sentence, word levels)

   Cognitive demands?

   Other?

3. What teaching strategies can support the learning process?

   Minilessons?

   Scaffolding language?

4. What computer and other resources can support the learning process?

5. What inclusive practices can support the learning process?

Figure 4.1. Form for planning projects.

This form was used to guide discussions in preparation for a third-grade animal report project as part of the science curriculum. As team members brainstormed, one person took notes. Many ideas were raised, particularly about the language and cognitive demands of report writing and how to handle the planning and organizing stages of the process. The team identified several student outcomes for the science project. At the discourse level, teachers wanted students to read texts for information and to take notes. They wanted students then to organize the information into paragraphs with a topic sentence followed by supporting details. At the word level, they expected students to understand and use specific vocabulary related to the study of animals (e.g., habitat) and to use colorful, descriptive language to describe their animals' appearances. At the conventions level, they wanted to introduce paragraph formatting and expected continued growth in use of sentence capitalization and punctuation.

The instructors voiced concerns that students would find report writing less engaging than previous narrative activities and identified reading sources and notetaking during the planning stage to be demanding new tasks for most of the class. The teachers also reflected on the keep it simple principle, recognizing that going from notes to an organized draft during the drafting process would be a new and difficult challenge for many of the students.

As an outcome of the planning discussion, the team listed lessons and supports that would be needed for this project. They assigned members to be primarily responsible for each, including:

- Minilessons introducing students to the parts of a book and ways to get information from reference books, notetaking strategies, and ways to organize paragraphs from written notes

- Ideas for locating books, magazines, and Internet resources about animals written at a range of reading levels so that all students could be challenged at an appropriate level

- Plans for developing a template with *Inspiration* (a children's software program by Inspiration Software that provides an organizational structure for student notes) to be printed and filled out in pencil or completed on the computer

To engage students in the animal report project, the instructional team introduced a range of available resources. After students were given an opportunity to review the resources, they were asked to choose an animal to write about. An early author chair experience also was scheduled for students to share interesting facts as they began their research. Together, the team designated members to provide extra support for students who were likely to need help reading their research sources. They also decided that some of the stronger student readers could provide support for those with lower reading skills. Based on the dynamic principle, further planning for this project was deferred for a follow-up meeting so team members would have the flexibility to change in response to the students' needs as the project developed.

Similar planning can be used to address any other genre. Figure 4.2 shows the results of group planning for a poetry project by an intervention team using the planning format shown in Figure 4.1. Notes added when the outline was revisited at the conclusion of the project reflect experience based on the research principle about what worked and what did not.

USING THE COMPUTER LAB

In setting up writing labs, we have worked directly with teachers in numerous elementary schools and indirectly with teachers in several middle schools and high schools (via after-school writing labs and summer institutes). All had one or more computer labs in their schools: some with enough computers for each class member, others with fewer computers than students. Many schools also had several computers in classrooms, often of varying vintage and quality but with a printer. When the total of computers in the lab and classroom does not support the goal of one computer per student, teams need to develop a system for sharing, although sharing a limited number of computers is not ideal.

In many schools, computer lab schedules are established by allowing teachers to sign up for an hour or so per week at the beginning of the school year. If so, it is important to sign up early to schedule mutually available team times—even signing up at the end of the prior school year if possible. When this has not been possible, our collaborating teachers have traded computer lab times with their colleagues (with administrator support) to accommodate limited mutual times.

The problem of too few computers should become less pressing in the coming years. In cases of inadequacy, however, teams should do everything they can to ensure that students with language-learning needs are allotted computers. A common problem occurs when computers are viewed only as publishing tools. In such cases, computers are made available first to students who are finished with the writing processes of planning, drafting, and revising. Students who are slower to finish, often those with language-learning risks, may be the last to gain access to motivating tools that they need to help them learn processes and create satisfying products.

Computer supports are for all stages of the writing process. Students who have produced little or no planning after a lab session devoted to planning still should have access to computers and software when the class moves to the computer lab. Helping students gain access to computers takes precedence as teams focus on behavior problems as symptoms of language-learning difficulties that require intervention. Students who struggle to complete work need additional supports and instruction for using self-regulatory strategies. As they develop inner reasons to attend to their work, most students increase their capacity for working for longer periods independently. Chapter 6 describes transitions in students' views of themselves as authors that can result when computer supports and instructor scaffolding are brought together to address the problem. Stories of individual student change within such supportive contexts also appear in Chapter 17.

When setting up the physical environment within a computer lab, teams need to decide where computer lab minilessons are to be conducted; how to assign students to computers; and rules for loading, saving, and printing work. In labs arranged with all students facing forward, computer lab minilessons can be conducted with students sitting at their computers, looking at a centralized large-screen monitor. This arrangement can save time and allow team members at the back of the room to see screens so they can make sure that all students are following directions in sequence, but it makes it difficult to move among the students. Space among computer stations can facilitate scaffolding and make it easier to work with students in small groups. Extra chairs in computer labs, preferably on rollers, also are helpful for allowing instructors to sit next to individual students to provide scaffolding.

To help students focus on goals and new techniques for a particular computer lab session, we generally start at a centralized computer station with a 5-minute group minilesson. Especially in labs where students are spread out, there are advantages to gathering students around a monitor rather than starting them out at their own computer stations. Computer keyboards can be tempting distracters for students who are eager to get started. Adjustable swivel chairs, sometimes a feature at computer workstations, also have high distraction potential. Therefore, bringing students to a central spot where they can view a teaching monitor may help them to sustain attention for minilessons about computer use. Later, when students are at their own computer stations, they can be led step by step through multistep procedures, such as loading, saving, and printing. Such procedural topics offer excellent opportunities to work on direction-following objectives, including an objective to wait until directions are completed before acting. Table 4.3 provides other recommendations for orienting students to computer-supported writing.

If sufficient computers are available, assigning students to specific computer stations generally is a good idea. Works in progress always should be saved on students' disks, but it is not uncommon for students to save their work inadvertently on hard drives. Predictable seating arrangements make it easier to retrieve missing documents in such cases. Assigning seats also makes it possible to place students next to classmates who are not distracting and can provide appropriate peer scaffolding.

1. What is the nature of the genre, or what makes a poem a poem?

    A group of words written in such a way that a mental picture or image emerges from reading it

    Thinking of language in a different way to make a mental picture

    Focusing on meaning and sound to capture a moment, feeling, or sensation

    Vivid images presented through simile, metaphor, and carefully chosen words

    Language that makes you think about something in a different way

    What sub-genres should we consider?

    Free form

    Structure with repetitive words and phrases

    List poem

    Acrostic

    Sensory descriptions

    Rhyming

    Haiku

    What key elements would we like to see as student outcomes?

    Patterns

    Interesting words, strong verbs, descriptive words, great sensory appeal

    Metaphorical thought, figurative language

    Line breaks

    Repeated phrases, refrains

    Sense of rhythm

    Choice meaningful topics, original thoughts

    Economy of language

    Use of language/cognitive skills to fit ability levels

2. What are the learning demands of the genre?

    Language demands? (discourse, sentence, word levels)

    Think of words to convey picture, sound, smell, ideas

    Variety of ways to say something: vocabulary and perspective

    Economy of language

    Abstract language, metaphor, figurative language

    Rhyming (but not necessarily)

    Cognitive demands?

    Organizing information to fit into a different mold

    Familiarity with a range of choices

    Real versus imagined

    Must read aloud attempts, knowing where to stop and start, and how to pause

    Must have heard other poetry read aloud

    Contrasts between prose and poetry

    Other?

    Connecting emotions and feelings to meaning

    Students become risk takers in using more than everyday language

Figure 4.2.   Team planning brainstorm for a project on poetry.

3. What teaching strategies can support the learning process?

Minilessons?

Prewriting, rhyming, topic choices

Sensory images, description, visualization, metaphor

How to use thesaurus or create a reference list for interesting words

Line breaks, centering, and spacing on the computer

Punctuation differences in poetry

Performance of poetry: eye contact, intonation, pausing

Scaffolding language?

How does it sound?

Can you think of a different word?

How could you change this from prose to poetry?

Close your eyes, and tell me what you see (feel, hear...)

4. What computer and other resources can support the learning process?

Hearing and seeing lots of poetry every day

Drafting and editing on the computer

Planning (word maps) with Inspiration

Illustrate with graphics

Teach centering early

Because poems tend to be shorter than prose, drafting on the computer is especially powerful

Kids' poetry pages on the Internet

5. What inclusive practices can support the learning process?

Group planning, choral reading

Reinforce minilessons and preteach some concepts in special education

More support and simplify tasks for some, using pictures to generate ideas

Practice with age/grade level peers, peer coaching/conferencing

Arrange to have students with disabilities in during minilessons that support content

Address oral language goals during discussions about poetry

Students should be taught routines for handling writing lab procedures independently. Procedures include routines for booting systems, finding and opening software programs, inserting and saving on disks, printing, and returning disks to a specified spot at the conclusion of the lab time. Instruction about organizational routines can be embedded in minilessons that also are used to target language and communication skills, especially listening, waiting for instructions, staying on task, sequencing and comprehending directional words. Younger students may benefit from directions to put their hands on their heads, ears, or noses interspersed with other instructions. This can keep them from using their mouse pointers to click impulsively around the screen and risk losing unsaved work. It also gives instructors time to walk around and make sure that all students' screens indicate they are on the right step.

It is helpful to have an attention-getting device, such as a bell (although flipping the light switch will work), to garner students' attention before giving instructions to print and save. We try to give students a 2- to 5-minute warning so they can come to a

Table 4.3. Orienting students to computer-supported writing

Orient students to computer components and related vocabulary (e.g., *keyboard, screen, disk drive, mouse, disk, CD-ROM*), how they function, and how to handle them (e.g., how to use buttons, how to point at the screen with the back of a fingernail to avoid fingerprints, how to hold and insert a disk to avoid damage).

Teach students computer use procedures for starting, saving, printing, using the Internet, and asking for help (e.g., students can be taught to place a plastic cup upside down on the computer monitor when help is needed).

Teach general word processing features and the names of keys and related vocabulary (e.g., how to *highlight, shift, move the cursor, insert, copy, cut and paste, backspace,* and *delete*), and demonstrate the danger of losing text by hitting any key when a block of text is highlighted. Teach the undo feature.

Scaffold self-talk as students learn the procedures of the writing lab.

Provide minilessons for navigating new software related to writing process decisions, with handouts for key words and definitions and procedural sequences.

Allow time to explore freely new software features such as *font, color, illustration, animation, sound, music,* and other *multimedia* options, with encouragement to share new discoveries with peers.

Dedicate a portion of computer lab time to developing keyboarding skills.

Select a keyboarding software program that is developmentally appropriate and intrinsically motivating and that includes settings for modifying the criteria for advancing through the program.

Consider whether the keyboarding program directly or indirectly assists literacy learning in addition to the motor patterns of typing (e.g., by presenting word family and word part lessons that instructors can use for scaffolding links between spoken and written language).

good stopping point. A system to amplify instructional language in the computer lab is extremely helpful. Even a toy microphone can improve the listening environment when students are spread out at individual computer stations.

Other organizational aids include alphabetizing and numbering floppy disks and keeping them together in a plastic box. When students know their disk numbers, individual disks can be pulled quickly from a storage box. Numbered disks also make it easier to check that all disks have been accounted for when leaving the lab. When CD-ROMs are needed to run a program, students on a particular row can be taught to keep their CD drawers open until all are filled at the beginning of the lab or until all are removed at the end, making the process more efficient. If lab assistants are available or parent volunteers can be identified, instructional team members can spend more time working with students and less time setting up the lab.

Computer lab jobs for students also can become part of the class's weekly job assignments. For example, students can be assigned rotating jobs to assist with CD-ROMs, floppy disks, printing, and gathering copies from the printer to take back to the class at the conclusion of computer lab time. It is important to prevent the chaos of everyone wanting to run to the printer to pick up his or her own product. Another student can be assigned the job of three-hole punching and date stamping printouts so that students can keep them in the Works in Progress section of their author notebooks for use in the next writing lab session. Such jobs should be assigned to all students regardless of ability level.

MINILESSONS

Minilessons provide a forum for direct teaching of writing lab procedures, writing processes, language skills, social interaction skills, and self-regulation. They generally are taught as whole class activities, but they may be used with smaller groups during peer conferencing or with individuals during one-to-one scaffolding. Minilessons often are

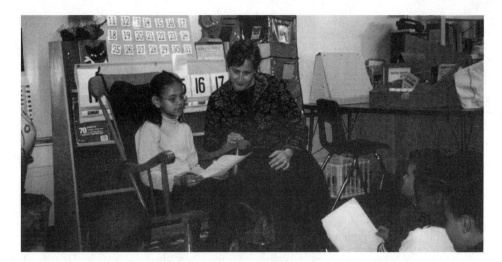

Figure 4.3. A minilesson in progress.

planned in advance to meet a particular need, but they may be introduced on the spot to respond to a need apparent at the moment. In this section, we discuss general procedures for minilessons and specific suggestions for each of their components. Then, we provide examples of minilessons for teaching a variety of knowledge, skills, and strategies. Minilesson support handouts are illustrated in the chapter appendix. Figure 4.3 shows a minilesson in progress.

Planning Group Minilessons

Whole-group minilessons establish shared concepts and vocabulary for writing processes and communicating about writing. Descriptions of minilessons across sources vary on such questions as duration and whether students should take an active role in them. We believe that there is no one right way to do minilessons, which is consistent with the dynamic principle. We also encourage teams to experiment with different approaches, which is consistent with the research and reflective practice principle. Following the constructive learning principle, we emphasize the importance of active student participation in all writing lab events.

In the writing lab approach, group minilessons typically are organized in two parts. First, instructors introduce concepts to the classroom as a whole, encouraging group participation. Then, they engage students in small group and individual practice activities that blend into the writing process. Within this broad structure, typical minilessons follow a predictable outline. Consistencies in procedures for group minilessons help students develop inner organizational schemas that allow them to participate more fully. Although minilessons tend to be teacher directed, they are planned explicitly to foster ownership for new learning. Some or all of the following components (each of which is discussed more fully later) are present in most group minilessons. Within the whole-group introduction, a minilesson is designed to

- Introduce the topic and create a framework

- Activate prior knowledge in a manner accessible to all

- Generate brainstorming to get all students thinking and participating

- Explain key content and vocabulary (calibrated to the general curriculum), with examples to encourage construction of new concepts or skills for students across ability levels

- Provide print supports to be kept in author notebooks as a reference and to aid review and retention

During individual and small-group practice, the minilesson is designed to

- Encourage students to apply new concepts and skills to authentic projects

- Provide opportunities for individualized scaffolding

- Help students develop higher-level writing processes, language abilities, and social interaction exchanges

Most researchers suggest keeping minilessons short—around 10 minutes—but keeping the "mini" in minilesson can be a challenge (e.g., Atwell, 1990; Hoyt, 2000; Muschla, 1993). Exceeding the recommended 10-minute time frame by 5 minutes or so may be needed on some days to provide adequate examples, encourage all students to participate, and help all students to construct new linguistic and cognitive connections. It is particularly important, however, to avoid extended whole-group lessons in which special service professionals spend the entire session standing at the back of classroom watching other teachers lecture and students act as passive listeners.

One reason that most minilessons can be relatively short is that they do not serve as stand-alone, one-time opportunities to focus on a topic. Rather, concepts and skills introduced with minilessons are revisited within and across sessions until students demonstrate competence with them. In addition, some writing lab sessions do not begin with a planned minilesson; rather, they begin with reminders about previous topics and reference to preexisting written supports in students' author notebooks.

During the application phase of minilessons, the extra adult attention that comes from the collaborative teamwork of the writing lab approach offers enhanced opportunities to scaffold individual students. At such times, many IEP and writing lab objectives can be addressed.

What Makes a Good Minilesson?

In our periodic reflections with colleagues during development activities and summer workshops, we have brainstormed what makes a good minilesson. The following qualities are often cited. Minilessons should

- Be student centered, fun, dramatic, active, quick, and recursive

- Address topics selected both in advance of projects and in response to immediate student needs

- Follow a predictable structure but remain fresh

- Involve active learning rather than passive listening

Instructional teams often divide responsibility for planning and teaching minilessons. Any team member may serve as lead instructor, but everyone should be present when a minilesson is introduced so all teachers can convey uniform expectations later. To keep students focused on the lead instructor, other adults in the room should use nonverbal strategies (e.g., eye contact, gestures) when necessary to redirect students' attention to that instructor.

All students should be actively engaged in both the whole group and individual practice activities. Generally, this means that students should not be allowed to move about the room during whole-group participation. Team members can take advantage of activities that require whole-group participation to observe and document behaviors related to attention, direction following, commenting, and other forms of classroom participation.

Introducing the Topic and Creating a Framework

A number of techniques can be used to introduce minilesson topics and to frame the questions each minilesson is designed to answer. The basic approach is to convey the purpose of the lesson in terms of how the topic will help authors answer key questions, solve procedural problems, and achieve their writing goals. If instructors have established themselves as members of the classroom writing community, they can communicate a minilesson's purpose by using self-talk to articulate their questions in a way that heightens interest in and comprehension of the targeted strategy or concept.

Concise statements are used to introduce minilesson topics and emphasize key vocabulary by producing it slower and with added stress. In some cases, groups are led in choral repetition. Examples of introductory comments are:

- "Last time we brainstormed some ideas about story topics. Today, we need to plan our stories. When I plan, I want to be sure that my story has all the important pieces. I also want to be sure that I have thought about how the pieces fit together and how my story will end. So what are the parts of a story I need to think about?"

- "This is a minilesson on doing research and taking notes. I am writing a report on kangaroos. I know something about kangaroos, but not enough to write my report. I need to brainstorm a list of questions I would like to answer about kangaroos. Then, I need to think about places where I can find the answers. What are some of the things I might want to know about kangaroos?" Student brainstorming contributions might include, "Where do they live? Why do they carry their babies in their pouches? How high can they jump? Can they live in Michigan?"

- "Last time, we worked on revising our work, but I want to know what others will think about my work when they read it. Today, we are going to learn how to use peer conferencing to make our writing better. I want you to all think about what a peer is, and when you think you know, raise your hand. I will wait until I see everyone's hand."

- "We noticed that some of you are starting to add dialogue to your stories. How many of you know what dialogue is? Think about it for a minute, and then raise your hand when you think you know." Take suggestions and help students frame the topic as writing the words their characters actually say. "Well, today we are going to have a minilesson about dialogue and how to tell the reader someone is talking by using quotation marks."

Activating Prior Knowledge

Once the topic has been introduced, it is expanded. Starting with introductory remarks, the goal is to activate prior knowledge so that all students can participate—not just those who raised their hands first. In fact, as the prior examples illustrate, it is important to design questions and to time the interaction to make it clear that all students are expected to be thinking all of the time. This may require a heavy dose of the patience principle. Communicating clearly that everyone is supposed to generate ideas means that instructors must be willing to wait until all (or most) students indicate that they have an answer. Wait time opportunities also must be balanced with efforts to keep the lesson active and short. Minilessons can be organized to provide immediate experiences that will stimulate ideas for opening discussions. Dramatization, modeling, and self-talk all support these purposes. Suggestions include

- Act out a problem and possible solutions, both good and bad.

- Provide examples of writing with and without targeted features.

- Embed humor and interesting content in examples.

- Involve individual students in planning and presenting lessons.

- Engage in self-talk to model self-regulation strategies.

Dramatizations with negative examples are particularly good for leading students to make observations they might miss otherwise. Students' observations and enjoyment are heightened particularly when teachers dramatize inappropriate actions. Students then can be scaffolded to describe desirable qualities that contrast with those that were demonstrated. For example, the SLP and classroom teacher might dramatize peer conferencing in which the author reads softly and never looks at the listener and the listener looks around, rummages in her desk, makes rude comments, and does other distracting things. Then, based on the constructive learning principle, the class can brainstorm what effective authors and editors would do in such circumstances.

Engaging a student in a demonstration is another effective way to begin a minilesson. For example, a lesson on peer conferencing might begin with an instructor and student sitting in front of the class, each with a current piece of work, to demonstrate good listening skills and what it means to ask a question that will help the author know what needs to be clarified.

Self-talk is another technique that can be used to activate students' schemas. When stimulating thinking about story idea generation, for example, the lead instructor might use an overhead transparency or marker board to map ideas solicited from the students into a semantic web. With self-talk, the instructor could demonstrate how one idea can lead to another while adding a branch to the web saying, for example, "Oh, that makes me think about other animal stories—I could write about the time my cat had kittens under my bed, or I could write about my dog who was afraid of fireworks" [adding bubbles for each]. Another example of using self-talk to activate schemas when demonstrating a computer software feature, such as "undo," would be for the instructor to say, "Oh my goodness, I didn't want to delete that phrase. What can I do?"

Brainstorming and Whole-Group Participation

In the process of introducing the minilesson topic and purpose and activating prior knowledge, instructors involve students in discussions about what they know and need to know. Note that these steps are not discrete but interactive—they blend, overlap, and support each other. The inclusive instructional challenge is to conduct discussions in a way that all students can participate. The goal in activating prior knowledge is to provide a foundation that will help all students construct new knowledge at a level that works for them.

In whole-group discussions, most students have subtle but fairly well understood expectations about which classmates always raise their hands and which rarely do. We have known students, for example, who stated explicitly, "I never raise my hand," and one who said, "I always raise my hand so others will think I know the answer even if I don't." Not surprisingly, this student's teacher said, "I never call on her because when I do, she never has an answer."

The first suggestion for breaking maladaptive patterns of nonparticipation is to pose questions that have more than one right answer. As mentioned previously, rules for brainstorming, in which all answers are accepted and listed without criticism or debate, can be the topic of an early minilesson (see chapter appendix). After students learn about brainstorming as a tool to generate lots of ideas quickly, brainstorming techniques can be used regularly. Instructors also should try to minimize known-answer or "teacher talk" questions, which are designed to yield the single answer the teacher has in mind. The goal in minilesson discussions is to ask questions that authentically seek students' input and lead them to construct higher-level meanings. Brainstorms or opinion questions are two good ways to do this.

Minilesson questions should be worded to be linguistically and cognitively accessible to students functioning at a range of ability levels. Students with cognitive limitations can provide answers that are more concrete to the questions designed to challenge students functioning at higher levels to draw inferences and make abstract connections among concepts. For example, in one of our class projects, students were debating the question of whether their school should continue a special "Lunch and Learn" program in which they ate lunch in their classroom and then engaged in activities they could sign up for once a week from a menu of options. One high-functioning student offered an argument for the pro side as an "opportunity to choose, based on the core democratic value, liberty." In the same discussion, a student with disabilities offered an argument for the pro side, as being able "to play with the big green ball on the playground." The important things were that both students were participating actively and that both students gained access to higher-level learning opportunities.

Timing and expectation encourage group discussion participation. These and other suggestions include

- Use wait time strategically by posing a question that allows multiple levels of response and indicating willingness to wait until all students have thought of an answer.

- Ask students each to write a response on paper, give them time to do so, then sample diverse responses and comment on how each fits.

- Phrase questions to communicate that whole-group involvement is expected—for example, instead of saying, "Who knows how to start a paragraph on the computer?" and calling on one student, say, "How many of you know how to start a paragraph on the computer?" then wait and say, "It looks like a lot of you have ideas about how to indent. What should I do? Everybody, I press the [pause to indicate expectation of choral response] tab key."

- Review new vocabulary, concepts, and procedures both within and across sessions so all can rehearse and everyone can participate actively.

Introducing Key Vocabulary and Explaining Concepts

Minilessons are designed to achieve specific instructional goals. Some are aimed at developing concepts and others at promoting skills or teaching strategies. In any case, teams should discuss which vocabulary and concepts are critical and which are likely to be new for all or some students. Then, they should plan how to make the new terminology explicit through examples and practice. When students and interdisciplinary professionals have a common vocabulary, it is easier to collaborate, communicate on a topic, and scaffold students to higher levels of competence.

Directly teaching new words and meanings is one way to accomplish this. Many students with special needs, however, have underdeveloped skills for figuring out word meanings and making semantic connections in novel contexts. They may require more experience with examples and more guidance to reflect on and retain language-based information. Discussions regarding word meanings may lead students to discover that they know part of a word's meaning or that they know a word with a related meaning. Multiple examples can help students develop generalized meanings that are not specific to one instance or referent. For example, when we introduced a second-grade class to the term *personal history* as part of preparing them to construct personal timelines, we asked them whether the words sounded like any they might know. *Person* was a familiar word, and it led to a discussion not only about the meaning of *personal history* but also of how word parts fit together to make new words.

It also is important to calibrate word use and word meaning across students and teachers. Students may have learned different terms to describe parts of a process or strategy. For example, in one of our minilessons, we discovered that what some of the students called a *draft*, others had learned to call *sloppy copy*. In another case, what we were calling *planning and organizing*, teachers were calling *prewriting*. When such discrepancies occur, groups should negotiate meanings and decide on common terminology. Metalinguistic discussions can help students develop the concept of synonyms in that multiple words may have similar meanings. Other metalinguistic discussions can teach the concept that single words may have more than one meaning. The goal of such discussions is to help students learn specific new academic content and vocabulary while also teaching broader concepts about language.

Providing Print Supports to Aid Retention

Most minilessons involve some type of print support or handout to make concepts more concrete. Minilesson handouts also serve as durable reminders of new concepts for review and future reference. Several examples are included in the chapter appendix.

We try to design minilesson handouts using the keep it simple principle. This means that instructors should keep handouts relatively uncomplicated both for themselves and for their students. In particular, it is wise to avoid putting too much content on the page. Often, when we are planning, one member of the team will sit at a computer and produce a handout for an upcoming lesson. Such handouts do not have to be elaborate, just clear.

When designing print supports, clear headings and larger fonts help students attend to important vocabulary. Adding clip art can make key concepts easier for all students to access and remember, particularly when students are in the earlier stages of literacy learning.

In some cases, print supports are introduced at the beginning of a minilesson. In others, handouts are reserved until most of the lesson is complete, then used to review important concepts or to provide spaces with instruction to add individual handwritten content. In still other cases, handouts are prepared *after* a brainstorming session so students' ideas and words can be incorporated into the handout, also supporting review in a follow-up session (see chapter appendix for an example).

Providing Immediate Application and Practice Opportunities

Minilessons should lead directly into practice activities as soon as main concepts are established and students have had opportunities to participate in whole-group discussions. Depending on the topic of the minilesson and stage of development of writing lab procedures, application might involve planning, peer conferencing, editing, note taking, author chair presentations, or any of the other writing processes or writing lab components.

Scaffolding Opportunities

Special educators or SLPs might preteach some concepts. Students who need more examples or other forms of support also can receive them during individual or small-group scaffolding. These are good times to ensure that all students have understood minilesson concepts. In addition, they are good times to address IEP goals and other written language and social interaction objectives.

To provide scaffolding, instructors move about the room observing evidence that students are incorporating new concepts as they begin their work. When necessary, instructors coach small groups about how to interact (e.g., waiting for turns, leading a discussion, listening to each other, using positive strategies to make each other aware of communication breakdowns). They also scaffold individual students to use the new knowledge, skills, and strategies targeted in the minilesson.

Planning Individual and Small-Group Minilessons

Individualized minilessons are designed to help particular students with missing knowledge or skills. This may seem the province of special service providers, but general education teachers using the writing lab approach seek such opportunities as well. It is part of the shared ownership principle that makes the writing lab approach so powerful. Having multiple adults available in classrooms can enhance teachers' opportunities to individualize instruction more than usual.

Individual minilessons may address any of a particular student's personal objectives, or they may address issues that arise at a teachable moment. Although they are not preplanned, these interactions can be supported with written content on a page in the student's author notebook. Examples are

- Individual minilessons focused on word families (i.e., the orthographic principle), such as *-at* and *-in* families for a student at earlier stage development and *-ought* or *-ould* families for a student at a later stage. Students having difficulty with such issues can be scaffolded to use emerging phonemic and orthographic awareness skills to generate multiple words following the pattern of the targeted orthographic family by using a page in the author notebook.

- Individual minilessons designed to help students disambiguate easily confused words that have been showing up in their work, such as *and* versus *in* (e.g., the boy "in" me); *are* versus *our* (e.g., we were in "are" car); or *there* versus *their* (e.g., they put on "there" coats). These lessons also can be supported with a special page in the spelling section of the author notebook.

- Individual minilessons related to spoken communication issues, such as articulation (e.g., production of a phoneme in isolation), stuttering (e.g., easy onset), or voice problems (e.g., preventing vocal abuse). Such speaking skills can be taught in occasional pullout sessions, if necessary, then practiced in writing lab contexts.

Teachable moments also arise for introducing or reinforcing knowledge, skills, or strategies in small groups. An example is a small-group minilesson designed to teach problem solving in response to a conflict in which group members are picking on and blaming one another, with the result that no work is getting done (see Box 4.2). The topic of a minilesson for such circumstances might be "communicating—not blaming." A discussion brings the concept of blaming to a conscious level, starting with student definitions of blaming, then setting a rule that when conflicts occur, the problem should be described from each person's point of view, but blaming is not allowed. With blaming set aside, small groups can be scaffolded to brainstorm what makes a group work well together and what makes a group have trouble.

This sets the stage for proactive targeting of any annoying pragmatic behaviors that may be displayed by a student who usually plays the role of victim at the same time that more cooperative behaviors are targeted for those who generally play the role of aggressor. Students can be scaffolded to describe such desirable behaviors as waiting for turns, taking turns leading the discussion, and listening carefully, in contrast to such undesirable behaviors as interrupting, name-calling, eye-rolling, and so forth. In this positive context, they can describe behaviors without blaming each other or attributing any negative behaviors to specific individuals. Then, they can set personal goals and be coached to practice the new behaviors in their own small-group interactions.

Minilesson Topics and Examples

Topics for minilessons may be curriculum-driven or selected in response to student needs. Table 4.4 provides a listing of possible minilesson topics. It includes lessons that address classroom procedures, writing processes, writing lab activities, discourse genres, computer supports, language targets, group participation, and oral presentations.

Box 4.2.   Triggering Event for Small-Group Minilesson

When third-graders Robert, Amir, and Rico entered the computer lab, it was clear that they had been in conflict once again. Each was playing out his well-rehearsed part in a familiar routine. Robert, in tears, assumed the role of victim. When asked what had happened, he said, "Amir kicked me. Rico thumped me in the forehead and called me names."

The three boys were taken into the hall so as not to disturb the rest of the class, which had begun a minilesson on a new piece of software. Rico, accustomed to the role of tough guy, volunteered, "I'm used to it. I was kicked out of school in kindergarten."

It was clear that something needed to be done to rewrite this well-practiced script or it was destined to be replayed over and over in more serious ways each time. The instructor said, "This is not about kicking you out. This is about you all learning some better ways to communicate. First, let's try to understand what happened. How did it start?"

The three boys all tried to explain at once about someone stepping on someone's foot and began to argue about whether the transgression was accidental or on purpose. The instructor commented on escalating violence and name-calling. "It may have started with an accident, but pretty soon is gets to be on purpose. Then, everybody is mad. What are some better things to say at the beginning to keep from getting to that point?"

Amir turned and reached over to Robert and volunteered, "I'm sorry, man."

The apology was a little too quick to have the ring of sincerity, but it was a starting point. The important thing was to move beyond the heat of the moment but not to forget the need for further intervention. Rico visibly relaxed but did not say anything.

Robert volunteered, "I'm sorry I called you names."

The scene ended, and the group returned to the computer lab with Rico apologizing for thumping Robert on the forehead. Removing this interaction from the drama of the moment and taking it to a higher plane involved planning a follow-up minilesson on communication skills for teaching a common vocabulary related to group problem solving. The follow-up minilesson was conducted, and the outbursts disappeared, at least in the writing lab context.

How Minilesson Topics Evolve

When planned as student-centered events, minilesson topics generally evolve with the group. For example, in one class students with LLDs were struggling with recognizing and marking sentence boundaries. Some used end punctuation and capitalization inconsistently and at odd places. Others avoided punctuation altogether, engaging the caps lock mechanism. A minilesson was designed to help students understand the communicative rationale for capitalization and end punctuation (so sentences will

Table 4.4. Minilesson topics

Topic area	Subtopics and example content
Classroom procedures	Classroom rules—where to sit, requesting to leave, how to listen, what to do with hands while listening, raising hands before talking, making sure everyone gets a turn, storing materials, permission to get materials, brainstorming
	Computer lab rules—assigned seats, asking questions, waiting for directions, saving and printing, helping neighbors without touching keyboards
	Jobs—passing out papers, printer monitor, computer disk manager, three-hole punch leader, library return leader, author notebook collector
Writing processes	Planning—topic generation, graphic webs, outlining, lists, planning for different discourse genres, coming back to planning later
	Organizing—numbering ideas in sequence to go in draft, changing notes in plan to sentences in draft, deciding what to include and leave out
	Drafting—using plans, thinking about audience, making good sentences to convey ideas, using interesting vocabulary, rereading while drafting
	Revising—thinking about content: Will others understand it? Is everything included? Is it clear? Is it interesting? How can I make it better?
	Editing—spelling, punctuation, capitalization, paragraph indents, typos, editors' notations, formatting. How does it look?
Writing lab activities	Author chair—what a good audience member does, how authors should hold their papers and read so others can hear them, making helpful comments, asking helpful questions, deciding who goes next, helping peers who want help
	Peer conferencing—author role, editor role, what to say
	Author notebooks—sections of notebooks, where to keep them, how to organize materials
Discourse genres	Narratives—parts of a story (characters, setting, problem, action, outcome, ending), interesting words, telling why things happen, telling what the characters are thinking and how they are feeling, making readers experience what the author sees and hears
	Expository—fact versus fiction, writing a report, doing research, taking notes, providing enough information, organizing ideas
	Poetry—what makes a poem a poem, how words are used, rhyming versus not rhyming, formatting a poem
	Letters—parts of a letter (date, greeting, body, signature), business versus friendly
Computer supports	Computer basics—keyboard, central processing unit, monitor, disk drives, mouse, cursor, shift key, space bar
	New software program—how to navigate, special features
	Tools for generating ideas, planning, organizing—clip art, stamps, graphic organizers
	Tools for drafting—picture symbols, word cueing and prediction, collaborative writing, speech recognition
	Tools for revising and editing—spelling checker, cut and paste, copy, delete
	Tools for publishing—illustrations, fonts, borders
Language targets	Discourse level—how to plan, how to check to see if the writing meets audience needs, macrostructures for different genres
	Sentence level—connecting sentences, knowing where sentences begin and end, adding interesting transitions
	Word level—interesting word choices, invented versus dictionary spelling, how to spell unknown words
	Writing conventions—punctuation, capitalization, paragraph indents, dialogue
Group participation	Paying attention—what it looks like, why it's important, what it helps people do
	Encouraging/discouraging—things people say or do to encourage or discourage themselves and others
Presentations	Reading in author chair or for a public presentation—eye contact, "public voice," reading with expression
	Reading poetry—Reading with meaning, rhythm, pausing
	Presenting multimedia computer shows—using technology, engaging the audience, pace

make sense to readers), to learn the connection between the two kinds of rules at the ends and beginnings of sentences, and to begin to use speech and complete idea cues to recognize sentence boundaries. The minilesson ended with editing practice focused on capitalization and punctuation in students' own compositions. The concepts and skills were reinforced over the next several sessions.

Within a few weeks, this group became more adept at writing and several students began to experiment with adding character dialogue in their stories. Soon, exploring dialogue became a group value. The need for information on punctuating and formatting dialogue evolved naturally. At this point, students responded favorably to lessons targeting punctuation of dialogue because the lessons addressed their needs. Other minilessons that evolved later included finding varied vocabulary as alternatives to *said* when leading into direct quotes and the difference between telling a story in first versus third person. A minilesson on "retired" words also appears in the chapter appendix.

Example Minilesson on Encouraging and Discouraging Talk

The minilesson on encouraging and discouraging grew out of a classroom experience in which some students harshly criticized their own work and the work of others. We were particularly concerned about one girl with Down syndrome who frequently called herself stupid or dumb. We also have used variations on this minilesson in situations in which a high proportion of reluctant writers or in situations in which students were being disrespectful to each other.

The purpose of the encouraging/discouraging minilesson is to help students focus on messages that people communicate to themselves and others. It is designed to 1) help students reflect on their feelings related to writing, 2) label talk in ways that can be referenced in future discussions, 3) teach students alternative ways to communicate ideas, and 4) introduce students to thinking about parts of words (morphemes) and their meanings. The lesson starts with an instructor writing the word *courage* in the middle of a marker board and asking students to brainstorm what the word means. A semantic web can be built from the phrases students generate, such as "be brave," "try hard," and "take risks" (see sample handout in the chapter appendix). The instructor then initiates a discussion of courage as it relates to learning new things and what it looks like in the writing lab.

After eliciting examples of how courage looks and sounds, the instructor introduces the word part (morpheme) *dis-* along with the idea that small parts can be added to words to change their meanings. Taking a different colored marker, the instructor adds *dis-* to form *discourage* and leads the group to think about how the small word-part changes the meaning. Many students know what it means to "dis" someone. When someone is *dis*couraged, it takes away the courage to be brave, try hard, and take risks; however, by changing the prefix to *en-*, as in *encourage,* all those things return. Again, using a different colored marker can help students visualize the differences between morphological word parts and how they affect meaning.

During the application portion of this minilesson, students make personal lists of discouraging things people say and do along with a contrasting set of encouraging things they can say and do. This page is inserted in the minilesson section of the students' author notebooks for consultation and later additions. When new writing lab activities are introduced, such as peer conferencing, for example, instructors can start by reminding the students to use encouraging talk. When negative comments are made, part of the classroom culture can be to remind students: "I am sure you can find a more encouraging way to make your suggestion." This message can be often repeated to build a writing lab culture as, "Here, we say encouraging things to ourselves and others."

Example Minilesson on Writing Processes

The introductory minilesson on writing processes might start with a series of questions to encourage discussions about the concept of author, including

- What is an author?
- What do authors do?
- For whom?
- How do they do it?

Out of this discussion, instructors can help students develop a list of the stages authors go through as they write. Many of the teachers we have worked with have had posters that display writing processes as including five or six stages depending on how they are combined and terminology choices within school districts and classrooms. Stages include 1) planning and organizing (or prewriting), 2) drafting, 3) revising, 4) editing, and 5) publishing.

In the minilesson, each stage is described and illustrated with examples (see sample handouts in the chapter appendix). A classroom support in the form of a poster board provides additional opportunities for reference and review. During the next few writing lab sessions, the stages are reviewed, and individual stages are examined in greater detail as they are practiced in an early project, chosen for its relative simplicity. The chapter appendix includes handouts for minilessons on stages of the writing process. One of these is an example of an author notebook page that can be used at the conclusion of each writing lab session to engage students in identifying where they are in the writing process and to discuss what they plan to do next.

In teaching the writing process, one group of teachers brought in a children's book author, who discussed the writing process and showed several drafts of her manuscript, including one that was returned by the editor with many edits. This made for a colorful example of the importance of revision even for established authors, and it showed the process of writing for a broader audience.

Example Minilesson on Narrative Discourse Structure

A minilesson on narrative macrostructure has the primary goal of teaching students to include all major parts in their stories. A story grammar template might be provided that includes a beginning with setting, characters, and problem; a middle in which the main characters make plans and take actions to solve the problem; and an ending that tells what happened, providing a good conclusion for the story. The chapter appendix includes a handout for planning a story. Alternatively, a template might be developed to encourage stories with five parts (one for each finger on a hand): setting (characters, place, and time), problem, action, outcome, and ending.

Minilessons on story writing vary with students' current developmental stages. For students in earlier stages of narrative development, discussion might focus on relating information temporally or causally. For those in later stages, discussion might focus on character motivation and planning. Numerous tools are available commercially to support analysis of narrative maturity (e.g., Hedberg & Westby, 1993; Hughes, McGillivray, & Schmidek, 1997; Mather & Roberts, 1995).

Instructor dialogue for minilessons on narrative structure can help students reflect on the parts of stories that work together to create interest. Strategies for activating prior knowledge and designing practice experiences include the following:

- Ask students to list and describe story grammar elements.

- Analyze story grammar elements in examples from trade books, specially created stories, or students' stories.

- Connect story grammar elements to writing process stages—planning (to include all parts), drafting (checking planning notes while writing), and revising and editing (making sure that all parts are included).

Example Minilesson on Taking Notes

When preparing to write expository discourse, two levels of questions are key: What do I need to know? and Where can I find the answers to my questions? A semantic webbing strategy can be used to generate questions (see Box 6.1 for an example). The introductory minilesson can then benefit from modeling the process of notetaking from a familiar text (see chapter appendix for example minilesson support).

In one third-grade classroom, students were introduced to the principles of notetaking using a familiar text on tornadoes that came from their language arts curriculum. Using this text, they learned a sequence that involved

- Having one or two questions in mind

- Reading until you find an answer

- Shutting the book

- Putting the words of the book author in your own words

- Writing the answer down (you don't have to use complete sentences—just get the main idea or important details)

After practicing with the familiar text, students selected an animal to study in depth. Then, they followed similar procedures to take notes from a variety of books their teacher had selected as approximately at grade level. An example minilesson handout on notetaking is located in the chapter appendix.

Notetaking generally needs to be followed by strategies for organizing notes prior to drafting. Depending on the age of students, that step may be more or less elaborate, but emphasis on the term *organization* may help students make the transition from planning to drafting.

Example Minilesson on Spelling

To activate prior knowledge about spelling, instructors might introduce the minilesson topic by commenting, then stimulating a brainstorming exercise. They might say, "Everyone has trouble spelling words some of the time. What are some of the strategies you could use to learn how to spell a word you do not know?" Student comments that follow generally include such contributions as ask someone, look it up in the dictionary, use the spelling checker on the computer, and sound it out (invented spelling).

The topic of spelling is not one that can be addressed in a single minilesson or even in a series of lessons. Some authors have commented on the linguistic bases of spelling (e.g., Kamhi & Hinton, 2000; Masterson & Apel, 2000). Any of the aforementioned strategies for figuring out how to spell unknown words can be the topic of its own lesson (see example minilesson handouts for spelling checker and spelling strategies in the chapter appendix). Suggestions for what to include are summarized in the following paragraphs. As discussed in Chapters 2 and 5, spelling is a function of sound and word knowledge. The skills underlying "sound it out" (also called *invented spelling*) are particularly rich for language learning. They are the essence of word-level literacy ability, differing across students in relationship to their phonemic and morphologic knowledge. Those with LLDs are especially likely to need individualized assessment and much tailor-made scaffolding to acquire them. Introductory minilessons, however, can serve an important role by developing a common terminology and set of strategies for use in a community of learners.

The dictionary strategy often is mentioned but less often successfully used. A lesson on how to use the dictionary can assist students to edit their work, but dictionary use can become a time-consuming, discouraging chore for students with multiple spelling errors. Alternatives include learning to use spelling checkers, word walls, or personal dictionaries or starting with well-founded invented spellings before looking up a word. Personal dictionaries can be produced using author notebook pages or may be built into a word-processing computer software program that includes a feature allowing the creation and editing of on-line dictionaries (see Chapter 9). Personalized supports also can include individual minilessons on spelling rules with examples kept in a differentiated section in the author notebook. They might include examples related to distinguishing homonyms or how to add suffixes (e.g., plural or past tense morphemes) to roots (see Chapter 2).

The spelling strategy of asking someone generally works, but it can become a habit, and it reduces ownership. There is a need to balance working independently and asking for help. The usual writing lab procedure is to scaffold students toward independent use of invented spelling and other self-regulated strategies rather than to tell words directly. At times, however, students have trouble moving forward unless someone gives them direct input. Some general education teachers also have historically told students spellings whenever asked. Taking away this support suddenly can be distressing. The provision of spelling supports is a good topic for team discussion. One suggestion is always to follow direct help with encouragement for students to add new words to their personal dictionaries.

Spelling checkers in computer software programs help authors monitor for spelling accuracy. Students can learn to use spelling checkers strategically to generate accurate spellings for words they are unsure about. Spelling checkers only work, however, when original spelling attempts are close enough to intended words to bring up the actual spelling among the choices. Therefore, students must be able to generate accurate invented spellings first. Then, when spelling checkers offer choices, students may be able to select the most plausible among them. If one is not plausible, some children's software programs offer opportunities to type in another alternative (e.g., *Ulti-*

mate Writing and Creativity Center, by The Learning Co., offers this choice). One teacher with whom we worked asked students always to attempt another spelling first before asking the software to provide alternatives.

To teach invented spelling strategies, a minilesson instructor might start by modeling invented spelling strategies for unknown words in a new composition. A sound-by-sound strategy with related letter-by-letter representations might be attempted first, emphasizing how to say target words slowly. The class can be engaged in a choral group production to demonstrate the value of stretching out sounds in words so as to hear and feel them better. The alphabetic principle also involves automatic and fluent associations between phonemes and letter combinations (digraphs), such as *ph*, *th* (voiceless), *th* (voiced), *sh*, and *ch*. Although the sound-by-sound, letter-by letter strategy works as a starting point, students also must be led to see the need for other strategies that involve chunking.

To go beyond a sound-by-sound approach, students can be led to compare the sounding out strategy with one for breaking a word into syllables or word parts (i.e., onset and rime, morphemes and their associated orthographs). In an early minilesson, they can learn about word families by thinking of words that sound the same (i.e., with the same rime) as the target word, and then changing the initial sounds (i.e., onset) to spell that word with different letters at the beginning. Later, they can learn the strategy of pronouncing a word (e.g., *restaurant*) as it is spelled (i.e., "*rest–a–ur–ant*") for the purpose of remembering how to spell it in the future.

Eventually, through examples and individualized practice, most students acquire the skills for using word chunks, syllables, word roots, and bound morphemes (e.g., *-ing, -tion, -ed*). For example, a child who spells *walked* as *walkt* can be taught a minilesson for using the past-tense *-ed* ending to words to tell about things that happened in the past, even if the word part sounds like /t/. The goal is to help students take advantage of the reciprocal interrelationships among speaking, reading, and writing to connect learning across modalities. This extended process can start with a minilesson, but ultimately, it is learned through repeated practice facilitated by individualized scaffolding. Special terminology (e.g., *onset, rime*) helps educators to clarify concepts for themselves. It is not usually taught to children.

AUTHOR NOTEBOOKS

Author notebooks serve as a tool for teaching students to organize their work and to learn self-regulation strategies. They also can be used to store minilesson handouts and other print supports, such as scaffolding reminders and spelling resource materials. They hold elements of individualized intervention, such as IEP language goals written in "kid language" and personal minilessons. They also can serve as a portfolio for documenting students' growth, although we do recommend that special service providers keep a separate folder of duplicated, dated examples of students' work for documenting change as well.

Author notebooks are introduced within the first few sessions of writing lab and are made available for all sessions thereafter and at free times when students want to work on their writing projects. Loose-leaf three-hole binders provide the greatest flexibility for adding pages and dividers for moving materials around. The minilesson in which author notebooks are introduced can be used to target direction following ability and such directional words as *top, bottom, left, right, before, after, tabs, dividers, abbreviations,* and so forth. In subsequent sessions, students can be asked to consult their minilesson handouts, spelling supports, works in progress, and other components in their author notebooks. They can be directed to store new materials in certain sections, and in the process can learn categorization and strategies for self-organization.

It may be necessary for adults to prepare the divider tabs for younger students. Older students (Grade 3 and above) can do this task themselves. One approach we have used is to write the names of the sections on the chalkboard for students to copy onto the divider pages, then to help them write abbreviations onto the small, perforated cards (often another new vocabulary word) that fit into plastic tabs. One role SLPs may assume on teams is to help members focus explicitly on new technical vocabulary that children need to learn, while also ensuring that language impaired students know basic vocabulary that may have been presupposed (e.g., *center, top, behind*), but that they may not have fully learned.

The sections of author notebooks can be personalized and the vocabulary calibrated to classroom routines of specific teachers. Typical sections include

1. Lab schedule—a single sheet taped to the front of the notebook or the first divider that includes days in the computer lab and upcoming publication deadlines. It helps students develop awareness of scheduling.

2. Goals and objectives—includes IEP goals for students who have them, preferably rewritten in collaboration with students in language at a level that they can understand. All students should have personal goals to convey that everyone has goals and that goals serve more than remedial purposes. Examples of individualized goals appear in Chapter 1 (Table 1.2) and Chapter 16 (Table 16.2). The goals and objectives completed with students help them to internalize stages of the writing process and to develop their skills for planning and evaluating their own work.

3. Minilesson handouts—serve to make main points more concrete and to give instructors and students something to refer to as they integrate new knowledge, skills, and strategies. Minilessons may include specialized vocabulary and procedural language for helping students to develop the self-talk to guide themselves through complex tasks (see chapter appendix). They assist students in organizing different discourse genres, as well as in proofreading symbols and describing roles for peers during conferencing.

4. Personal minilesson supports—blank paper that can be used for individualized minilessons in the moment, as well as existing practice materials that have been developed in therapeutic interactions with individual students. All students should have a personal minilesson section.

5. Works in progress—used to store the student's plans and drafts for group projects the class is working on.

6. What I did today—dated journal entries in which students indicate the stage of the writing process worked on that day and establish personal goals for the next session (see Figure 4.4 for an example form and also Figure 16.9, in Chapter 16, for an example of this form completed by a fourth-grade student).

What I did today…

_____ Topic _____
     date

(Circle all you did today.)

Researching/Planning   Drafting   Revising

My comments: _____

Teacher comments _____

_____ Topic _____
     date

(Circle all you did today.)

Researching/Planning   Drafting   Revising

My comments: _____

Teacher comments: _____

_____ Topic _____
     date

(Circle all you did today.)

Researching/Planning   Drafting   Revising

My comments: _____

Teacher comments: _____

The Writing Lab Approach to Language Instruction and Intervention, by Nickola Wolf Nelson, Christine M. Bahr, and Adelia M. Van Meter
Copyright © 2004 Paul H. Brookes Publishing Co., Inc. All rights reserved.

Figure 4.4.   Example notebook page for guiding "What I did today" self-assessments.

7. Free writing—stocked with paper and previous free writing efforts. Students also can keep lists of ideas in this section for future writing.

8. Completed works—when projects are completed, they can be moved into the section for completed works. It is helpful to keep all stages of a finished project and to date them to show this progression. When completed works still need copyediting to meet school district standards, the last drafts can be identified as "independent" and "edited with adult assistance."

9. Spelling supports—grade level lists of spelling words arranged alphabetically. Spelling support dictionaries also can be purchased at teacher supply stores. It is helpful if such lists have room to add additional personalized words. As an alternative, we have prepared personal dictionary pages for students by printing letters with spaces between for students to write in their own words.

In summary, author notebooks provide a concrete tool for assisting students to organize themselves and their work. Author notebooks also can be used to keep students in touch with concrete supports for assisting them to meet their personal goals related to writing processes and products and for meeting social communication targets.

PEER AND TEACHER CONFERENCING

A community of authors is enhanced when peers have opportunities to conference with each other as well as with their instructors. Author groups, peer conferencing, and teacher conferencing all provide contexts in which special service providers can address IEP goals while working with students in the general education classroom. Such activities provide rich opportunities for instructional teams to target advancing social interaction and audience response and revision skills for all students (Stoddard & MacArthur, 1992).

The routine for peer conferencing generally is introduced in a minilesson dedicated to the topic. This is a special opportunity to build the concept of an immediate authentic audience. The opinions of peers are particularly important to students. When students learn to attend to the attitudes and values of their peers, they gain an important skill for building audience sensitivity and social communicative competence.

A minilesson on peer conferencing often begins with dramatic role play between general education teachers and special service providers. The goal is to help students picture themselves interacting with peers and to identify facilitative and nonfacilitative interaction techniques. The immediate goal is to introduce author and editor roles, with the accompanying expectations for each. The chapter appendix includes an author notebook handout that was designed for students to use when practicing these roles. It introduces the general rules of peer conferencing. More specific rules can be developed for other projects, such as those in which students interview each other for compare-and-contrast essays or for other special purposes.

Author groups form an alternative to peer conferencing. Students in author groups work together over an extended period of time. They might be grouped based on assigned seats or to meet IEP requirements for time with a special service provider; however, students without disabilities should be grouped with those with special needs to take advantage of inclusive environments. Author groups get to know each other's works in progress when they meet on a regular basis. Therefore, less time is required to go over previous work, and authors can focus on what has been added since last meeting (McAlister et al., 1999). Students also can take turns serving as author group leader. This can build self-regulation skills and ownership for the process of interaction.

Teacher conferencing can also add to students' sense of themselves as authors. Although conversations between students with disabilities and their special education teachers and SLPs are important, interactions with the general education teacher set the stage for students with disabilities to view themselves as full members of the classroom (Anderson, 2000). Anderson suggested that these conferences start with such open-ended questions as "How's it going?" "What are you doing today as a writer?" "What work are you doing as a writer this period?" and "What do you need help with today?" (2000, p. 29). Such questions can guide the student–teacher conference to focus more on students' ideas than the need for editing. This focus is particularly important for students with disabilities.

AUTHOR CHAIR AND OTHER PRESENTATIONS

In the author chair, students read from their own work, listen constructively, develop group-speaking abilities, and benefit from and provide supportive input as members of a community of authors (see Figure 4.5). Other writing lab presentation experiences can enhance the role of parents as appreciative audience members and can further students' confidence as public speakers. The author chair is the original presentation experience, however, and one of the most powerful.

The routine of the author chair may vary, but generally it includes the following:

- Students are selected in turn to sit in a special chair and read all or part of a work in progress.

- Peers act as the audience by listening attentively and thinking of comments they might make on parts they like or questions they might ask the author to clarify aspects that need elaboration.

- After reading, the author calls on fellow students to make comments and ask questions (one or two of each, depending on time).

The author chair routine is established via a minilesson in which instructors act out the roles of author and audience. To highlight the importance of the author's role in reading clearly and making eye contact with the audience, the instructor in the role might violate such expectations. This can bring effective communication behaviors to students' attention for mention in initial brainstorming. Two things authors need to keep in the forefront while writing are focus on the content of what is written and its effect on the audience. That is the real value of author's chair, which can heighten the sense of audience so authors will carry it with them into the writing experience. To highlight the importance of the audience's role in paying close attention, expressing appreciation, and offering suggestions, a member of the instructional team might play this role as well, perhaps starting with a negative version, then switching to positive

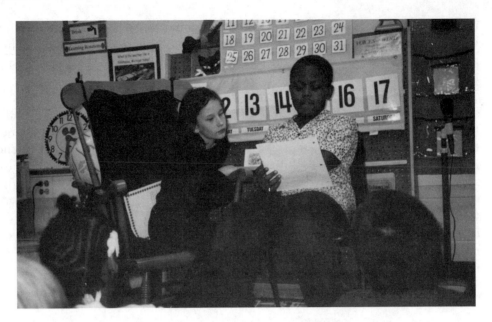

Figure 4.5. Students in author chair.

role modeling after soliciting students' brainstormed comments about how the audience should behave and respond (as opposed to the negative model).

The chair used for author chair might be one that teachers have decorated or one generally reserved for the classroom teacher's use, such as a stool or swivel chair. The author selection process might take place through an objective method, such as drawing wooden sticks with names from a jar or having each student select the next student to go. In those cases, however, scaffolding should be provided to ensure that students with special needs are chosen. Participation in the author chair is voluntary, but all students are encouraged to take a turn. For some, this requires a heavy dose of the patience principle and support either from an instructor or a peer. For example, Chapter 17 tells the story of Steven, who was dependent on peers to read his early works but who could read works independently by the end of the school year.

Although the author chair works best for works in progress (so students can benefit from the input in making revisions), other presentations may be planned to celebrate and perform final works in front of broader audiences, such as other classrooms of students and parents. In our after-school activities, we have held publishing parties with student presentations and awards to recognize their work. Our recommendation in making such awards is to personalize them in ways that genuinely compliment each student's efforts and to avoid such backhanded compliments as "Justin hardly ever gets off topic any more." Instead, the award might be worded as "Developing topics with many interesting details."

It is important to display work in ways that are attractive and accessible. It is particularly important that display methods put the work of students with special needs on equal footing with the work of their typically developing peers. Publishing parties are not "separate but equal" presentations for students with special needs. Rather, they provide opportunities for all students to feel the magic of accomplishment and success that an appreciative audience can bring. In inclusive presentation opportunities, students' original works are presented in print form or as live or videotaped performances. During such events, parents can browse and feel pride in their children's works, and students can experience being part of a productive community of authors.

SUMMARY

The process of designing instruction starts with a decision for general and special education instructors to work together as a team in the context of an inclusive writing lab experience. In this chapter, we consider the logistics of coming together to design intervention and the initial decisions that must be made about schedules and projects. The chapter also offers an overview of the major instructional components of the writing lab, including minilessons, author notebooks, peer conferencing, and the author chair, and other presentation experiences.

Appendix
Minilesson Handouts for Author Notebooks

The following pages contain example handouts for topics listed in Table 4.4.

Classroom procedures
1. Our lab schedule
2. Rights and responsibilities
3. Brainstorming (simple version for younger students)
4. Brainstorming (more complex version for older students)
5. Tips on raising your hand

Writing processes
6. The writing process (simple version for younger students)
7. The writing process (more complex version for older students)
8. Planning
9. Plan, organize, draft
10. Revising
11. Editing your article

Writing lab activities
12. Peer conferencing
13. Partner conferencing
14. Author groups
15. Your notebook

Discourse genres
16. Planning a story
17. Animal report
18. Notetaking
19. Parts of a book
20. Mystery
21. Color poem

Computer supports
22. Spelling checker
23. Illustration

Language targets
24. Student self-evaluation
25. Retired words
26. Spelling strategies

Group participation
27. Encouraging/discouraging
28. Oral presentations (simple version for younger students)
29. Giving oral presentations (more complex version for older students)

Our Lab Schedule

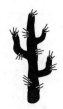

Tuesday

4:00 – 4:25   Newspaper time

4:25 – 5:05   Homework—School skills

Thursday

4:00 – 4:15   Large-group minilesson

4:15 – 4:50   Homework—School skills

4:50 – 5:05   Newspaper report

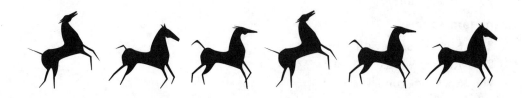

The Writing Lab Approach to Language Instruction and Intervention, by Nickola Wolf Nelson, Christine M. Bahr, and Adelia M. Van Meter
Copyright © 2004 Paul H. Brookes Publishing Co., Inc. All rights reserved.

RIGHTS AND RESPONSIBILITIES

Rights	Responsibilities

1. Respect
  • Body
  • Feelings
	Treat everyone respectfully.—CR*
	 Take care of people's things.—NP
	 Act respectful.—JV
	 Take turns.—CN
	 Be nice to others. (Share)—AP & PP
	 Be friends.—SP
	 Be careful about touching other people.—CR
	 Keep objects to yourself.—MJ
	 Don't hit.—SP
	 Don't say bad stuff about others.—CR & SP
	 Don't grab.—BT
	 Don't talk out real loud.—PP
	 Don't be a space invader.—RG
	 Don't laugh at mistakes.—SP

2. To learn	Take turns.—SP Don't goof off.—SJ Don't distract others.—SJ & CR
3. Clean and safe environment	Take care of your stuff.—CR Pick up.—SP & JV Recycle.—PP Join "Big Help."—MJ Don't tap on computer.—CR Don't mess up books.—BT

*Initials refer to students who offered specific contributions in a prior group brainstorm.

The Writing Lab Approach to Language Instruction and Intervention, by Nickola Wolf Nelson, Christine M. Bahr, and Adelia M. Van Meter
Copyright © 2004 Paul H. Brookes Publishing Co., Inc. All rights reserved.

Brainstorming

1. Think of as many ideas as possible.

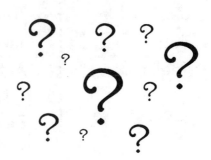

2. Which ideas will work?

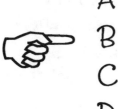

A
B
C
D

3. Pick the ideas you want to use.

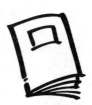

4. Keep all your brainstorming ideas for another day.

The Writing Lab Approach to Language Instruction and Intervention, by Nickola Wolf Nelson, Christine M. Bahr, and Adelia M. Van Meter
Copyright © 2004 Paul H. Brookes Publishing Co., Inc. All rights reserved.

Brainstorming

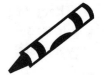

Rules for group brainstorming:

1. Only one person talks at a time.

2. All ideas are accepted (no ideas are dumb.)

3. Share all of your ideas.

4. Everyone's ideas are important.

Rules for brainstorming on your own:

1. Write down all of your ideas.

2. All ideas are good ideas at this point.

3. Later, you can decide which are best to meet your goal.

The Writing Lab Approach to Language Instruction and Intervention, by Nickola Wolf Nelson, Christine M. Bahr, and Adelia M. Van Meter
Copyright © 2004 Paul H. Brookes Publishing Co., Inc. All rights reserved.

Tips on Raising Your Hand

There are many different reasons why you raise you hand in your classroom. Here are three reasons and some questions you should ask yourself.

1. Raising your hand to answer a teacher's question

   Questions I Should Ask Myself

   - Do I have an answer to the question?
   - Have I had too many turns?

2. Raising your hand to ask a question

   Questions I Should Ask Myself

   - Is my question on the topic the teacher is talking about?
   - Is the teacher in the middle of an explanation?
   - Is another student in the middle of talking?
   - Is the teacher pausing?

3. Raising your hand to share a comment

   Questions I Should Ask Myself

   - Have I heard or seen a signal that it is appropriate to share a comment now?
   - Is my comment about the topic the class is discussing?
   - How long is my comment?

      * Question: What is the best way to raise your hand?
        * Answer: Quietly

What questions do you ask yourself before you raise your hand? Think of a time when you raised your hand in class. Write down why you raised your hand and what questions you asked yourself.

The Writing Lab Approach to Language Instruction and Intervention, by Nickola Wolf Nelson, Christine M. Bahr, and Adelia M. Van Meter
Copyright © 2004 Paul H. Brookes Publishing Co., Inc. All rights reserved.

The Writing Process

A. Prewrite
- Think
- Plan

B. Draft

C. Revise
and Edit

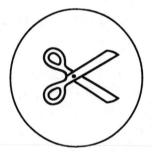

D. Publish

The Writing Lab Approach to Language Instruction and Intervention, by Nickola Wolf Nelson, Christine M. Bahr, and Adelia M. Van Meter
Copyright © 2004 Paul H. Brookes Publishing Co., Inc. All rights reserved.

The Writing Process

1. Planning and organizing

    *   These are things you *do* before you begin writing.

    *   Make a "map" or a "story web."

2. Story writing/drafting

    *   Put all of you ideas into sentences that make a story.

    *   This is the "sloppy copy" or "rough draft." It's okay to make mistakes.

3. Revising and editing

    *   Make changes in your story.

    *   Fix punctuation and capital letters.

    *   Learn spelling rules.

4. Publishing

    *   Make a final copy of your story, and put it in a book.

5. Presenting

    *   Share your work with an audience.

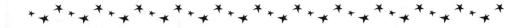

The Writing Lab Approach to Language Instruction and Intervention, by Nickola Wolf Nelson, Christine M. Bahr, and Adelia M. Van Meter
Copyright © 2004 Paul H. Brookes Publishing Co., Inc. All rights reserved.

Planning

Questions you must ask yourself:

1. What is my GOAL?

2. What parts should I include in my plan?

3. What *do* I NEED to accomplish my goal?

4. Where can I get what I need?

Always recheck your list. Did you forget anything??

The Writing Lab Approach to Language Instruction and Intervention, by Nickola Wolf Nelson, Christine M. Bahr, and Adelia M. Van Meter
Copyright © 2004 Paul H. Brookes Publishing Co., Inc. All rights reserved.

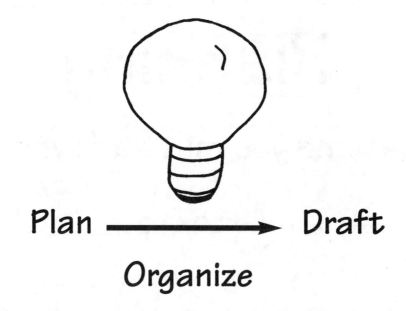

Plan ——————▶ Draft

Organize

- What goes together?

- What is important?

- What should go first?

- How should I say it?

- What goes next?

- How should I end it?

The Writing Lab Approach to Language Instruction and Intervention, by Nickola Wolf Nelson, Christine M. Bahr, and Adelia M. Van Meter
Copyright © 2004 Paul H. Brookes Publishing Co., Inc. All rights reserved.

Revising

Authors revise their work to make sure their ideas are clear and interesting to readers. Follow these steps to revise your paper.

1. Read your paper aloud.

2. Ask yourself,

   "Is this clear?"

   "Is this interesting?"

3. Ask yourself, "Can I make this paper better by:

   - Adding more details?

   - Using interesting words

   - Changing sentences?

   - Moving ideas?"

4. Try ideas talked about in your peer conference.

5. Check your planning guide to make sure you included all your information.

The Writing Lab Approach to Language Instruction and Intervention, by Nickola Wolf Nelson, Christine M. Bahr, and Adelia M. Van Meter
Copyright © 2004 Paul H. Brookes Publishing Co., Inc. All rights reserved.

EDITING YOUR ARTICLE

THERE ARE MANY THINGS TO LOOK FOR WHEN YOU ARE EDITING AN ARTICLE OR STORY YOU HAVE WRITTEN.

SOME QUESTIONS TO ASK YOURSELF ARE:

- IS MY ARTICLE CLEAR TO THE PERSON READING IT?

- IS MY ARTICLE INTERESTING FOR OTHERS TO READ?

- DOES MY ARTICLE PROVIDE GOOD INFORMATION?

- ARE MY SENTENCES FULL OF DETAIL AND DESCRIPTION OR ARE THEY SHORT AND PLAIN?

- DOES MY ARTICLE FLOW EASILY WHEN YOU READ IT OR DO MY THOUGHTS JUMP AROUND?

- HAVE I GIVEN GOOD DESCRIPTION AND DETAIL TO SUPPORT MY IDEAS?

SOME THINGS TO LOOK FOR IN EDITING ARE:

- SPELLING

- PUNCTUATION – PERIODS, COMMAS, QUESTIONS MARKS, EXCLAMATION POINT/MARK

- CAPITALS

- USE OF CONJUNCTIONS (AND, BUT, OR) TO JOIN SENTENCES THAT ARE LINKED WITH THE SAME IDEA. (I WENT TO THE STORY. I BOUGHT SOME MILK. / I WENT TO THE STORE AND BOUGHT SOME MILK.)

- USE OF TRANSITION WORDS (FIRST, SECOND, NEXT, LAST, FINALLY, IN THE END) TO MAKE DIFFERENT SENTENCES FLOW.

YOU CAN ALSO EDIT OTHER PEOPLE'S ARTICLES:

LOOK FOR EVERYTHING YOU WOULD IF IT WAS YOUR OWN PAPER AND BE ABLE TO TELL THE WRITER:

- CHANGES, IF ANY, IN SPELLING, CAPITALIZATION, PUNCTUATION, ETC.

- WHAT YOU LIKED ABOUT THE ARTICLE.

- WHAT YOU MIGHT ADD TO MAKE IT MORE CLEAR IF IT ISN'T CLEAR.

The Writing Lab Approach to Language Instruction and Intervention, by Nickola Wolf Nelson, Christine M. Bahr, and Adelia M. Van Meter
Copyright © 2004 Paul H. Brookes Publishing Co., Inc. All rights reserved.

Peer Conferencing

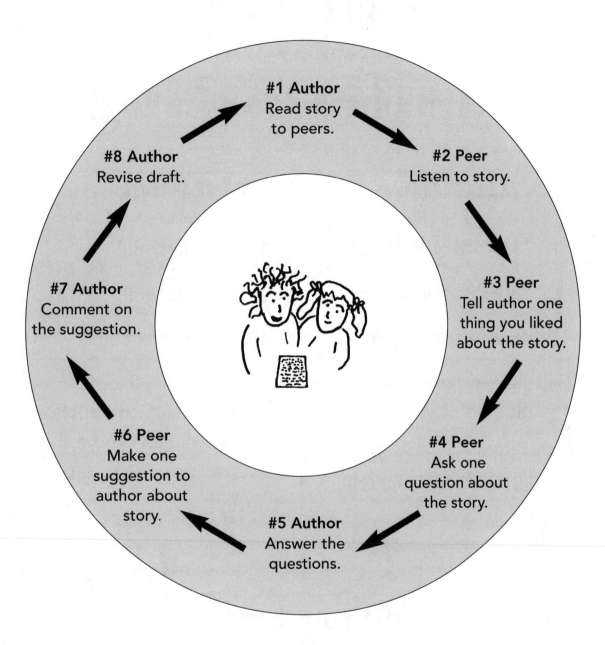

- **#1 Author** Read story to peers.
- **#2 Peer** Listen to story.
- **#3 Peer** Tell author one thing you liked about the story.
- **#4 Peer** Ask one question about the story.
- **#5 Author** Answer the questions.
- **#6 Peer** Make one suggestion to author about story.
- **#7 Author** Comment on the suggestion.
- **#8 Author** Revise draft.

The Writing Lab Approach to Language Instruction and Intervention, by Nickola Wolf Nelson, Christine M. Bahr, and Adelia M. Van Meter
Copyright © 2004 Paul H. Brookes Publishing Co., Inc. All rights reserved.

Partner Conferencing

Author

1. "My story is about . . ."

2. Read story to partner

3. Read story again!

4. Listen to what partner has to say.

5. Begin to make your story even better!!!

Listener

1. Just listen!!!

2. Just listen!!!

3. Listen and think!

4. Tell what I liked and what the author could improve on.

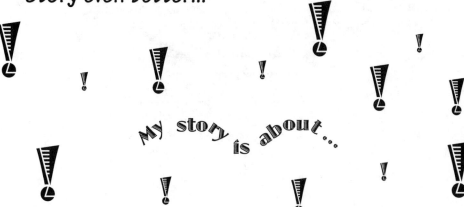

My story is about...

The Writing Lab Approach to Language Instruction and Intervention, by Nickola Wolf Nelson, Christine M. Bahr, and Adelia M. Van Meter
Copyright © 2004 Paul H. Brookes Publishing Co., Inc. All rights reserved.

Author Groups

During Author Group meeting time, everyone takes a turn being the Author. Other group members are Editors.

 ## The Author

1. Tells about the topic

2. Reads the article or explains the notes

3. Takes note of listeners' ideas and suggestions

4. Revises the article or expands the notes after the group meeting

 ## The Editors

1. Listen to the author

2. Share ideas about the topic

3. Share ideas about resources

4. Share ideas about organization

5. Write, "Something I really like about your article is…"

6. Write, "You could try…"

The Writing Lab Approach to Language Instruction and Intervention, by Nickola Wolf Nelson, Christine M. Bahr, and Adelia M. Van Meter
Copyright © 2004 Paul H. Brookes Publishing Co., Inc. All rights reserved.

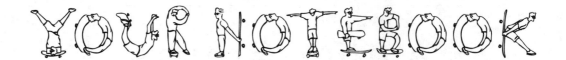

Section

1. My reminders

2. Minilessons

3. Planning and research

4. Drafts

5. Daily log

6. Keyboarding

Where does this go?

Write where you think each item should go in your notebook.

- Instructions for making a cover sheet
- This paper
- Paper about encourage/discourage
- Rights and responsibilities
- Notes from what you have read
- The title of a book you want to read
- Extra paper
- Your first draft of a paper
- A "web" of ideas
- The second draft of a paper

The Writing Lab Approach to Language Instruction and Intervention, by Nickola Wolf Nelson, Christine M. Bahr, and Adelia M. Van Meter
Copyright © 2004 Paul H. Brookes Publishing Co., Inc. All rights reserved.

Planning a Story

Setting	Where?
	
	When?
	
	Who?
	
	    Main characters:
	
	    Other characters:

Problem	What happened to make the story interesting?
Action	What did the main character decide to do to try to fix the problem?
Outcome	How did the plan work?
Ending	How does the story end?

The Writing Lab Approach to Language Instruction and Intervention, by Nickola Wolf Nelson, Christine M. Bahr, and Adelia M. Van Meter
Copyright © 2004 Paul H. Brookes Publishing Co., Inc. All rights reserved.

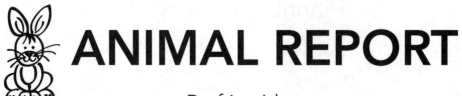

ANIMAL REPORT

Drafting Ideas

Introduction: At the beginning of a report, tell readers what you are writing about.

- Grab their attention.

- Tell them something interesting.

- Use exciting words.

Paragraphs: A paragraph groups related ideas together.

- Paragraphs have sentences about the same main idea.

- You can write a paragraph about each section on your planning form (example: habitat, food, survival adaptations).

- Start each paragraph with a topic sentence (tell the reader what your paragraph is about).

- Report main facts and descriptions.

- Use complete sentences (remember capital letters and periods).

Conclusion: At the end of your report, tell readers what you want them to remember about your animal.

The Writing Lab Approach to Language Instruction and Intervention, by Nickola Wolf Nelson, Christine M. Bahr, and Adelia M. Van Meter
Copyright © 2004 Paul H. Brookes Publishing Co., Inc. All rights reserved.

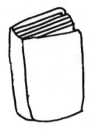

Notetaking

1. SKIM the material to make sure it is something you can use.

   • Does it give me information about my topic?

   • Does it discuss the specific things I want to know and write about?

2. Read the information to make sure that you UNDERSTAND it.

   • If you don't understand what you are reading, ask a friend, a teacher, or a parent to read and talk it over with you.

   • Ask yourself, "What is important?"

3. Read a PARAGRAPH OR TWO, then stop.

4. CLOSE the book or magazine, and cover the computer screen. Record what you learned in your OWN WORDS.

   • Paper and pencil

   • Notecards

   • Computer

5. Don't waste time writing a whole sentence. Write down a FEW WORDS or a PICTURE to remind you of YOUR IDEAS.

6. When you are done, REREAD your notes.

   • Do I have enough information?

   • What do I need to know more about?

   • Can I understand my notes?

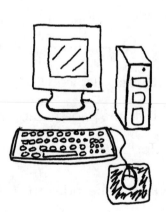

7. Organize your notes and ideas.

   • Map

   • Outline

   • You may not use ALL of your information!

The Writing Lab Approach to Language Instruction and Intervention, by Nickola Wolf Nelson, Christine M. Bahr, and Adelia M. Van Meter
Copyright © 2004 Paul H. Brookes Publishing Co., Inc. All rights reserved.

Parts of a Book Can
Help You Find Information

TABLE OF CONTENTS

Where is it, and what information does it provide?

- Located in the front of the book

- May list units, chapters, and sections within chapters

- Lists page numbers of units and chapters

- Shows how the book is organized

I could use the table of contents to answer the following questions:

- What are the main topics in this book?

- What order are these topics in?

- What are the units in this book?

- What are the chapters in each unit?

- What are the sections in each chapter?

INDEX

Where is it, and what information does it provide?

- Located in the back of the book

- Gives a detailed list of topics in the book

- Lists the page numbers for each topic

- Topics are organized alphabetically

I could use the index to answer the following questions:

- Is this topic mentioned anywhere in this book?

- On what pages is there information about this topic?

The Writing Lab Approach to Language Instruction and Intervention, by Nickola Wolf Nelson, Christine M. Bahr, and Adelia M. Van Meter
Copyright © 2004 Paul H. Brookes Publishing Co., Inc. All rights reserved.

Mystery

What's the mystery?

_____

_____

_____

Who are the detectives?

_____

_____

Who did it?

_____

Where did it happen?

_____

How did they do it?

_____

_____

_____

How do the detectives solve the case?

_____

_____

_____

What are the clues?

_____   _____

_____   _____

_____   _____

The Writing Lab Approach to Language Instruction and Intervention, by Nickola Wolf Nelson, Christine M. Bahr, and Adelia M. Van Meter
Copyright © 2004 Paul H. Brookes Publishing Co., Inc. All rights reserved.

COLOR POEM

1. CHOOSE A COLOR TO WRITE A POEM ABOUT.

2. DESCRIBE THE COLOR USING YOUR FIVE SENSES.

- LOOKS

- SMELLS

- TASTES

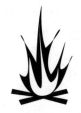

- FEELS

- SOUNDS

   (USE ADJECTIVES!)

RED

RED IS A HOT CANDY
THAT BURNS YOUR MOUTH.
RED IS A BRICK IN A BUILDING.
RED IS THE CRACKLING
OF A FIRE IN THE WINTER.
RED IS THE APPLE PIE
BAKING IN THE KITCHEN.
RED IS THE WARM SUN
ON YOUR BACK.

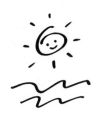

The Writing Lab Approach to Language Instruction and Intervention, by Nickola Wolf Nelson, Christine M. Bahr, and Adelia M. Van Meter
Copyright © 2004 Paul H. Brookes Publishing Co., Inc. All rights reserved.

Spelling Checker

1. Finish typing your work.

2. Press TOOLS.

3. Press Spell CHECK.

4. Look at the yellow word. Press SUGGEST WORD.

5. Look in the white box, and find the right word.

6. Click the right word.

7. Press CHANGE WORD.

8. If your word is right and the computer doesn't know it (such as your name), press SKIP WORD.

The Writing Lab Approach to Language Instruction and Intervention, by Nickola Wolf Nelson, Christine M. Bahr, and Adelia M. Van Meter
Copyright © 2004 Paul H. Brookes Publishing Co., Inc. All rights reserved.

ILLUSTRATION

DID I REMEMBER TO...

☐ **MATCH MY PICTURE WITH MY STORY?**

☐ **USE THE WHOLE PAGE FOR MY ILLUSTRATIONS?**

☐ **INCLUDE THE PARTS OF MY STORY IN MY ILLUSTRATION?**

- **SETTING**
- **CHARACTERS**
- **EVENTS**

The Writing Lab Approach to Language Instruction and Intervention, by Nickola Wolf Nelson, Christine M. Bahr, and Adelia M. Van Meter
Copyright © 2004 Paul H. Brookes Publishing Co., Inc. All rights reserved.

Student Self-Evaluation

About my story	First story	Second story
	Number of sentences: Number of words:	Number of sentences: Number of words:
Setting	Where? When? Who? Main Characters: Others:	Where? When? Who? Main Characters: Others:
What was the problem?		
How was it solved? How did it end?		
Special words and facts that made my story interesting:		

The Writing Lab Approach to Language Instruction and Intervention, by Nickola Wolf Nelson, Christine M. Bahr, and Adelia M. Van Meter
Copyright © 2004 Paul H. Brookes Publishing Co., Inc. All rights reserved.

Retired words*	New and improved words
Nice	Gentle
Good	Satisfying
Happy	Thrilled
Fun	Exciting
Pretty	Beautiful
Said	Yelled

*Words that get used too much. They should be "retired" or replaced with new and improved words. Some examples are given here, and more possibilities can be added.

The Writing Lab Approach to Language Instruction and Intervention, by Nickola Wolf Nelson, Christine M. Bahr, and Adelia M. Van Meter
Copyright © 2004 Paul H. Brookes Publishing Co., Inc. All rights reserved.

Spelling Strategies
Hard Words

Say – Listen – Feel – Check

1 Say the word in broken syllables.

2. Listen to the first syllable.

   • Is this a chunk I know?

   • If so, write it.

3. If not, say the sounds in the syllable slowly.

   • Listen to each sound.

   • Feel each sound in your mouth.

   • Write a letter for each sound.

   • Read what you wrote. Check if it matches.

4. Say the word in syllables again.

5. Listen to the next syllable.

   • Is this a chunk I know?

   • If so, write it.

6. If not, *Say – Listen – Feel – Check*

   Keep doing this until the word looks like it sounds!

The Writing Lab Approach to Language Instruction and Intervention, by Nickola Wolf Nelson, Christine M. Bahr, and Adelia M. Van Meter
Copyright © 2004 Paul H. Brookes Publishing Co., Inc. All rights reserved.

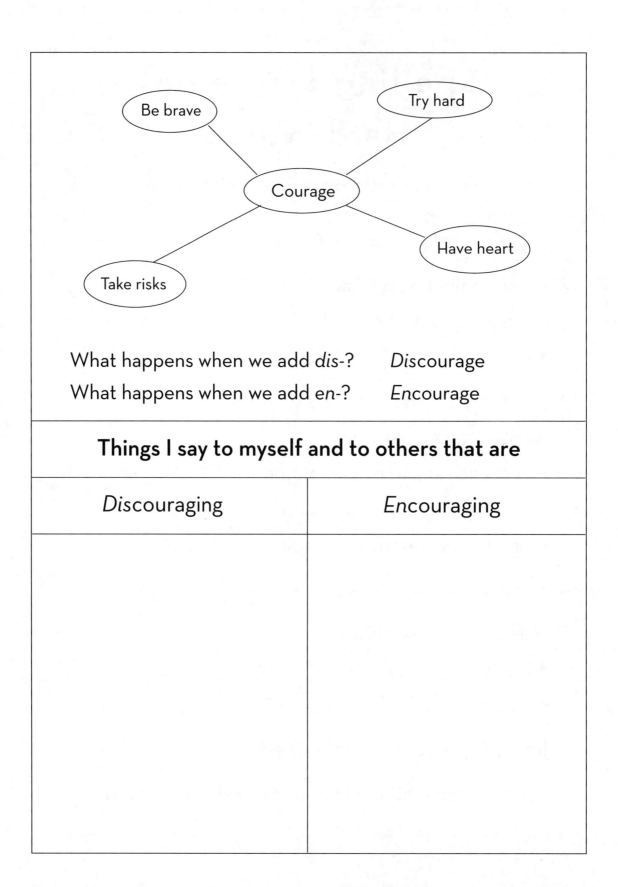

What happens when we add *dis*-?   *Discourage*

What happens when we add *en*-?   *Encourage*

Things I say to myself and to others that are

Discouraging	*Encouraging*

The Writing Lab Approach to Language Instruction and Intervention, by Nickola Wolf Nelson, Christine M. Bahr, and Adelia M. Van Meter
Copyright © 2004 Paul H. Brookes Publishing Co., Inc. All rights reserved.

Oral Presentations

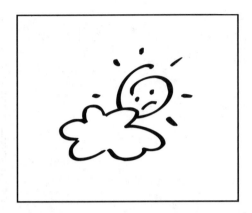

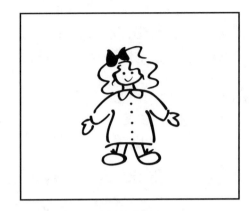

1. Don't hide your face while you are talking!

2. Try to stand up straight, show us your face, and look at the audience!

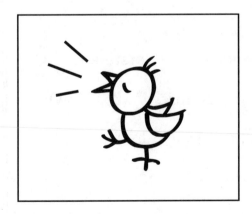

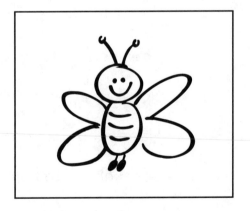

3. Use your public voice!

4. Smile and have fun!

The Writing Lab Approach to Language Instruction and Intervention, by Nickola Wolf Nelson, Christine M. Bahr, and Adelia M. Van Meter
Copyright © 2004 Paul H. Brookes Publishing Co., Inc. All rights reserved.

Giving Oral Presentations

What is an oral presentation?

An oral presentation is when one person speaks in front of a small or large group of people in order to share information.

Why would someone give an oral presentation?

- To give a report of what he or she learned.

- To share a story or paper he or she wrote.

- To tell others about something new.

- To share information.

What things should the speaker do to help the listeners hear and understand the message?

- Make eye contact with people in the audience.

- Speak loud enough so the audience can hear.

- Speak clearly so the audience can understand.

- Speak at an easy speed (not too fast, not too slow).

- Have good posture (stand up straight, look proud).

What can a speaker use to help the listeners?

- Handouts

- Overheads

- Props (pictures, graphs, models)

The Writing Lab Approach to Language Instruction and Intervention, by Nickola Wolf Nelson, Christine M. Bahr, and Adelia M. Van Meter
Copyright © 2004 Paul H. Brookes Publishing Co., Inc. All rights reserved.

Scaffolding, Self-Regulation, and Author Profiles

5

THE BASICS OF SCAFFOLDING

The primary instructional technique of the writing lab approach is scaffolding. Most pediatric SLPs and general and special education teachers are familiar with the term, *scaffolding,* but our experience has been that few are confident about their ability to do it well. Scaffolding, in its literal sense, is an adjustable support used by a construction worker to reach a level higher than otherwise would be possible. Scaffolding as an instructional strategy also provides constructive adjustable support for individual learners. When scaffolding, instructors respond to students' needs to focus selectively on informational cues in integrated learning experiences, to construct new meanings, and to develop self-regulatory strategies for future learning. The outcome is that learners reach higher levels than would be possible without support. Ultimately, the goal is to create successful and independent learners.

The metaphor of scaffolding applied to language development is generally attributed to Jerome Bruner (1975, 1977). Bruner elaborated a theoretical perspective that had been introduced earlier by Russian psychologist Vygotsky (1978). Vygotsky explained the social origins of self-control and the development of the mind as phenomena in which mediation by a more mature learner contributes to cognitive-linguistic development by a less mature learner. Bruner applied this theory to the support parents give to their toddlers in the "games" of early language acquisition and cognitive development. Bruner noted that at first mothers take responsibility for the entire interaction script, but over time, variation in the games is critical to lead the child to independence. In extending the concepts to school-age populations, Cazden (1988) described scaffolding in a way that applies equally to the writing lab approach:

> The adult so structures the game that the child can be a successful participant from the beginning; then, as the child's competence grows, the game changes so that there is always

something new to be learned and tried out, including taking over what had been the adult's role . . . this is a very special kind of scaffold—one that self-destructs gradually as the need lessens and the child's competence grows. (p. 104)

Silliman and Wilkinson (1994) differentiated scaffolding that occurs from developmental and intervention perspectives. From a developmental perspective, they described supportive scaffolds as "the process by which control is gradually transferred from the adult to the child for task planning, strategy selection, monitoring of effectiveness, and the evaluation of task outcomes" (p. 38). From an intervention perspective, they described scaffolds as "the discourse mechanism by which clinicians demonstrate their primary role as a working model for the elaboration of students' thinking" (p. 38). In the writing lab approach, the two roles merge in transdisciplinary teams who collaborate in the intentional processes of helping students gain language and literacy skills and employ them independently.

Scaffolding supports are temporary. Schuler and Wolfberg indicated that the art in scaffolding "lies in the construction and intentional dismantling of flexible, transparent, and child-centered structures that provide children not only with an anticipatory set but also with enough room for initiation" (2000, p. 263). Scaffolds may be nonverbal, but most are built through social-dialogic transactions (Gaffney & Anderson, 1991; Pressley & Wharton-McDonald, 1997). Through transactional dialogues, students construct problem-solving strategies they can apply more broadly. When children absorb the dialogic elements of scaffolds into their private speech, they gain access to the invaluable tool of self-talk to control their planning and actions (Diaz & Berk, 1992). In this way, students learn not only specific tasks but also how to learn.

Applebee and Langer (1983) listed five features to strive for when scaffolding: 1) intentionality, 2) appropriateness, 3) structure, 4) collaboration, and 5) internalization. These criteria are consistent with our recommendations:

- Start by being student centered.

- Build a scaffold.

- Don't forget to take it down.

Scaffolding that leaves a learner dependent on a particular instructor is not really scaffolding at all. Rather, effective scaffolds enable students to reach higher levels of competence, stay there independently, and benefit from even higher-level scaffolds to reach beyond. In Section II, we suggest that some of the features of children's writing software tools can serve as scaffolds for supporting students in their self-regulated learning. In Chapter 4, we describe how author notebooks, word walls, and similar environmental supports can support students to become increasingly independent. None of this is likely to occur, however, unless it is preceded by deliberate, intentional transactions in which more mature learners use discourse and other focusing techniques to show less mature learners how to use tools effectively to scaffold themselves.

Scaffolding, Executive Functions, and Self-Regulation

Scaffolding permits instructors to target and achieve individualized objectives in partnership with students. The writing lab culture conveys a message that teachers and students are in this together, side by side and shoulder to shoulder (Tattershall, 2002).

Scaffolding to learn independent strategies is not effective until learners can internalize the questions and other techniques of their mentors. Brown, Campione, and Day (1981) described effective strategy instruction as involving three aspects: 1) training in specific strategic skills; 2) metacognitive training in the self-regulation of those strategies; and 3) instruction in skills for implementing, monitoring, maintaining, and generalizing the strategies.

Executive functions are defined as the metacognitive "decision-making and planning processes that are invoked at the outset of a task and in the face of a novel challenge" (Singer & Bashir, 1999b, p. 266). These are the control processes that involve attention, working memory, and instructions to self. Executive functions are applicable across multiple contexts and content (Denckla, 1994). They apply to general problem solving and learning. Their existence implies that an individual has benefited from and internalized prior scaffolding.

Berninger (2000) reviewed literature on the typical development of executive functions and noted that although elements of self-regulation can be detected during early childhood, executive functions require considerable scaffolding from adults until early adolescence. Executive functions are at risk for failing to develop in the presence of disabilities, particularly such developmental conditions as attention-deficit/hyperactivity disorder and such acquired conditions as traumatic brain injury. Ylvisaker and DeBonis (2000) listed problematic executive functions as affecting

- Awareness of one's strengths and limitations relative to specific task difficulty

- Ability to set reasonable goals and to plan and organize actions to achieve them

- Ability to initiate acts for achieving goals and inhibit acts that are incompatible with goals

- Ability to revise plans flexibly and to solve problems strategically when encountering difficulty or failure (i.e., to profit from feedback efficiently)

Interventions for individuals with disabilities should be designed to promote executive control and self-regulatory abilities but too often, therapeutic practices usurp them instead. Ylvisaker and DeBonis cautioned against "anti-executive function routines," in which "professionals act as prosthetic frontal lobes" by assessing students, setting goals for them, creating instructional or treatment plans, monitoring and evaluating progress, and implementing strategic alternatives to adjust when insufficient progress is noted (2000, p. 43). The problem with all of these activities is that they remove the ownership from individuals who need to assume greater control and responsibility for their own growth and change. Writing lab contexts can be used to turn this process around. That is, students can be involved in evaluating their own writing, setting goals for themselves, monitoring progress, and deciding what they want to work on next.

Self-regulation is the ability to use preestablished routines to scaffold oneself through new and more difficult problems. Some researchers equate executive functions and self-regulation; others differentiate them (Singer & Bashir, 1999b). Our sense is that the term *self-regulation* may be viewed as a special aspect of executive functioning. It involves learning to use one's inner voice to mediate problem solving and to regulate choices and behavior (Nelson, 1995).

This more specific meaning is consistent with intervention literature in which the self-regulated strategy development (SRSD) instructional model is given a particular meaning. The SRSD model is one that is supported by a number of research studies conducted in a variety of writing process contexts by Graham and Harris and their colleagues (see Graham, Harris, & Troia, 2000, for a review). Most of these studies were conducted with fourth- through eighth-grade students with learning disabilities. The SRSD model also has been found to be effective in inclusive environments (Danoff, Harris, & Graham, 1993).

The general framework for SRSD training involves six steps. Instructors 1) develop the student's background knowledge about the strategy to be learned; 2) use an initial conference with the student to establish the significance of the strategy and to set personal goals for learning it; 3) model the strategy for the student; 4) provide a mnemonic to help the student memorize the strategy (although paraphrasing is allowed as long as meaning is maintained); 5) provide collaborative practice opportunities; and 6) provide independent practice opportunities and teach the student to use new self-talk supports.

The following are examples of mnemonic acronyms Graham, Harris, and Troia developed for specific written language genres (except where noted, these were summarized by Graham, Harris, & Troia, 2000; Harris & Graham, 1996):

- POWER was the acronym Englert (1992) developed to support students learning stages of the writing process: *plan, organize, write, edit, rewrite, and revise.*

- W-W-W, 2 Whats, 2 Hows is a mnemonic device for reminding students to include in their stories answers to the following questions: *Who* is the main character, and who else is in your story? *When* does the story take place? *Where* does the story take place? *What* does the main character do or want to do? (and what do the other characters do?) *What* happens when the main character does or tries to do it? (and what happens to the other characters?) *How* does the story end? *How* do the characters feel?

- SPACE is an acronym for reminding students to write stories with *setting, purpose, actions, conclusion, emotions.*

- TREE is an acronym for reminding students to write opinion essays in which they develop a *topic* sentence or premise, generate *reasons* to support their topic sentence, *examine* each reason to see if it makes sense, and develop an *ending.*

- STOP–DARE is an acronym for reminding students to write argumentative essays in which they *suspend* judgment to brainstorm ideas for each side before taking a position, *take* a side, *organize* their ideas into an outline, and *plan* more as they write. The plan step includes reminders to *develop* a topic sentence, *add* supporting ideas, *reject* possible arguments for the other side, and *end* with a conclusion.

Structured sequences like these are helpful in outlining the organizational requirements of particular curricular tasks, serving as an important first step in scaffolding. The sequences can be introduced in minilessons, with planning sheets based on the acronyms to remind students of primary genre traits or writing processes. Alternatively, planning sequences can be built into "frozen text" computer software templates, in which the instructor embeds prompting text that students cannot alter, to support planning and organizing (see Chapter 7).

We are cautious, however, about requiring students to memorize mnemonic acronyms. Memorizing can carry unnecessarily high learning costs. We encourage teaching students strategies for asking themselves whether their communicative goals are being met. Such awareness can lead logically to the construction of dynamic self-regulation strategies that make sense in the context because they achieve desired communicative functions. These strategies are controlled internally and contribute to broader executive functioning. They do not have to be memorized because they can be reconstructed later in similar circumstances to serve similar purposes. Some children and educators, however, benefit from using mnemonic acronyms to aid recall.

Englert and Palincsar contrasted how reading and writing are represented in scaffolded learning, "as a means of communication" with how reading and writing are presented in traditional teaching, "as the mastery of a sequence of mechanical skills" (1991, p. 226). Teachers scaffold writing processes when they think out loud strategically but without rigid scripting (Englert et al., 1991). Pressley and Wharton-McDonald also distinguished scaffolding in the form of "transactional strategy instruction" when they noted that "there are no restrictions upon the order of strategies execution and fewer restrictions about which students can participate and when they may do so" (1997, pp. 457–458). In their later work, Graham et. al. (2000) emphasized a need for greater flexibility as well.

Scaffolding and Dynamic Assessment

Flexible and dynamic teaching does not mean that instructors should not plan ahead. "An important part of the teaching equation is teachers' moment-to-moment responsiveness to their students, and their abilities to make bridges between what their students know and need to know" (Englert & Palincsar, 1991, p. 228). Effective scaffolding requires preplanned, ongoing, and immediate analyses of students' current states of knowing, based on students' actions and responses to tasks, as well as to the varied dynamic assessment techniques instructors employ during scaffolding.

Scaffolding and dynamic assessment are not the same, but they are integrally related. Dynamic assessment uses a pretest–intervention–posttest format to assess a student's learning potential (Lidz & Pena, 1996; Palincsar, Brown, & Campione, 1994). We might call this assess–scaffold–reassess. That is, instructors use scaffolding strategically during dynamic assessment to vary intervention and test hypotheses about the student's learning capabilities. Responses to scaffolding can yield important diagnostic information that supports further intervention.

Feuerstein (1979) generally is credited with introducing dynamic assessment as part of his Learning Potential Acquisition Device (LPAD). LPAD was designed to assess children whose IQ scores underestimated their intelligence or potential to learn. Although LPAD has been criticized for using tasks that bear little resemblance to school-like activities, it provided an early model for dynamic assessment that can be adapted easily to relevant curricular contexts (Nelson & Van Meter, 2002; Palincsar et al., 1994).

In our opinion, Feuerstein also provided one of the best descriptions of scaffolding as "framing, selecting, focusing, and feeding back environmental experiences" to produce in the child "appropriate learning sets and habits" (1979, p. 179). We use those descriptors to outline scaffolding techniques in the following section. These are the techniques that instructors can employ to assist students to pay attention to relevant cues they might otherwise miss, to discover new connections, and to reach higher levels of independent learning.

The contributions of dynamic assessment to this process are that, in order to know what cues to frame, instructors must experiment with varied scaffolding techniques. They start by analyzing language and learning skills mature learners would bring to targeted tasks. Then, they analyze what a less mature learner would do when attempting those same tasks (Nelson & Van Meter, 2002). The strategic application and evaluation of scaffolding techniques is what constitutes the dynamic part of cyclical assessment and intervention processes.

Scaffolding Directness and Cultural Diversity

Scaffolding language is communicative and designed to leave the ownership for change in the hands of the learner. Like any act of communication, it should be suited pragmatically to the needs of a particular audience. In some cases, scaffolding that is intended to foster ownership is too indirect for learners to benefit. Students with disabilities, in particular, need input and feedback that is clear and explicit (Graham & Harris, 1994, 1997).

Communicative directness has cultural variants (Delpit, 1995). Knowing something about the communicative style of diverse populations helps scaffold students of different cultural backgrounds. Native American students, for example, may have difficulty accepting attention on their work before they are ready to share it (Robinson-Zanartu, 1996). Scaffolding for them may require patience and a style that is more indirect. Some African American students may respond better to scaffolding that is more direct (e.g., "Put those books back, please," instead of "Those books need to be reshelved").

Instructors who use dynamic assessment techniques to check their students' understanding by scaffolding strategically and monitoring change are in a position to modify the directness and degree of support in their scaffolds as they implement them. Scaffolding proceeds in recursive cycles of more- to less-direct instructional discourse. Instructors can learn to provide scaffolds that are sensitive to students' cultural experiences and expectations, as well as to their individual differences.

SCAFFOLDING TECHNIQUES

Scaffolding and mediation frequently are mentioned in the literature of general education, special education, and language intervention. Skill at scaffolding, however, is difficult to acquire just from reading about it. Skillful scaffolding requires practice. Scaffolding also can be viewed as an art. Indeed, masterful scaffolding does seem artful in the hands of expert teachers and therapists. Scaffolding follows basic principles and structures, however, and these can be learned. With practice and reflection, instructors can improve their skills.

To be successful, scaffolding instructors must first have a thorough understanding of the developmental phenomena they are trying to help students learn. Writing lab contexts allow instructors to focus balanced attention on three mutually facilitative developmental systems:

1. Social-emotional security, without which, it is difficult for a child to learn at all (Greenspan, 1997)

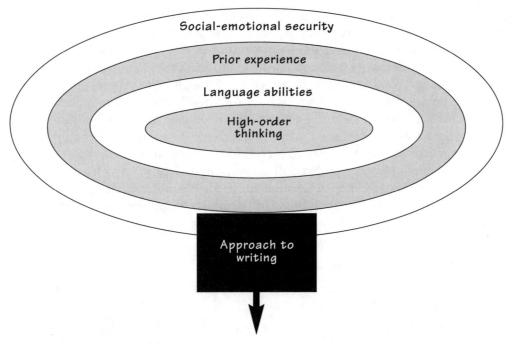

Figure 5.1.   Model of traits successful authors bring to the task.

2.   Language ability, both spoken and written (see Chapter 2)

3.   Higher order thinking skills, with executive functions including self-regulation

As illustrated in Figure 5.1, a successful approach to writing requires interactions of these systems with prior experience and current knowledge states. Successful scaffolders rely on the balance principle to help them decide what to address and what to leave alone at any point in time.

The primary tool of scaffolding is the *strategic question.* It contrasts with questions in the predictable exchanges of teacher talk, which are sometimes characterized with the acronym IRE. It stands for the pattern in which a teacher *initiates* with a test-like, known-answer question; a student *responds*; and the teacher *evaluates* the response as correct or not, usually based on whether it matches what the teacher had in mind (Cazden, 1988). Clinicians also use IRE discourse in therapeutic exchanges. Questions in IRE discourse have a place in education and therapy to check comprehension or to activate existing knowledge, but they are not scaffolds.

In contrast, the questions of scaffolding are designed to guide students to attend to cues that previously were undetected in order to make cognitive, linguistic, and social connections to support further learning. The goal is to help students stretch their understanding and use of language by creating a link between the observed response (what students are doing now) and the expected response (what they must do to reach the next higher level of maturity) (Nelson & Van Meter, 2002).[1]

---

[1]The terminology of *observed response* and *expected response* was introduced by Goodman (1969) to differentiate a miscue a student makes while reading a word aloud (the observed response) in contrast to the word printed on the page (the expected response). Nelson and Van Meter (2002) expanded the meaning to represent other mismatches between what a curricular task requires (the expected response) and what a student does in attempting the task (the observed response).

Scaffolding discourse focuses students on missed cues to make them more concrete and accessible. It is structured more as communication than correction. For example, an instructor might comment to a student, "The computer doesn't know where to stop when it reads your story." The idea is to encourage self-questioning, asking only if necessary, "What could you do to tell it?" Later, a more general question might be used, such as, "What should you ask yourself here?" Success can be celebrated when students begin to self-monitor, generate their own questions, and initiate changes independently. For example, a student might move the cursor on a computer screen to insert periods as end punctuation, even before a question is posed, indicating the onset of self-regulation strategies that will sustain the student in other learning.

Instructors start with background knowledge about language systems (as in Chapter 2) to analyze the cognitive-linguistic demands of specific tasks. They follow with dynamic assessment techniques to analyze how a student deals with those demands. The steps of the procedure are

1. Observe the student attempting the task independently.

2. Form hypotheses about critical cues and skills the student may or may not be using.

3. Test the hypotheses by framing, focusing, or feeding back selected cues to see what helps.

4. Decide whether to press an issue, be patient and wait, or switch to other needs that may be more amenable to scaffolding.

5. Pull back, and observe whether the student is able to apply new learning with a growing degree of independence.

The goal is to achieve a balance between supports that are the least intrusive but the most challenging for a particular student at a particular point in time. The dynamic decision-making and patience principles are required particularly when a student is simply not ready or willing to work on preestablished targets. The scaffolding approach then is to find some other aspect of the writing process, a target at a different language-level, or another aspect of communication to which the student is open and ready to learn (an example is provided in Box 5.2 later in this chapter).

Peers can scaffold, too, although it may take instructional scaffolding to show them how. For example, they may need to be reminded that they should help their peers but not do their peers' work for them. Peers are particularly effective in the role of authentic audience. A community of writers shares responsibility for supporting each others' efforts to achieve authentic, effective, literary purposes, such as to inform, entertain, or enlighten. The magic of the writing lab occurs when students begin to view themselves as authors who want to improve their writing for the sake of communicating better with their peers, not just to meet teachers' expectations.

A summary of general suggestions for scaffolding in the writing lab includes

- Intentionally target objectives while recognizing teachable moments.

- Support students to see what they do know before attempting to bridge to the next higher level.

- Using the scaffolding "sandwich" by providing positive comments specific to targeted features, scaffolding a child to higher levels of competence, then leaving the interaction with another positive comment (e.g., "I love this character. You make him sound so interesting by describing how he looks. I wonder what he is thinking." Pause. "Do you have some ideas about that?" Wait, listen, and affirm. "I can't wait to see what you write next.").

- Take the role of authentic audience to help students see their work from another's point of view.

- Provide feedback about syntactic and semantic anomalies by "tripping" over errors.

- Model thinking aloud and self-talk, such as "I wonder . . . "; "What if . . . "; and "Wait, let me think."

- Scaffold peer-to-peer discourse so students can improve at giving and receiving constructive feedback from their peers.

- Teach new vocabulary to aid understanding and organization.

- Calibrate scaffolding language to curricular, teachers', and students' language, using those words to support inner dialogues likely to transfer across contexts.

- Provide written scaffolds and other environmental supports, and teach students to return to them independently.

- Take advantage of computer software features as scaffolds.

These are just a few general recommendations for scaffolding in writing lab contexts. Scaffolding is most effective when it is customized for individuals and situations. In the sections of this chapter that follow, we suggest techniques for scaffolding students with differing views of themselves as authors. In Chapter 6, we describe techniques for scaffolding students to gain skill for achieving specific language targets. No single formula or strategic mnemonic device works for all students. Teachers need reflective practice in order to understand what students are thinking and experiencing and also to envision how to scaffold students to the next higher step. Scaffolding does improve with practice. To work on scaffolding, along with our graduate students, we have kept reflective journals on our scaffolding attempts and their effects. Many of the examples in this book have been drawn from the data in those journals.

The Framing Scaffold

The framing scaffold is used to highlight aspects of the learning or writing problem needing the student's attention. For example, framing techniques might involve teaching students to ask such questions as "What am I trying to do here?" or "What is it I need to know?" Minilessons can be used to introduce concepts of goal setting and self-talk and to provide initial practice. Then, individual scaffolding at a student's desk or computer station can be used to establish independent use of the self-questioning strategy. Teacher conferences, in which students indicate the stage of the writing process on which they are working, also can be built into the writing lab's daily structure. This procedure frames the features of the writing process and helps students integrate them into self-sustaining routines.

Within writing lab sessions, a good framing technique is to direct students to open their author notebooks to a page on which their IEP objectives are written in kid-friendly language. Before starting to work, students might be asked in a group or individually to think about the stage of the writing process they are working on and look at their personal goals. Which of those can they work on today? If a student is working on planning and organizing, for example, and is gathering information for an expository article, a desired response might be "Read about my topic and put the ideas down in my own words."

In the context of author groups, instructors might frame social interaction issues by rehearsing students chosen to be author group leaders of the day, which might consist of such questions as "Are you ready to lead the author group today?" and "Let's think about what you might ask first."

At the computer, when students seem to be moving the mouse around and clicking randomly on the screen, the instructor might ask, "What is your goal here? What are you trying to do?" Helping students articulate immediate purpose goals for themselves gets them set to follow through on a series of steps to achieve those purposes. This is the essence of the framing scaffold. When students begin to ask themselves goal-directed questions such as "What should I do next?," instructors can take it as a sign that the scaffolding has worked.

The Focusing Scaffold

Once a problem has been framed, educators can focus students on salient features to help them take the first (or next) step toward solving it. Both instructors and computer software can provide scaffolds to focus students on discriminative features of problems. The focusing scaffold involves tuning students' sensory perceptions to consider strategically informative pieces of data, while ignoring uninformative or extraneous data.

When a student's writing does not make sense, for example, focusing might involve selecting a bit of text (e.g., pointing to the text, using the mouse to highlight the selection on the computer screen); then conveying interest in, but confusion about, the meaning. Or, if a student has typed a sentence with anomalous syntax, the instructor might frame the sentence by highlighting it and then having the speech synthesis feature of the software program read it back. Another example would be to focus a student on phonological sequence for a word that is misspelled by asking the student to say the word slowly out loud and listen to its final sound. Then, the instructor might say, "Let's look to see if all of those sounds are in your spelling."

Some writing software programs include revising and editing features that highlight problem areas for an author's attention (see Chapter 9). Once students have the language and self-regulation abilities to use such features, they can achieve greater independence. Isolating relevant data requires knowing about language. Simply knowing how to activate a spelling or grammar checking feature is not enough. Linguistic judgment is needed to select among the choices that are presented.

The Feedback Scaffold

Feedback scaffolds are aligned closely with focusing. Strategic feedback, in fact, can be used to help students focus on critical missing information. One way to do this is to read back what a student wrote and to "trip" over any errors, showing befuddlement and confusion over aspects of the student's language that do not make sense. We sometimes refer to this as our "Columbo routine," in honor of the television detective. When students begin to internalize self-reflective strategies, they can use synthetic speech feedback features independently to notice problems they might not otherwise hear in their mind's ear.

Feedback scaffolds focused on aspects of writing *processes* provide cues aimed at helping students identify why a particular approach to a problem was not effective. For example, "Hmm, we tried that but it didn't work so well. How about if we try this?" Feedback scaffolds focused on aspects of written *products* provide cues aimed at helping the student ask such evaluative questions as "Did I get it right?" In some cases, application of the feedback scaffold requires heavy doses of the patience principle as well. We worked with one student who often said, "I know I could say that differently, but I like it this way." When possible, we recommend leaving such decisions to the author, even if the result is not immediately "correct" language. With ownership and additional feedback that comes directly from instructors and peers, we have found that such individualists eventually do respond to feedback. Over time, this student began to make choices to use more literary language on his own. He learned to make strategic improvements to his work in ways that allowed him to retain his unique voice. Individualism is part of what makes written language work so delightful.

The Guiding Scaffold

Students may need more direct guidance to construct new meanings and connections. Guiding scaffolds include modeling, telling, and giving the rationale for taking certain actions. Showing and telling constitute heavier scaffolding, but they sometimes are needed to get students started on the road to constructive learning.

Examples of guiding scaffolds aimed at writing processes, self-regulation, and social-interaction targets include the following:

- "Let me show you how to sit at the computer so that you don't get a backache."

- "Would you like me to show you how to use cut and paste to make your revisions?"

- "We are running out of time. You need to get some of these good ideas down on paper so you'll be ready for author chair."

- "Do you have some tools in your author notebook that might help you?" Pause. "How about your personal dictionary?"

- "I cannot allow you to say any more discouraging things to your neighbor."

- "Susan knows how to add borders. You could ask her."

Examples of guiding scaffolds aimed at language and literacy "discoveries" to improve students' written products include the following:

- "I love this character. In fact, I am trying to picture her. Could you help me see her better?"

- "I'll bet you can think of a more interesting word to fit here."

- "When something doesn't sound right to me, I ask myself, 'Is there another way to say this?'"

- "Take another look. I think you left something out of your sentence right here." Point to text.

Recursive and Dismantling Aspects of Scaffolding

Scaffolding is not considered successful until a student's new learning can stand on its own. As a part of a scaffolding cycle, dynamic assessment techniques are used to check for new learning at a later time. Instructors can simply observe the student as an on-looker and look for evidence of independent use of the targeted knowledge or skill. The instructor can comment or not depending on a student's individual style (e.g., "Look at you—rereading on your own to see if you need to revise. You really are an author").

In other cases, students need more explicit instruction before they can use self-regulatory strategies rather than relying on an instructor or peer. Depending on the maturity of students, we have described this step as transplanting questions. We might say, for example, "What would I usually ask you here? See, you can ask yourself that. We just transplanted that question from my brain to yours. That means you can do this by yourself."

Summary of Scaffolding Techniques

To summarize, knowing how to frame, focus, guide, and provide feedback regarding missing cues rests on background knowledge and dynamic assessment insights into language systems and writing processes. Effective scaffolders recognize interactions of language and literacy needs with social-emotional factors, cultural and educational experiences, world knowledge, and self-regulatory strategies.

In writing lab contexts, instructors select elements for more intensive scrutiny and help students to frame aspects of specific individualized problems. They then assist students to focus on previously missed cues identified with dynamic assessment. They hold students responsible for making use of feedback, drawing conclusions, and planning next steps. If necessary, they model desired behavior or otherwise guide students to construct new meanings. The cycle continues as effective scaffolders make sure that students apply the new knowledge and skill independently in similar contexts on another day. In this way, the instructional team ensures that learning is stabilized and students acquire the executive functions to support their growing independence.

SCAFFOLDING STUDENTS TO MORE MATURE AUTHOR PROFILES

Watching students at work can reveal important information about how they view themselves as learners and authors. As represented graphically in Figure 5.1, combinations of personal social-emotional tendencies, spoken and written language abilities, and prior knowledge and experience come together to prepare students to approach early writing experiences differently.

When writing processes are introduced, students approach them differently, depending on their prior experiences both with writing processes and with their personal histories as learners. The descriptions that follow portray author profiles we have observed in our work and scaffolding techniques we use to help students advance.

We caution readers not to treat profiles as stereotypes, but as guides for preparing students to get the most out of writing lab. Some students evolve through several profiles on the path to becoming competent and confident communicators. Although the sequence of profiles represents a continuum from less to more desirable, students start at different points and take different routes toward independent learning. Individual differences and personal traits never disappear but become integrated into the creative processes of a delightfully diverse community of authors.

Paper Wadder

The paper wadder, when asked to write, seems to convey, "I hate this," by wadding or otherwise destroying preliminary authoring attempts. Students with this profile also may refuse to work at all. Other characteristics include

- Having a history of failure

- Getting frustrated easily

- Displaying inadequate language and literacy skills (although not always)

- Conveying perfectionist tendencies

Students who wad and throw their papers need an appreciative audience, someone to focus on their ideas rather than their technical correctness. We urge caution, however, because such students may be particularly sensitive to adult compliments that seem insincere. Some put up barriers to fend off adult attention until they can feel successful in a new realm. Others use the delete key on their computers as a substitute for paper wadding, erasing an entire session of hard work with one keystroke, much to their teachers' dismay. Some have well-practiced acts for avoiding productivity or getting in trouble rather than working for any extended period on a project. These students may be skilled at triggering adults to issue authoritative commands or to set ultimatums. Prior experiences for such students often are full of red marks, low grades, incomplete assignments, and trips to the principal's office.

Before attempting to scaffold paper wadders, instructors first must try to understand the sources of students' frustration. Second, they should avoid being drawn into any well-practiced behavioral routines, which may have become games the student cannot help and the adult cannot win. If historical approaches have not worked, then it is time to try something new.

In mild cases, the novelty of working with computers to prepare unique and attractive products appreciated by peers may nudge students out of a paper-wadding phase. We suggest scheduling a publishing party and celebrating phase fairly soon after introducing the writing lab approach (see Chapters 1 and 4). Students with extroverted

---

Box 5.1. Scaffolding a Paper Wadder to Relinquish a Maladaptive Act

Jeremy's early writing lab attempts were frustrating for him. During the first probe, he wadded and threw paper. Jeremy was uncomfortable with his writing abilities. He did finally arrive at a topic about attending a football game that led him to produce a temporal sequence. One technique that helped Jeremy was to know that he was producing a rough draft. He was told that he was not expected to be able to spell all words correctly, and in fact, he should choose his words without worrying about spelling. If he was unsure of how to spell a word, he could indicate his uncertainty by putting "(sp?)" after it or circling it. Jeremy wrote,

> I went to a football Game (sp?) and I had a good time. I saw
> someone get hert (sp?). I ate (sp?) good. we won the Game (sp?)
> two time.

Although he was not entirely happy with this composition, Jeremy was able to leave his paper intact and turn it in as representative of his work.

---

tendencies may respond best to the authentic audience principle. They seek social attention from peers and adults and are motivated to improve their work so it will have the desired effect on their audience.

Extreme paper wadders present major challenges. Some particularly bright students, with or without LLDs, have perfectionist tendencies that lead them to become easily frustrated and to act out when things do not go as planned. Other students have issues with control that make them angry and unresponsive when teachers or parents try to get them to do something. They would rather go to the principal's office than to comply. Jeremy is a student who started out as a paper wadder then moved through a perfectionist stage on his way to becoming an individualist. Scaffolding for Jeremy involved helping him to understand his perfectionism in order to help him learn inner control and self-regulatory strategies. This approach is illustrated in Box 5.1.

Other recommendations for scaffolding students who are paper wadders, say they hate writing, or destroy their efforts include

1. Use strength areas (e.g., drawings, spoken dictation) to plan and draft.

2. Keep early projects simple and short, and use dynamic assessment to identify genres that appeal to the student.

3. Engage the student working at a computer as soon as possible, and teach formatting and revision features to produce interesting illustrations and presentation formats.

4. Support wobbly language skills by providing environmental supports (e.g., word walls) and heavier scaffolding (e.g., spelling as requested).

5. Provide opportunities for the student to take the author chair early, but do not insist that the student participate in this way.

6. Scaffold peers to share what they like about the student's work in author chair and other contexts.

7. Introduce the discouraging-encouraging minilesson (see Chapter 4).

8. Acknowledge the student's feelings of anger and frustration, and provide self-talk alternatives (e.g., Sometimes when I feel frustrated, I say to myself, "I'm getting angry, I just have to leave this part of the work alone until I feel better about it. For now, I will work on a different part")

9. Find specific elements that justify sincere positive audience feedback (e.g., "Your illustrations have the nicest sense of color and design; I can't wait to find out what happens next in your story")

Fragile Beginner

Fragile beginners seem to want to write, but they are scared. Their approach to the writing task seems to convey the message, "This is scary." Other characteristics associated with the fragile beginner profile are

- Having low self-confidence

- Pulling back under the slightest hint of criticism

- Demonstrating emerging language skills

- Having limited experience as a successful learner

Fragile beginners need optimal scaffolding to keep working. That is, they need assistance, but overbearing instruction or even excessive enthusiasm can cause them to shut down because they may perceive any feedback as criticism. Again, all of the BACKDROP principles and writing lab components apply.

Andrea was a fifth-grade student with learning disabilities who entered our after-school writing lab as a fragile beginner. Andrea had a difficult time accepting even gentle scaffolding at first. When instructors approached, she used computer software features to turn the font to hieroglyphics or to make it yellow. This made the text impossible to read and discouraged scaffolding for written language improvements. Therefore, we focused our early scaffolding on building Andrea's social-emotional trust in herself and us. We wanted her to trust that we valued her ideas as primary over technical correctness. We also encouraged Andrea's mother to focus on the interesting ideas in Andrea's stories when she arrived to pick Andrea up after each session, rather than pointing out errors in the day's printout or asking how many new words Andrea had produced.

As illustrated in Box 7.1, Andrea used software clip art and listing strategies to plan and organize her early stories. The instructional team established a discourse-level objective for Andrea to produce narratives that included a problem. After several months in the writing lab, Andrea no longer was as fragile, but she continued to need scaffolding that was sensitive to her need for internal control. Box 5.2 tells the story of one scaffolding session. Gradually, Andrea learned to enjoy her audience and to draw readers into her reflections on important fifth-grade social problems.

Box 5.2.   Scaffolding a Fragile Beginner by Using Dynamic Decision-Making

Andrea was a fifth-grade student with learning disabilities who was a fragile beginner early in her after-school writing lab experience. Andrea wrote willingly at her computer, but resisted scaffolding. She tended to use a listing approach to story writing, often including her girlfriends and occasionally their pets. An early example of one of Andrea's picture-based stories appears in Box 7.1. During the latter half of her fifth-grade year, she wrote:

> The fight of friends and food
> Once upon a time there were nine girls and there names were
> Alicia, Susan, Juanita, Andrea, Carolyn, Danielle, Jen, Maria, Penda.
> They were all ways mad at each other so they had a food fight.
> They got all messy and got even madder at each other. They had a
> water fite and got wet. Now they got even madder at each other
> and had a animal fite. They were sad and sorry and made up and
> hugged.
>
> The End
> By Andrea

By the beginning of her sixth-grade year, Andrea was more fluent in her writing, and she was prepared with topics when it was time to write. Although she was still sensitive to too much scaffolding, she was able to express her goals in a way that gave her more control. At one point, Andrea announced that she had planned her next story on the topic "the boys in my class." Her instructor planned to use this story as a context for targeting an intervention goal at the discourse level to include more story grammar elements than were evident in Andrea's previous simple reactive sequences.

Andrea began her story and had reached the description of the fourth boy when the instructor inquired, "Will there be a problem in your story?" to which Andrea replied, "There are 14 boys in my class." Andrea made it clear that she was on a roll toward an authoring goal of her own and that it was one that did not include story grammar. This goal-directed behavior, while it still did not invite scaffolding, signaled an emergence from Andrea's earlier stage as a fragile beginner. She was becoming an autonomous writer, but she still could benefit from mediation by an instructor with intentions to help her develop her skills.

Guided by the ownership and dynamic instruction principles, the team came to the conclusion that this was not the time for a discourse goal aimed at plot development, but it certainly was an opportunity to work on rich character description. Andrea's story shows her experimentation with several literary and figurative language techniques, some more elegant than others, especially as she ran out of time for drafting, revising, and editing. We were particularly delighted with Andrea's wonderful description of a classmate from Vietnam, "He has hair like the night and eyes like the dark sky when it rains." The complete story read:

The Boys in my class

Today I was thinking about a story for this class so I thought about the boys in my class and I thought it would be nice to write a story about them. Well there's Raul he has blond hair like the sun and his blue eyes are like the sky. He has glasses and he is a kindergarten safty like me and in the same room but he is in the afternoon. He is a very good basketball player and a good football player. He mixes with the kindergarteners very very well even thow I'm not with him! He has lots of friends and he sits in row five. Thats four rows down from me.

Then there's Phil he has brown hair is like the drit and brown eyes are like choolet chip. He has a littel sister named Kasie she so cute. He is very good at basketball and he is really funny. He sits in row three. Thats one row down from me.

Then there's Emil. He is in row five. Thats four rows down from me. He has brown hair like the ground and his blue eyes are like the sky. He is very good at football. He is very scared of me because I kick him. He is really nice to me but some times he gets mad at me and chases me a lot.

Then there's Connor. He has frackels and he has red hair. His hair is like fire and his glasses are plane glasses. He is a very good soccer player he runs like the wind. I know because we were on the same soccer team for two years!

Then theres Cam. He is from Viet Nam. He is realy funny. He has hair like the night and eyes like the dark sky when it rains. He has dark skin is really nice. He sits in row five. Thats four rows down from me.

Then theres Jacob he has brown hair like drit and eyes like mud he is from Pennyslvainea. He sits in row five. Thats four rows down from me.

Then theres Neil. He has brown hair and blue eyes. he sits in row five. Thats four rows down from me.

Then theres Billy he has bloond hair and blue eyes he sits in row theer. Thats one row down from me.

Then theres Greg. He ha brown hair and blue eyes he sits in row two. Thats right next to me.

Then theres Alex he has brown hair and blue eyes. He sits right next to me.

Then there's my dear techer Mr. Jenson. He has brown hair and blue eyes.

The End

By Andrea

Recommendations for fragile beginners, who pull back when scaffolding becomes too intense, include the following:

1. Provide gentle scaffolding to support the successful production of early works.

2. Scaffold the student's ideas and writing content first, before focusing on form and correctness.

3. Scaffold parents and other important adults to minimize criticism and to emphasize their role as an appreciative audience for the student's ideas. Reassure them that editing skills will be taught as soon as the student becomes more comfortable getting ideas on paper.

4. Scaffold invented spellings, but spell words for the student if the need seems urgent.

5. As the student develops confidence, up the ante on scaffolding, giving the student more responsibility.

Avoider

Avoiders have well-rehearsed procrastination routines, sometimes taking avoidance to the extreme, conveying "I'd rather do anything than write." We have even known students to run around the room or hide under desks. More subtle avoiders spend inordinate amounts of time at the pencil sharpener, selecting just the right piece of paper, or helping their classmates. In the computer lab, avoiders play computer games or search the Internet when other students are starting to work. Avoider profile characteristics include

- Employing a rich repertoire of avoidance strategies (e.g., acting out, making excessive preparations, being overly concerned with helping others, inactivity)

- Having a possible history of failure and criticism from peers or adults

- Displaying limited language skills (although not always)

Avoiders require a liberal application of the patience principle, balanced with determined instruction, to help them experience the satisfaction of ownership on the road to becoming constructive learners. Some respond particularly well to the publication and presentation phases of the writing process. Their avoidance strategies fade as they learn to anticipate presentations and related feelings of completion and success.

For many, however, avoidance patterns are well established and difficult to overcome. They may require persistence, as well as patience, along with deliberate strategies to help them discard old patterns. Some students who have historically been placed in special education classes are particularly good at avoiding. Refusing to work may have been one of the primary areas in which they could exert control in the past. An example of this appears in Box 5.3.

Box 5.3.   Scaffolding an Avoider to Be Willing to Try

Nino was a third-grade student with significant cognitive limitations. He spent most of his day in a special education room but was included in a general education classroom for writing lab activities. Nino's classmates viewed him as different, and he avoided interacting with them at first, even hiding under the desk. A turning point (see Chapter 13) came for Nino one day when his general education class was in the school's computer lab, and he was among the first to learn how to put an artistic border around his work. Nino, who generally required heavy scaffolding to complete any academic task, learned this feature in one trial and with minimal scaffolding.

When one of Nino's fellow students noticed his border and wanted to try the feature, she asked for help from an adult. We pointed out that Nino could show her what to do. She looked surprised but allowed him to come to her computer and demonstrate. The adult was prepared to scaffold Nino to find the toolbar menu where the feature was located, but he did not need help. He independently showed her how the feature worked, leaving the classmate (and adult) both amazed. Nino left with enhanced confidence and willingness to try new things, and his classmate had new respect for Nino as a full-fledged classmate.

Suggestions for helping avoiders get down to work include recommendations to:

1. Use computer software features to provide motivating activities that differ from prior associations with failure. For example, early in the drafting process, assist the student to find and use illustration and publication software features (e.g., clip art, sound effects, attractive borders).

2. Provide heavier scaffolding initially to support weak language abilities (e.g., the "shared" pencil or keyboard and dictation can be used to get the student's words on paper). Fade these as the student becomes more invested in producing interesting products.

3. Set up opportunities for publication and presentation as soon as possible.

4. Help the student establish goals for writing a certain number of words each day, and create a chart in the author notebook for use in daily conferences to document and celebrate progress toward the goal.

Reluctant Writer

Another pattern of avoidance is the reluctant writer. These students actually may put into words the message, "I can't." In fact, we sometimes tally the number of times a student says, "I can't," within a unit of time to serve as a baseline index against which to measure progress. Reluctant writer profile characteristics include

- Having low self-expectations
- Stopping periodically while working

- Being unwilling to take risks

- Feeling afraid of failure

- Having limited language skills (but only suspected because it is difficult to assess them due to the student's hesitance to try new activities)

Students who say, "I can't," frequently and who are afraid of failure are similar to avoiders, but they avoid more passively. Their unwillingness to take risks limits their learning opportunities and tries the patience of their instructors. Reluctant writers need scaffolding to see what they can do. They benefit from the application of the keep it simple and authentic audience principles, particularly in early writing lab activities.

It is tempting to get drawn into a game of "I can't"—"Oh, yes you can" with reluctant writers. Stacy was a third grader with Down syndrome who had mastered this routine. In response to Stacy's "I can't," we created the discouraging-encouraging minilesson that is described in Chapter 4. Box 5.4 describes how Stacy responded to scaffolding.

Recommendations for scaffolding reluctant writers into investing themselves more actively in the writing process include

1. Teach the encouraging-discouraging minilesson, and assist the student to find encouraging alternatives to the discouraging "I can't," such as "This is hard, but I can try."

Box 5.4.   Scaffolding a Reluctant Writer to Take Learning Risks

Stacy was a third-grader with Down syndrome. She had been included in general education classrooms since she entered public school in kindergarten. Goals had been set for Stacy to keep her in the general education curriculum, and indeed, her reading and writing abilities far outdistanced those of many other students with Down syndrome. In contrast to past practices, in which such students routinely attended special schools or were institutionalized, Stacy had been taught directly to read and write.

Even so, Stacy had concerns about her abilities. She often made statements like "I can't," or "I'm stupid," in response to which we were tempted to say, "Oh, yes you can," or "Oh, no you aren't." It did not take long, however, for us to realize that we were being drawn into a familiar game that was not productive for anyone. That is when we developed the discouraging-encouraging minilesson and used it for the first time.

The intention was to give us some positive, preemptive ways to address the problem of how Stacy was communicating with herself and others about her abilities and attempts. Once we had established a common vocabulary for and some examples of "encouraging talk," it was easier to set the stage for helping Stacy use encouraging talk (e.g., "This is hard, but I can try") as a bridge to feeling better about herself and persisting in problem solving.

2. As recommended for the fragile beginner, provide sincere and enthusiastic, but gentle, audience appreciation focused on ideas.

3. Use the computer to provide a unique learning environment where success can be realized quickly.

4. Provide heavy guiding strategies in the early stages, using dictation and other techniques to bridge from "can't" to "can," to help the student experience some success, and to take more risks in subsequent sessions.

5. When trust grows, conduct more complete assessment activities, and tailor intervention to address low-level skills.

Perfectionist

Perfectionists often start out as paper wadders or fragile beginners. They transition into a perfectionist stage as their preliminary concerns are addressed and they are able to produce longer texts. Perfectionists continue to need scaffolding, however, to overcome their concerns that "this is not good enough," even when others try to tell them it is. Other characteristics associated with the perfectionist profile are

- Holding unreasonably high standards for one's own work

- Stopping periodically while working due to frustration (may start out as a paper wadder and transition into perfectionist)

- Demonstrating language skills in highly supportive contexts, but hesitating to use them to take academic risks

- Resisting scaffolding

- In extreme cases, having compulsive needs for certain elements to be included in processes or products

Perfectionists may become stymied and frustrated by their inability to meet their own standards of perfection. Getting them to accept certain elements of the writing process is challenging. Asking them to accept invented spelling during drafting and strike-through and insertion during revision may be particularly distressing. In Chapter 1, we described how Bill could not stand to leave a story incomplete at the end of a writing lab session and how a serial chapter writing strategy enabled him to work more than one day on the same piece. Bill later benefited by learning to use a "to be continued" phrase when it came time to stop work for the day. Ultimately, he was able to give up both of these strategies and work for extended periods on the same piece. (See also Box 3.1 for a description of Serena, a kindergarten student with compulsive needs for stories to include more than one character.)

Previously in this chapter, we noted how Jeremy, in his paper-wadding phase, and Andrea, in her fragile-beginner phase, both had perfectionist tendencies associated with those patterns. In its milder forms, perfectionism is not a bad thing and can lead an independent author to keep polishing a piece and to make sure that all details are in place. When perfectionism paralyzes progress or completion of products, though, it needs to be given special attention. Box 5.5 exemplifies this pattern.

Box 5.5.   Scaffolding an Extreme Perfectionist by Using the Patience Principle

Jeremy began as a paper wadder, but unlike some students with that profile, he had many written language strengths. Jeremy's low tolerance for frustration seemed to stem from his perfectionist tendencies more than from deficient abilities. Jeremy's perfectionism put him in great jeopardy as a learner, nevertheless. Many days, when it was time for writing lab, Jeremy was in the principal's office because of an outburst earlier in the day. Jeremy's general education teacher tried several approaches to deal with the problem, including separating him from his classmates to give him space, positive encouragement, and behavioral ultimatums. The problem was difficult, however, and it kept interfering with Jeremy's ability to learn.

Finally, the team decided to address the problem by confronting it directly. Jeremy was drawn aside. He was asked to think about his choices, and he was introduced to the term *perfectionist* which was written on a page of his author's notebook. We told him that a perfectionist is someone who has to have everything perfect and who gets upset when it is not. The problem is that a perfectionist has a hard time thinking anything is ever perfect, so the perfectionist feels upset most of the time. This is a real problem if it keeps the perfectionist from doing his best work, and it is even a bigger problem if it leads to outbursts and trips to the principal's office.

We asked Jeremy whether he thought he might be a perfectionist, at least some of the time. He agreed. Then, together, we constructed some goals in his author's notebook for dealing with his perfectionism:

- I will tell myself it is okay not to be perfect.
- I will concentrate on my ideas and not worry if I make a mistake and have to cross out or start over.
- If I start to get frustrated, I will take a break and come back in a few minutes without having an outburst.

Several elements led to improvements for Jeremy. Establishing goals and terminology to deal with the problem helped move it beyond a behavioral issue for him. Although Jeremy continued to have high and low days and occasional outbursts, he was able to reach a more even keel and to produce some excellent work in the writing lab. One particularly helpful discovery was finding that Jeremy had a passion for poetry. He especially benefited from an approach that asked the students to think about their five senses. In December, he wrote this poem in his very tiny, handwritten script. The script was tightly controlled, but the words showed that Jeremy was getting in touch with his feelings and the joy of writing.

Blue Green

Blue green is the warm sky that macks you feel good inside. Blue green is the sound of the sea that fish live in. Blue green smells like a blue green marker that people write with. Blue green looks like a lovele crayola that boys and grils color with. Blue green is the tastes of blue barry pies cooking in the kitchen.

> A little later Jeremy produced this poem about football during free writing. It shows his adoption of the five senses approach to expressing himself poetically and represents his greater sense of control over the writing process:
>
> Football is fun to play
>
> football is a fun game
> it feels soft
> some footballs do smell
> I can hear someone kicking a football
> I can hear a football whistling.
> I can see someone throwing the football.

Suggestions for working with perfectionists include

1. Start with a simple project that results in a computer-supported published product relatively soon.

2. Assure students that they will receive help to make the published version correct.

3. Label the characteristics of each phase of the writing process to contrast drafting and publishing standards (e.g., sloppy copy versus publication copy; invented spelling versus dictionary spelling).

4. Provide a bulletin board that shows how a student's work changes through stages of the writing process.

5. During scaffolding transactions, never mark on a perfectionist's paper (or as a good rule, any student's paper) without asking permission first.

6. Acknowledge the need for perfection, and model self-talk that will help the student feel ownership and control over editing decisions (e.g., "When I start feeling like a perfectionist, I ask myself, 'Do I have to fix this now or can it wait till later?'")

7. Teach revising features on the computer as soon as possible (e.g., how to use mouse and arrow keys to highlight, cut and paste, delete selectively, and insert new text).

8. Have the patience to give the student space when perfectionist needs seem overwhelming.

9. Explore different genres, and encourage free writing in a genre the student prefers.

Quick to Finish

The student who is quick to finish is the opposite of the perfectionist. Such students apparently have low standards for their work, often asserting prematurely, "I'm done," and resisting further attempts at scaffolding. Characteristics associated with this profile are listed on page 183.

Box 5.6. Scaffolding the Quick to Finish Student to Keep Working

Tyrone was a third grader who received services from a consultant for the hearing impaired to work on speech perception problems and language comprehension. He had a unilateral hearing loss but did not use an aid. Tyrone had some highly practiced avoidance strategies, including writing a few words, erasing them (or deleting them at the computer), writing a few more, and then announcing that he was done. His first story was

I playfootball

I love to play football. This is my favorite sports. Sometime Jaleel,
Chuck, Rich, and. I play football sometime. The kides akros the hall
paly to

The End

Tyrone's speech was not always clear to his peers, but he was sociable and well liked. He loved an audience, and it did not take him long to recognize the power of the author chair. One trial, and Tyrone was ready to set goals to write more. Before reading, Tyrone said, "I play football (that's the title). And I got some more to write, but I don't think Mr. G. is gonna let me. And I'm fixin' to put in some big words at the end."

After Tyrone read the story, students asked questions:

Kisho:	"What team is you on?"
Tyrone:	"Northside 49ers"
	[Kisho asked for repetition]
Tyrone:	[more clearly] "Northside 49ers"
Tim:	"Did you play at school?"
Tyrone:	"What?"
Tim:	"Where we're at."

Several class members chimed in to point out to Tim that Tyrone had just said he played at the "Northside," which they recognized as a youth club, not the school.

Tyrone needed less scaffolding to produce his next story, "Two Dogs that Like Football." The first part was

I have two dogs that like football. They come to me all the time.
Their names are Face and Goldie. The first dog likes to kick the ball.
The second one likes to catch the ball.

Although the entire story was not a lot longer than his previous story, there was more to it. It was two pages long and included a section where he talked about taking his dogs for a walk.

This time the author group discussion went as follows:

Tyrone: [Starts to read without reading title] "Can I start over?" [Gives title with a big smile; reads story]

Kira: "How long was your walk?"

Tyrone: "About 50 minutes or an hour."

James: "Does one of your dogs play like the Detroit Lions?"

Tyrone: [showing a little confusion about sports teams] "No, they don't play basketball. They play like the Green Bay Packers."

Adrian: "Why does they play football?"

Tyrone: "Because I like the game."

Kevin: "Oh, can I ask a question? How did they catch the ball?"

Tyrone: [Pantomimes dogs running and jumping up to catch a football between chin and front paws. Calls on Dennis.]

Dennis: "I forgot."

Tyrone: "Okay, I'll call on you in a minute. Are you thinking?" [then he adds, almost to himself] "So many people want to talk about my story!"

- Stopping before completing a project and resisting encouragement to continue

- Demonstrating few executive control and self-reflection strategies

- Being willing to leave errors in work even after recognizing them

- Having limited experience with the joy of completed, self-motivated projects

Students who claim to be done after limited effort often test the instructors' patience to balance acceptance of the young author's ownership with challenge to reach higher levels of performance. Yet, patience in the first few projects generally pays off by showing the student that the ownership principle is real. It is also important to determine how the student's prior experience might be influencing the "I'm done" position. One sixth grader seemed arrogant at first about saying "I'm done," but later admitted to a trusted teacher that he was reluctant to try because he felt stupid when trying to write with pencil and paper. The computer gave him a stronger sense of success and made him willing to keep trying. The publication phase of the writing process is particularly important for these students. They also may benefit from having direct help from a teacher to edit their work, showing them what changes are needed and why.

Students who are quick to finish also need to learn to use self-talk to become constructive learners. Tyrone was a third-grade student with unilateral hearing loss who illustrated quick-to-finish behavior (see Box 5.6). Suggestions for working with students who are quick to finish include

1. Engage the student in a publication and presentation celebration as soon as possible so that ownership becomes focused on producing a better product for sharing rather than stopping prematurely and claiming completion.

2. Interview the student about areas of interest, and seek ways to integrate those into writing lab projects.

3. Maximize authentic audience elements, inviting peers and parents to enjoy the student's work as well.

4. Teach the student to evaluate his or her own work and to set personal goals.

5. Model self-talk strategies aimed at specific components of writing genre (e.g., "What is the conflict in my story? What will my audience want to know about my topic?"), and provide scaffolding supports as necessary.

6. Make sure that the student confers with his or her general education teacher, who officially is in charge of classroom standards, before considering a work ready to publish, and work to show consistency as a team (see Chapter 13).

7. Take advantage of the motivating power of the computer to encourage sustained effort.

Individualist

Some students are individualists who seem to say, "I'm different." Previously, we considered how students like Jeremy and Andrea might start out as paper wadders or fragile beginners and transition through periods where their perfectionism stands in the way of progress. Eventually, such students can reach a point of maturity at which they can establish that they are different, yet still fit in with their peer group and meet general education expectations. Characteristics of individualists include

- Perceiving self to be different from other students

- Having limited language abilities or having dialectal or second language issues

- Being a divergent thinker who resists story starters or overly controlled topic setting and writing requirements

Students who feel they are different from their peers need to be in a safe, trustworthy, and respectful environment where diversity and creativity are celebrated. The ownership principle is particularly important for such students, as well as patience for letting them find their own voices in writing.

Students whose language is mainstream but whose ideas are divergent may need encouragement, and even bargaining, to complete highly structured teacher-directed writing projects. They do better with projects that offer more degrees of freedom in topic selection, discourse structure, and writing style. These students can benefit, however, from learning how to conform to nonnegotiable mainstream expectations while still expressing their individual creativity. Emphasis on the constructive learning principle can be used to teach students self-regulatory strategies for responding to their teacher's requirements in creative, unique ways. Box 5.7 provides an example of a fourth-grade student, Scott, with language impairments who wrote several stories before integrating story elements after his instructors began scaffolding them.

Suggestions for individualists, who take a different approach to the writing process, include

1. Focus early scaffolding on audience appreciation for the student's unique ideas and interesting information.

2. As the student progresses in expression at the discourse level, implement higher standards for technical correctness, and make explicit criteria of particular projects, allowing room for creativity within the boundaries.

3. Enjoy the student's uniqueness, learn from it, and scaffold peers to appreciate it.

4. Keep the dynamic principle in mind as adjustments are made in instructional expectations.

Risk Taker

Students who are risk takers convey a sense of, "This is fun!" as they work. Risk takers may or may not have disabilities, but they do demonstrate socioemotional security and a positive approach to the writing process. This security serves their learning well and makes them fun to teach. Characteristics of risk takers include

- Being willing to try new things

- Making some mistakes while experimenting with higher-level language

- Setting goals and making plans to achieve certain audience effects

- Attempting to write in new discourse genres

Some risk takers start out that way. Others evolve from earlier profiles. When a student shifts from one of the previous patterns to begin taking risks and attempting to use higher-level language structures and vocabulary, the team can quietly celebrate. This is an important point in the instructional process. Learners who take risks are open to new learning and are responsive to scaffolding on all language levels. Instructors should understand, however, that when students attempt more complex language and writing strategies, many produce more (rather than fewer) errors in their work. This is a good time to remember Weaver's (1982) advice of "welcoming errors as signs of growth."

Some students enter the writing lab experience as risk takers by nature, even though they have significant language-learning needs. Chandler, a third-grade student who scored low on both language and cognitive tests (and thus, did not qualify for special education), was such a student. Chandler's expressive language (both spoken and written) was disorganized and difficult to follow. His language comprehension problems led to unusual responses to questions that sometimes made his classmates giggle. For example, one day when his teacher asked who was interested in joining the Girl Scouts, Chandler raised his hand. His teacher said, with sensitivity, "Chandler, I think you might be thinking of the Boy Scouts; we'll have to look into that." Chandler was not easily embarrassed, however. He was a risk taker from the start. He sought out and benefited from his teachers' scaffolding, and he always started working immediately and wrote without encouragement both in the classroom and the computer lab. Examples of growth in Chandler's work related to his willingness to take risks and attempt new strategies appear in Box 5.8.

Box 5.7. Scaffolding the Individualist to Conform to Some Expectations

Ownership and creativity are highly valued in the writing lab, but there are moments when authors need to listen to the members of the audience in order to meet their information needs. Scott was a fourth-grade student with special language learning and literacy needs. He did not much care for reading, except comic books. Scott had a fertile imagination and a dry wit. He was good at creating pictures in his mind, but not as good at putting his vision into words that his audience could understand. His early story attempts were mostly isolated descriptions with insufficient detail and no clear character development or temporal sequence.

> Beast was the X-,men,s ferball. gambit was lost. jonhh was a boy. Cyclops was lost too. the X-MEN were lost all but beast and Sunspot. magnto was the one who took the X-men. \ Beast fond a file in a labry [laboratory] . . . . to be cunnud

Goals were established for Scott to add character description and to relate his ideas temporally. Scaffolding strategies included

- Involving him in an author group discussion of story grammar elements
- Encouraging author group members to ask Scott questions about unclear portions
- Helping Scott focus on his peers' stories and provide suggestions for them in author group
- Asking questions at the computer to clarify information about Scott's interesting ideas

In a session a few weeks later, Scott added the name of a city in a response to a question asked by one of his author group mates. In this story, he also showed some sensitivity to the need to explain his characters to those uninitiated in cartoon character lore:

> Cop hit Tyrow. Tyrow fell off the John Hancock building in Chicago. Cop and Thunder saw Tyrow die. Cop and Thunder are the 2 best superheros paired up. Fireball hit Gwcript off the John Hancock building. He died.
>
> by
Scott

Scott's next story was one of our favorites. Although it was at the level of action sequence, with only a hint of cause and effect, Scott used this story to introduce his "Mortal geezer" character. At first, we were not sure that Scott had a conventional concept of what it means to be a "geezer," but when asked, he pantomimed for us as a bent-over old man using a cane. Then, he added the detail of "flammable dentures," which confirmed for us his grasp of the concept. For this story, Scott responded to the instructors' frequent requests for more information by including a paragraph labeled "information" at the bottom of the page.

(continued)

Box 5.7. *(continued)*

Mortalgezzer

One day Mortalgezzer threw flammable dentures at Fireball. Fireball died. Mortalgezzer is cool. Mortalgezzer threw a bomb at Inton. Inton died. Thunder shot Mortalgezzer. Mortalgezzer got a scar. the end
[printed at the bottom of the same page]
information Mortalgezzer was born may 31rst in the year 1. he is bald. He has no legs no left arm in worldwar 1, 2 he has a wheelchair he is deadly.

Box 5.8. Scaffolding Risk Takers to Meet Higher Standards

Some students approach writing with attitudes of self-direction and positive expectation even though their skills lag considerably behind those of their peers. Chandler was a third-grade student whose language skills were affected by comprehension difficulties. Pragmatic concerns, such as off-topic comments in classroom discussions, sometimes made his classmates giggle. His general education teacher (who also was certified in special education), however, was making efforts to help Chandler fit in. She was able to scaffold him to participate both actively and appropriately with a natural, quiet style. In his first piece, which was intended to be "About the Author," Chandler wrote about his interest in banjo and drums, showing some of his difficulty in discourse organization.

Chandler is a musician Chandler play banglo Chandler like siwm and brither day is September 18 I am 8 year old and I live in Kalmlazoo the bandglo is a Drom to play with be careful with the bandglo no play with the bandglo and do not touch the Drom or the bandglo I will do my best to play the Drom is a best beat to play with the head Drom is less to catch with you.

Like all students, Chandler brought with him some particular strengths. In his case, a positive attitude and an ability to attend to tasks that interested him made him a willing student. Whether at his desk in the classroom or at a computer in the lab, Chandler always seemed to be focused on his work. Chandler scored low on tests, especially those requiring language comprehension, but he did not qualify for special services because of a lack of discrepancy between his language and cognitive abilities. Yet, in the writing lab, Chandler picked up a strategy to organize his work by creating a numbered list (with very little scaffolding) for his second project that helped him straighten out many of the confusing elements that characterized his first story. His risk-taker attitude served him well.

Instructional suggestions for students who are risk takers include

1. Take advantage of the student's positive attitude to engage actively in all components of the writing lab approach.

2. Take advantage of the student's fluency, and encourage the student to challenge him- or herself to attempt higher-level language and communication skills for planning, organizing, drafting, revising, and editing.

3. Scaffold self-evaluation and self-regulatory skills for reflecting on progress and planning further improvements.

4. Introduce the full range of computer software features as soon as possible.

Independent Learner

Students who are independent learners are self-directed but still willing to respond to instruction. They exude confidence and may even state explicitly, "Here's what I'm planning next." Characteristics of the independent learner include

- Using strategies for generating content from memory and external sources
- Using knowledge of basic text structures to organize writing
- Developing goals for writing and plans to achieve those goals
- Holding appropriately high standards
- Working independently but calling for assistance when needed
- Having competent language skills, but continuing to seek ways to improve
- Being aware of audience needs
- Using stylistic devices to achieve desired effects to entertain, inform, and so forth
- Balancing attempts at new language forms and discourse structures with high standards of technical correctness

Scardamalia and Bereiter (1986) called students who exhibit such traits *expert writers*. Students with disabilities can be independent learners as well, even though they continue to need language intervention. Independent learners can benefit from deliberate, intentional scaffolding to reach higher levels of proficiency. One of the advantages of the writing lab approach is that it works well for all students and can take their compositions and spoken communication skills to the next higher level. When students with LLD or other educational risks reach the level of independent learner, the possibilities for further growth are exciting. When students start to assume ownership and responsibility for their own learning, the possibilities for further growth are optimized.

By the end of her second year as a member of the after-school computer-supported writing lab, Andrea was in sixth grade and had become an independent learner. Box 5.9 illustrates a story she produced when she had entered this stage.

Box 5.9.   Scaffolding Independent Learners to Keep Growing

Andrea spent 2 years in the after-school computer-supported writing lab. Her early work, when she was in fifth grade, appears in Box 7.1 and the start of Box 5.2. By the autumn of her sixth-grade year, Andrea had been exerting her power as a writer to meet her own goals, as in her "Boys in My Class" story, during which she was willing to work on character description, but declined to put in the elements of story grammar. By the following February, Andrea was more ready to attempt stories with the discourse structure of complete episodes. She also worked on goals related to variation in sentence structure, the inclusion of dialogue, conventional spelling patterns, and editing—all evident in the following story.

The First Dance That Andrea Went Too!

ONCE there was a girl named Andrea and she was very shy around boys. One day her friend Maggie told her that there was a dance coming up. Maggie asked her if she wonted to go to the dance with her and Andrea asked if boys were going to be there. Maggie said "yes" , then Andrea said "let me think about it" but Maggie said "you have to go." So Andrea went and a lot of boys asked her to dance, but no one asked Maggie to dance with her because all the boys liked Andrea and Andrea said "yes" to all of them! Then in the middle of a song Maggie ran in to the bathroom and Andrea went running after her and when Andrea got there she asked Maggie what the matter was and Maggie said "its not fair!" Then Andrea asked what wasn't fair and Maggie said "that all the boys are asking you to dance with them and they are not asking me to dance."

THEN Andrea promised to say no to the next boy that asked her to dance. Then the cutest boy there asked Andrea to dance and remembering what she told Maggie, she said "no" he was very mad. Then she told him to come back in one second and he did. Then they danced the rest of the night and other boys asked Maggie to dance and she was very happy! When the dance was done Maggie, Steve Andrea, Omar went out to for ice cream.

Then after they went out for ice cream the boy took the girls home and when they got to there homes the boys kissed them and said good night to them and said told them that they were going to see them to marrow at school.

The End

By Andrea

Suggestions for scaffolding independent learners to higher levels of competence include

1. Provide opportunity for maximal freedom in topic selection and other author choices.

2. Provide scaffolding aimed at continued improvement in language and literacy skills.

3. Encourage the use of a journal or a section of the author notebook to keep lists of writing ideas and plans for upcoming projects.

4. Help the student become a supportive peer for students who have not yet reached the independent-learner stage.

Summary of Patterns of Student Approaches to the Writing Process

Profiles of individual approaches to the writing process vary depending on personality traits and prior experience. Different scaffolding strategies are needed for different students. Students who start out wadding their papers have the potential to become independent learners. Students who are reluctant writers may demonstrate active patterns of avoidance or more passive patterns characterized by frequent use of the phrase "I can't." Other students enter the writing process without avoidance, but prematurely insist they are done. Still others indicate a sense of being different, either in their divergent language use or their manner of topic selection and discourse organization. As students gain confidence, they become risk takers. As they gain competence, they become independent learners. No student is too advanced for scaffolding. Intentional goal setting and scaffolding can be used to take all students to the next higher level of maturity, no matter where each starts. In this section, we have encouraged the appreciation and celebration of diversity, along with acceptance of responsibility to help all children achieve higher levels of competence.

SUMMARY

This chapter describes the basics of scaffolding, which is the primary tool of instructor–student interaction in the writing lab approach. The chapter relates scaffolding to dynamic assessment and to self-regulation and executive control, which are accomplished as students learn to use self-talk to scaffold their own higher-level learning. The chapter describes general techniques of scaffolding as framing, focusing, feeding back, and guiding students to make new linguistic and cognitive connections. Nine profiles of student authors and their varied approaches to the writing process are then presented, along with associated scaffolding techniques. Individualizing instruction by scaffolding student growth within the inclusive writing lab makes it possible for all to develop higher-level academic and social-communication skills and a deeper sense of confidence in themselves as learners, which results in increased participation for all.

6

Scaffolding Writing Processes and Language Targets

Scaffolding techniques (introduced in Chapter 5) can support students to become independent within all stages of the writing process. In this chapter, we describe scaffolding techniques for helping students become competent at each stage of the writing process. We also describe scaffolding techniques to address language targets at levels of discourse, sentences, words, and for writing conventions and spoken communication.

SCAFFOLDING WRITING PROCESSES

The writing process includes planning, organizing, drafting, revising, editing, and publishing and presenting.

Planning and Organizing

The focus of intervention aimed at planning and organizing is to teach writers to approach the writing task more mindfully (Wong, 1994). Scaffolds should be designed to help students to use their knowledge of text structures "actively, deliberately, and analytically" (Roth, 2000, p. 22). The context for such abilities is established through group minilessons, then reinforced with individualized scaffolding.

Brainstorming is an important tool used by authors in the initial stages of generating ideas. Chapter 4 suggested some of the elements that should go into a minilesson on brainstorming. Chapter 7 describes idea generating software features. After teaching one group of fifth-grade students with LLDs to brainstorm, Troia, Graham, and Harris (1999) documented increased time planning and increased number of written plan statements.

Drawing is a skill used by some students to support their brainstorming or other planning efforts. Ukrainetz (1998) described how children's stick drawings can be scaffolded to perform this function. We also have worked with students who preferred using clip art or sound effects to stimulate their planning of original stories. Chapter 7 describes the use of computer drawing tools to help scaffold planning and organizing.

Generating ideas is only the tip of the iceberg for planning and organizing. Like all writing processes, planning is recursive. Scaffolding aimed at teaching students metacognitive strategies for guiding themselves reflectively through planning, drafting, and revising processes is at the heart of this intervention. These elements are reflected in many of the SRSD routines developed by Graham and associates (2000), and in Englert's (1992) POWER acronym, reminding students to plan, organize, write, edit, rewrite, and revise (described in Chapter 5).

Wong (2000) described how to scaffold high school students to plan opinion and compare-contrast essays. The intervention started by activating general planning schemas, such as what to do when planning to attend a rock concert. The brainstorming heightened awareness that planning requires thinking about what a problem entails first, then designing a series of steps to address it. Wong and her colleagues next helped students use planning sheets outlining the organizational elements of opinion and compare-contrast essays to address such age-relevant topics as whether teachers should allow students to use personal stereo systems in class. Students were grouped into planning dyads, worked to come up with arguments of equal weight for opposing views, then shared those arguments with the broader group.

We have used a similar approach with third- and fifth-grade students in our writing lab experiences. In a project motivated by district and statewide testing formats, we required students to brainstorm pro and con arguments, pick a stance (i.e., "take a stand"), and write an essay supporting their decisions, in which they cited core democratic values. In the third-grade version, the instructional team planned a debate on whether the student's elementary school should return to a traditional lunch and recess program or keep their innovative lunch-and-learn program where students could choose from a menu of extracurricular learning options and eat their lunch in conjunction with those activities.

We started by dividing the class into two groups and clustering them around two instructors on opposite sides of the computer lab using the *Inspiration's* (Inspiration Software) "RapidFire" feature to brainstorm arguments for each position. Then, we printed out the group-generated results of brainstorming, making a copy for each student. For the debate, the two groups lined up across from each other in the computer lab, and another adult member of the team scaffolded a group discussion on opposing opinions on the topic. Students were told that they would get to take a stand about their position next. Then, the group discussed what "take a stand" might mean. The hour session ended with students moving to the pro or con side of the room depending on the personal "stand" each decided to take.

Drafting

Scaffolding for the drafting process should focus on content as a starting point. When parents scaffold their young children to tell a story, they do it with the primary motivation of getting the message straight, not of eliciting more complex language. Nevertheless, the outcome is the same. Children acquire more mature language to convey more elaborate ideas (Wells, 1986).

Similarly, SLPs often advise parents of children in speech therapy to "listen to your child; what your child says is always more important than how he says it." Writing lab contexts should foster trust among students that they are in the presence of adults who care more about the content of their ideas than about identifying their mistakes. More complex and correct forms generally result from successful communication experiences and contribute to them. As noted in Chapter 5, editorial correctness is targeted after building a foundation of confidence and willingness to write.

The content of a student's draft language can be the object of joint focus by the student and a supportive adult either at the student's desk or at a computer station. The scaffolding approach is to first read a section of the draft aloud or to ask the student to read it. The instructor might begin by expressing appreciation for a particular feature of the draft, often an instructional target the student has started to use independently. Then, the adult frames a problem in a remaining area of difficulty, focuses the student on a miscue, provides feedback, or guides the student to an issue that will lead to higher-level learning. The exchange ends with another positive and encouraging comment. Always, the instructor conveys the role of interested audience. It is not really a role. In fact, students' ideas are interesting and entertaining when they are original.

Author groups, author chair, and peer conferencing activities can provide peer supports for making the authentic audience principle explicit. Peers, in fact, often are perceived as the most important audience by their fellow students. The interaction of students with and without disabilities is one of the major benefits of an inclusive writing lab approach. A few students seem to have natural scaffolding talents for assisting their peers. Many others benefit from minilessons and individual scaffolding to help dyads of peers or author groups learn to support each other. For example, when a peer whispers, "I can't hear him," the instructor can scaffold the peer to deliver the message directly (e.g., "Tell him. Let him know that you want to be able to hear him.")

For young students or others with emergent literacy skills, drafting scaffolds might include dictation at first and shared pencil strategies later. Students who need heavy scaffolding supports to draft their written products still can exert independence by learning to activate speech synthesis features on their computers to read back the drafted language word by word. Other computer software features that support students in encoding skills are described in Chapter 8. As students advance, scaffolding can be used to help them develop invented spelling capabilities. This involves a focus on phonemic awareness. Techniques aimed at scaffolding such word-level skills are described later in this chapter. Students with more drafting capabilities can participate in setting personal drafting goals (e.g., to add three new ideas). Then, instructors can scaffold them toward independence by saying, "I'll let you work on that and be back in a few minutes." Such scaffolds make the expectation of independence explicit.

Revising

Scaffolding revision processes has goals to increase frequency, extent, and skillfulness with which students attempt to improve their discourse by revisiting it (Roth, 2000). Revision supports can come in the form of checklists with questions about desired features for a particular discourse genre. Teams can design revising checklists for any genre based on their school district's general education curriculum and scoring rubrics. For example, a revising checklist for narratives might include

- How does my story begin? Describe my characters and setting.

- What is the problem? What do my characters decide to do about the problem?

- What happens?

- How does my story end?

When devising such checklists, we suggest minimizing yes/no questions because students will sometimes just check "yes" without reflecting on their writing. It is better to ask students to indicate actual content from their composition. In fact, many students assume that ideas in their heads have been communicated to their audience when such presupposition is not justified. Instructors may have to teach the metalinguistic and pragmatic skills explicitly. Students must learn that if they want others to know what they mean, it is not enough for the idea to be in their heads; it also must be in their words on paper. To scaffold this concept, instructors can ask strategic questions about missing details and then assist authors to identify where such details should be inserted in the text.

Many students initially confuse revising and editing, especially students with disabilities, who are likely to become overly focused on the mechanics of editing at the expense of more substantive revising to improve the content, organization, or clarity of a piece (MacArthur & Graham, 1987; MacArthur, Graham, & Schwartz, 1991). To differentiate the process of revising from editing, instructors can set publication deadlines and make copyediting the goal of the last day prior to publishing. Then, earlier sessions can be devoted to true revising in which goals are set to improve the substance of students' written products. During revision, which most students resist at first, it is tempting to think that students are bored with the project and that it is time to move on. When this occurs, instructional teams should remind themselves that the benefits of reflective learning will last longer than the completion of a single project and are worth the effort. The students are learning how to learn, particularly how to self-monitor and guide their own actions, not simply how to finish.

Scaffolding students to revise involves helping them to take multiple points of view. This starts with scaffolding to consider their own points of view first, using self-regulation questions, such as "Is my writing clear?" and "Is it interesting?" Then, students are scaffolded to consider others' points of view in contexts of author groups, peer conferencing, and computer-station discussions. In these contexts with a focus on perspective taking, students can be scaffolded to develop other social-communication skills as well. As described in Chapter 4, a minilesson is used to introduce peer conferencing. Handouts describing author and editor roles, along with a script for initiating peer conferencing discourse, remain available in students' author notebooks, including "One thing I liked . . . " and "One suggestion is . . . ."

Author chair experiences also offer an excellent means for building sensitivity to others' points of view. In this routine, after classmates listen to an author read a current draft aloud, the author has the opportunity to call on one or two classmates who have comments about the work and one or two who have questions. Timing this experience to occur with ample time before a publication date makes it possible for the author to use the peer input to revise. We sometimes give students clipboards to take notes from their peers' suggestions to help them remember the suggestions they want to use while revising. Although initially all peer input may sound the same or focus on irrelevant details (e.g., "What is your mother's name?" "How old was your cat?"), over time instructors can scaffold the group to provide more original and relevant feedback by commenting on desirable features (e.g., "Asking *why* the character decided to go back home was an excellent question. Do you see how it really helps the author to know when an important piece of information is missing?"). If necessary, instructors can discourage redundant comments or questions of a particular kind (e.g., "It seems that everyone is interested in characters' names so let's make a note to include them. Now, let's see if we can ask questions about other things").

Ultimately, instructional teams should seek evidence that students are beginning to develop independent revising strategies and to notice needs for revising on their own. This is where the ownership principle makes a particular impact. For example, when one eighth-grade student with attention-deficit/hyperactivity disorder, a hearing impairment, and pragmatic communication issues reread his story about video game characters, he commented, "I forgot to put Chung on there." Such reflective comments are cause for celebration.

Editing

Even young students can benefit from learning to use proofreader symbols to edit print-outs or handwritten drafts of written products. The editing features of computers (see Chapter 9) make editing more palatable. As noted in the previous section, establishing publishing deadlines also can make the need for editing more salient.

When a publishing deadline looms due to expectations of the general education curriculum, several techniques can be used to facilitate completion. For example, adults can take a turn at the computer keyboard and use heavier scaffolding and think-aloud techniques to talk a student through the process. This allows publication in a timely fashion while still focusing on student learning. Individual student–teacher conferences can be used to achieve similar goals by having an instructor sit with the student and enter copyediting symbols directly on the next-to-final draft. Although it is best to use lighter scaffolding to support a student to make edits more independently, we prefer either of these heavier scaffolding approaches to the no-scaffolding approach sometimes used in elementary schools for expediency's sake. Sometimes, parent volunteers are brought in to retype students' stories, correcting errors in spelling and punctuation without the student being present. Such practices drastically reduce student ownership in the work. When the ownership principle is honored through the publication stage, final drafts may still include imperfections in spite of scaffolding. In such cases, students' products may be stamped "works in progress" (teacher supply stores generally carry such stamps), or two versions of a student's may be placed side by side in folders, with the student's "best independent work" labeled as such.

Most students resist revising and editing in their early authoring experiences. To be good at editing, authors need to develop metalinguistic abilities to reflect on their own work. To be able to identify cues that signal the need for edits, students also need strong syntactic, semantic, and pragmatic language skills, as well as awareness of the conventions of writing. These elements are targets of the writing lab approach, as discussed later in this chapter. Scaffolds in the revising and editing stages may focus students on missed cues in accord with particular language intervention objectives. For example, when students have weak metalinguistic concepts for sentences, scaffolding focused on final punctuation can help them increase this awareness.

Publishing and Presenting

Scaffolding aimed at publishing and presenting should focus students on the surface features of their products or performances while keeping them in touch with deeper meanings and authentic audience concerns. This includes visual presentation elements for printed representations of students' works and voice quality and body language elements for spoken presentations of those same works.

The authentic audience principle can become particularly salient on such occasions, making self-regulation motivation particularly high. This is the payoff for everyone's hard work. Some students with disabilities may be included in such events or have their work posted on the wall with classmates for the first time. Seeing tears of pride in parents' eyes as they acknowledge such landmark occasions provides the best reward to teachers and clinicians.

Preparing work to appear in a book or getting ready for a public reading offer opportunities to work on such goals as louder voice production and appropriate eye contact. These events can lead to generalization of new skills in a few months that otherwise might take years in traditional therapy sessions. Figure 6.1 shows how this opportunity was used to work on IEP goals related to eye contact for a third-grade student with an autism spectrum disorder. Her SLP helped her think about ways to remember to look at her audience during her author chair, and the student drew eyes on the paper to remind herself to look up.

Videotaping technology allows students to critique their own performances and establish personal goals for improvement. Teachers may need to help students understand that they will not look or sound like themselves at first on videotape and to help shy students begin to take increasing risks. Students who do not want to participate, of course, should be given that option. Author chair and small-group presentations generally are less threatening than videotaping. They can be used to desensitize students who find public presentations too frightening (Nelson et al., 2001). Chapter 13 also describes turning points in learning to take one's turn in the author chair.

When computer supports include ready access to printers, students can fuss with their products and gain more ownership for the appearance of final published versions of their work. Chapter 10 describes software features that support publishing. Being allowed to review and revise printed copies helps students learn to make deliberate, self-regulatory decisions about presentation, formatting, and illustration. Print preview features also are helpful for this purpose. We recommend saving the privilege of printing in color for the final copy.

Teachers we have worked with have been creative in displaying their students' work and creating presentation opportunities. Examples have included posting products artistically in hallways, helping students prepare written products for schoolwide events such as poetry slams and science fairs, and setting up book review displays for other students to see as they enter the school library. The possibilities are endless. Students are

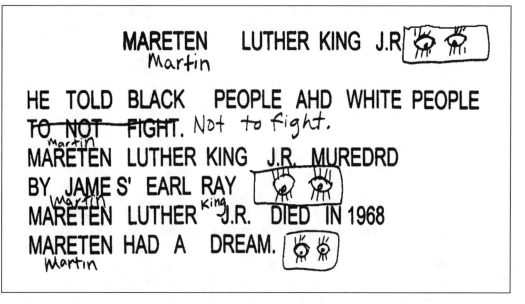

Figure 6.1. Scaffolding eye contact during the presenting process.

particularly thrilled when an actual book binding technique is used to make their work look like a real book. They also like to share animated or multimedia presentations they have created with computer software supports with their parents at publishing parties, with students in different grades, or with students in a companion class.

For students in the early elementary years or students with severe disabilities, a class book can be made with a combination of pictures and captions (e.g., "Our Trip to the Aquarium," with each student responsible for generating vocabulary and text for a single page within the book). A digital camera is helpful for supporting these efforts. Digital cameras also can be used for creating About the Author pages that can be attached to other works. Students' actual drawings are delightful, and computer-scanning technology can be used to add them to written products. Illustration activities should be preceded by minilessons focused on what makes a good illustration.

Presentations provide a particularly powerful context for including students with disabilities in education experiences with their typically developing peers. Students with disabilities may require extra supports, such as peers, to assist them in reading their works, but over time, these students become increasingly independent.

Summary of Scaffolding Techniques for Stages of the Writing Process

The writing lab approach takes advantage of all stages of the writing process to address students' personal goals. These can include a student's IEP goals as well as goals of the general education curriculum. Scaffolding can be designed for activities that involve planning, organizing, drafting, revising, editing, publishing, and presenting. In this section, we have highlighted some of the writing lab opportunities to address social interaction, language and literacy, and self-regulatory controls associated with each of these phases. The techniques have emphasized the use of instructor and peer discourse, minilesson handouts, computer software supports, and other environmental and technology supports. Possibilities are endless. Both instructor and student creativity grow in the process of establishing an inclusive community of authors.

SCAFFOLDING LANGUAGE TARGETS

Spoken and written language use depend on abilities to construct 1) morphemes from one or more phoneme or letter; 2) words from one or more morpheme; 3) sentences from one or more word; and 4) discourse from one or more sentence (as discussed in Chapter 2). In the writing lab approach, this part-to-whole view can be balanced with a whole-to-part description, which focuses on language organization in the progression of discourse, sentences, words, and sounds. Chapters 14 and 15 describe how to use such an organizational framework for conducting individualized assessments and creating individualized intervention plans. This approach is supported by Berninger, who demonstrated that "individual writers vary as to whether they have relative strengths and/or weaknesses at the word, sentence, and text levels in translating ideas into visible language" (2000, p. 67).

In our analysis system of language targets and "language levels," we include writing conventions, as well as spoken communication. These language-level divisions are somewhat artificial, but they contribute to individualized planning. They guide team members to know what to scaffold for a particular student at a specific point in time.

Discourse Level Targets and Scaffolds

When discourse macrostructures become part of a person's intrinsic knowledge, the old, or background, information enables the person to concentrate on the new, or foreground, information, which, in turn, enhances comprehension. Scardamalia and Bereiter (1986) found that expert writers use 1) knowledge of basic text structures to help organize their writing, 2) strategies from memory and external sources to generate content, and 3) goals and plans for their writing to achieve those goals.

Scaffolding Narrative Discourse

In the process of teaching students to construct their own written discourse, instructors focus students on the structures of texts they listen to or read themselves. This practice leads to new organizational possibilities for writing. In reciprocal fashion, as students learn to organize ideas to achieve communicative purposes, they develop higher-order thinking and language abilities they can use for understanding more complex texts.

In Chapter 15, we offer several strategies for assessing the developmental maturity and structural complexity of students' discourse macrostructures. We suggest using a classic European story grammar to characterize advancing narrative maturity and to establish intervention targets for movement to the next higher level (Hedberg & Westby, 1993; Stein & Glenn, 1982). In the following paragraphs, we describe scaffolding techniques to support these developments.

Scaffolding Isolated Descriptions

When students are working on isolated descriptions of people, places, or events, instructors can use the authentic audience principles to scaffold more elaborate descriptions. They do this by expressing their interest in the students' ideas and getting them to provide more detailed oral descriptions of main characters and other aspects of settings, such as "What did the snake look like?" Then, they can scaffold students to put more of this detail in writing.

Scaffolding Temporal Sequences

When students are producing isolated descriptions, instructors scaffold them to connect events temporally into sequences. Such stories often have a dominant "And then . . . " quality. A scaffold that can lead students to this level is, "I wonder what happened next."

Scaffolding Reactive Sequences

To reach the level of reactive sequences, students must include cause–effect relationships. Instructors assist students to express causal relationships by asking *why* questions such as, "Was there a reason why the men were going into battle?"

Scaffolding Abbreviated Episodes

To reach the level of abbreviated episodes, students must clearly state a problem and imply or state their characters' aims or intentions to solve it. To scaffold these, instructors ask strategic questions to encourage students to think about problems their characters are facing. The process might start with a simple question such as, "Does your story have a problem?" Scaffolds also can probe the landscape of consciousness for characters, for example, "I wonder why the kids decided to go into the haunted house."

Scaffolding Complete Episodes

To reach the level of complete episodes, students must clearly state their characters' plans to achieve goals and solve their problems. Complete episodes also include an ending that brings closure. Scaffolds for these elements involve deeper prodding into the landscape of consciousness, focused on goal setting and planning. For example, the instructor might ask, "How did they decide to go on?" Scaffolding also can ask students to think about a good ending for their stories. A minilesson on the topic could involve a brainstorm about what makes a good ending. Students also could be directed to think about the endings of favorite stories and to tell what they like and dislike about those endings. Older students could be asked to debate the relative merits of happy endings.

Scaffolding Complex/Multiple Episodes

To reach the level of complex or multiple episodes, students must add obstacles to the goal path or write more than one abbreviated or complete episode. To scaffold such elements, the instructor asks, for example, "Is that the end or is there more? What if something else happened? What if it weren't so easy to solve the problem?"

Story grammar templates also can be used to help students include all critical components and elaborate their written narratives (Graves & Montague, 1991; Roth, 2000). We have used a variety of story grammar supports, including some generated with computer software (see examples in Chapter 4). Our research has shown positive effects of such supports in helping students to plan and organize their narratives strategically (Bahr, Nelson, & Van Meter, 1996). Such supports might consist of a graphic organizer, list of desired elements, or on-screen templates prompting students to include characters, setting, problem, plan, outcome, and ending. We also have added notes to students' notebooks that say, "Feelings make my story interesting." The transaction around the meaning of a particular narrative, however, is most likely to trigger higher levels of thinking, not just providing a list of desirable parts.

Scaffolding Expository Discourse

Expository texts, regardless of subgenre, share the general purpose of providing information. In order to do so, authors first must organize existing information and plan a strategy for gathering new information. Gathering new information implies research. Options for conducting research include reading about a topic in books, searching the Internet, or using CD-ROM encyclopedias. Other options include interviewing others or experimenting first hand. Any of these elements presents learning opportunities for addressing other IEP and general education goals and objectives.

Reading for a purpose and taking notes can be a particularly powerful technique for building reading comprehension skills within the context of expository writing lab activities (Westby, 1999a). Scaffolding in such cases includes skills for isolating a topic, organizing a set of questions to address a purpose, finding sources that might help answer the questions, skimming the text to look for key words and phrases that suggest possible answers, reading carefully to see if the sections do provide useful information, then closing the book (or darkening the computer screen), and putting the information in the author's own words. Chapter 4 provides a minilesson handout for use in teaching notetaking skills.

Once an initial set of notes is collected, organizing is used as a transition to drafting. It involves taking main ideas and turning them back into sentences. Although the cognitive-linguistic demands of these activities are multiple, so are the learning opportunities. As students develop their drafts, they can be scaffolded to use all stages and tools of the writing process to evaluate their growing compositions. Print and instructor scaffolds can focus them on such characteristics as completeness, transitions, and how well their work is meeting its purpose for a particular audience.

Discourse-level organizational scaffolds should be aimed at helping students abstract the macrostructures of the particular subgenre being targeted. Expository discourse subgenres vary widely. Exposure to variations in expository textbook examples, with scaffolding to make structures explicit, can provide students with background schemas for completing the writing tasks that many high-stakes districtwide and statewide tests employ.

In order to scaffold students to competent uses of expository subgenres, instructors first need to analyze key characteristics of the targeted type themselves. They then scaffold students to discover those key features as well. Instructors can use computer software (e.g., *Inspiration*, Inspiration Software) or generate their own templates as guides for features of expository subgenres that should be incorporated into authors' plans. Mnemonic acronyms such as TREE and STOP–DARE (Graham et al., 2000) were designed for similar purposes to assist students in the process of SRSD to organize and evaluate expository texts.

As noted in Chapter 5, we think students should learn to play an active role in constructing discourse features, not just to memorize mnemonic devices. In our experience, this is more conducive to making the learning more accessible over time. Such instruction involves framing the problem as addressing a particular audience for a specific purpose. If students can learn to ask themselves such questions as "What am I trying to do here?" and respond with a clear statement of purpose, they have a more flexible and dynamic tool for generating questions to guide their research than a memorized mnemonic device provides.

Scaffolding techniques for supporting students to produce varied expository discourse subgenres are described in the sections that follow. To organize this discussion, we use the list of expository genres and associated functions provided by Westby and Clauser (1999, p. 191). This set differs from the set for narratives, however, because this list is not a developmental sequence. Rather, scaffolds are suggested to help students make developmental advances in expository texts as evidenced by the "five facets or traits: organization, content, written language style (syntax, cohesion, vocabulary), written conventions, and sense of audience" (Westby & Clauser, 1999, p. 271).

Scaffolding Descriptive Texts

Descriptive texts tell what something is. Framing scaffolds for descriptive texts should be designed to help students appreciate the goal of using specific, interesting words to help their readers form mind pictures that match what the author was thinking. Actual drawings may help young children or those with severe disabilities learn how to describe. We have encouraged children with limited vocabulary, such as kindergarten children who are deaf and hard of hearing, to draw first. Clip art and scene depiction software tools (described in Chapter 7) could be used by any child but are specifically helpful to children whose motor control issues make them single switch users (see Chapter 11).

Following the constructive learning principle, when students generate their own ideas, they are primed to connect new vocabulary to represent them. In such contexts, older students might be scaffolded to use more descriptive vocabulary for different parts of speech (e.g., more interesting verbs, adjectives, and adverbs, as well as nouns). Such metalinguistic terms typically are not used in scaffolding until they are introduced in the general curriculum. Earlier, scaffolding language is chosen to trigger questions that would lead the child to find better words to describe each grammatical role. For example, to scaffold better action terms, the instructor might say, "Close your eyes, and see your fish moving through the water. What does that action look like? How could you describe it to me so I will see the same thing?"

Students can be asked to generate words related to a category of ideas in order to keep them in the constructive role. For example, when a class of third graders we worked with was engaged in a social studies project to plan a business and to describe the human resources they would need to run it, we had numerous occasions to help students in small groups associate new vocabulary with partially developed concepts. First, they had to contemplate the meaning of *human*. Then, they were helped to describe and label such jobs as cashier for *the person who takes the money* and chef for *the person who cooks the food.* The result is richer concepts.

Scaffolding Enumerative Texts

Enumerative texts use a listing format to elaborate on a topic. Brainstorming guided by a graphic organizer, either with pencil and paper or computer, is a good strategy for generating lists. Then, items are evaluated for goodness of fit. Some software programs (e.g., *Inspiration*, Inspiration Software) include features to support this activity. As students grow in competence and have names for the strategies they have been learning (e.g., *brainstorming, webbing*), they can be given examples of enumerative texts and be asked what tools they know that would help them with this kind of writing. The goal is to help students use all of their tools and strategies independently.

One of the fifth-grade students in our after-school writing lab, Shena, was a natural list generator. When we prompted her to pick a topic and write about it, she generated a list of uses for balloons (see Box 6.1). A peer scaffolded Shena to elaborate her planning web by adding another level of subordination, which served as a reminder to us of the immense power of peer mediation. Shena immediately integrated this technique into her repertoire and was able to use it independently in subsequent writing.

Scaffolding Sequential/Procedural Texts

Sequential/procedural texts tell about events or instruct how to complete a task. To scaffold such texts, instructors can support students to select topics that tell about familiar experiences or can provide the experiences themselves. Early childhood teachers and clinicians often use cooking or art exercises to activate procedural knowledge. Then, they support groups of students to generate language to communicate the experience to others. A feedback scaffold might include following the student's directions exactly, without inferring any missing steps. The results of following inadequate instructions exactly can help students identify areas where their procedures need a more detailed description. One activity that might serve a dual function would be to have teams: 1) learn a new software feature, 2) write an instruction manual to teach classmates to use the feature, and 3) test it out.

In a variation on sequential texts, we have addressed a general education curriculum goal by helping third graders to develop personal timelines. This activity requires support from home, but we have used it in communities where that support is not always forthcoming. Students take home a structural scaffold about important life events designed for parents and their children to complete together. Alternatively, teachers or school social workers may use student records, older siblings, and other known information to help gather background data. Then, students use the notes to connect ideas sequentially and to select clip art to illustrate them. Their parents' or guardians' words serve as scaffolds for the drafting process, and students begin to learn something about paraphrasing. Computer-software features that allow users to connect ideas in a particular sequence make the sequencing feature more salient for students still grasping that concept. Box 6.2 shows the final product of one student who had been struggling earlier in the year to get any words on paper.

Box 6.1. Effects of Peer Scaffolding During Planning for Expository Description

When Shena began planning her expository piece on balloons, her idea of semantic webbing was to put one idea in the center and to connect all other ideas to it. At one point, her friend, Kayla, looked over and showed her how to map a third level of ideas, adding to the complexity of her simple report (see Figure 6.2)

A few months later Shena was able to use the more complex planning schema independently when generating questions to guide her research for an expository report on planets with rings (see Figure 6.3).

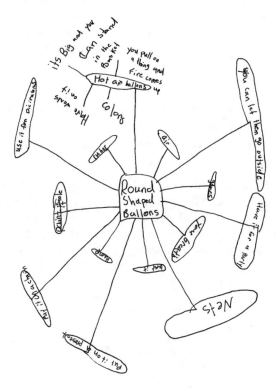

Figure 6.2.   Effects of peer scaffolding during planning for expository description.

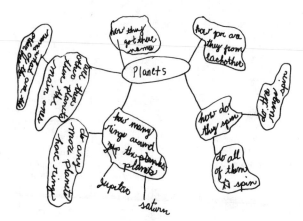

Figure 6.3.   Planning for sequential-procedural discourse and changes following scaffolding.

203

Box 6.2. Time-Line Sequence Produced with Scaffolding by a Third-Grade Student

Randy started his third-grade school year as a reluctant writer with many negative behaviors who combined avoidance and "I can't" strategies. He said he could think of no topics for his first baseline story, and he did not want to write. With heavy scaffolding supported by partial dictation, he produced a story at the level of temporal sequence with 8 T-units and 53 words.

Randy's goals included interacting appropriately in social conversation, initiating ideas for writing, producing sentences with minimal scaffolding, and working independently. As the school year progressed, Randy's behavioral issues were channeled into more positive activities of peer assistance when he assumed a special helping role with a classmate with special education needs. Toward the end of the year, Randy wrote a trip story with minimal scaffolding about a vacation to Mexico with his family.

> I like going on vacation because it is a lot of fun. I have been to
> many states. My favorite is Texas. I have even been to a different
> country—Mexico. There are a lot of Spanish people in Mexico.

He also produced a time line that is shown in Figure 6.4. By the end of the school year, Randy's final probe showed him capable of producing a story at the level of a complete episode, which included 28 T-units and 208 words. A special moment came for Randy when he was scaffolding Filip, his peer, to read his final story from author chair. Filip, who had needed almost complete scaffolding to read aloud earlier in the year, was reading independently. Randy turned to his instructor and said, with delight, "He's reading it by himself!"

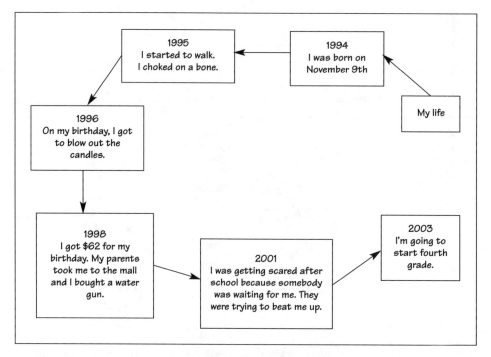

Figure 6.4.   Time-line sequence produced with scaffolding by a third-grade student.

204

Scaffolding Compare–Contrast Texts

Compare–contrast texts show how two or more things are the same or different. Figure 6.5 provides an example of how a peer dyad made up of a special education student and general education peer completed a compare-contrast activity. We have repeated this activity with success in several early elementary classrooms as an introduction to the compare–contrast genre. The activity is designed also to facilitate social interaction discourse, as students need to interview each other to identify their similarities and differences.

Compare–contrast texts lend themselves to various other curriculum-based activities as well. For example, students can learn to compare and contrast different books. Depending on their ages and prior learning, they might even be able to generate their own self-scaffolding tools for categories that could be used to structure the essay, (e.g., purpose of the book, type of story, setting, problems the characters faced, how the characters solved their problems, endings, how well the author told the story, how the student felt about each book). Then, they can learn to contrast two books on each feature.

Scaffolding Problem–Solution Texts

Problem–solution texts state a problem and offer solutions. Scaffolding is enhanced when students start with a problem that draws on their experiences. In one third-grade classroom, the students were addressing a general curriculum goal of writing business letters. They brainstormed problems about which they could write to the principal and decided that their building was looking shabby. Once the topic was selected, the class brainstormed possible solutions, such as replacing stained ceiling tiles and repainting rooms. Then, they learned the features of business letters and wrote individual letters sharing their suggestions with their principal. As on outcome, they were allowed to paint the ceiling tiles.

Scaffolding Persuasive Texts

Persuasive texts require the author to take a position on some issue and to justify it. K. McAlister (personal communication, 1999) worked with students and their elementary school special education teacher to review products (e.g., favorite pens or pencils, snacks, or other foods) and persuade others why they should like them as well. Later, the students did movie reviews. In the process of completing both projects, students were scaffolded to notice that their arguments worked better if they first introduced a product, then gave several good reasons why the audience should like it, and finally closed with a summarizing statement. The students used this discourse framework to construct scripts. Then, they videotaped their persuasive essays, using the products as props to make their arguments. They worked on their performances to improve them, and their final performances involved a real audience of students from other classes who responded by telling how the persuasive arguments made them want to try the products or go see the movie.

Scaffolding Cause–Effect Texts

Cause–effect texts describe causal relationships. Topic selection again is important to set the stage for writing cause–effect texts. For younger students, cause–effect elements might be targeted first within narratives. Older students might be scaffolded to select research topics about matters of personal interest (e.g., "Why did dinosaurs become extinct?" "What are the causes of pollution in a local river?").

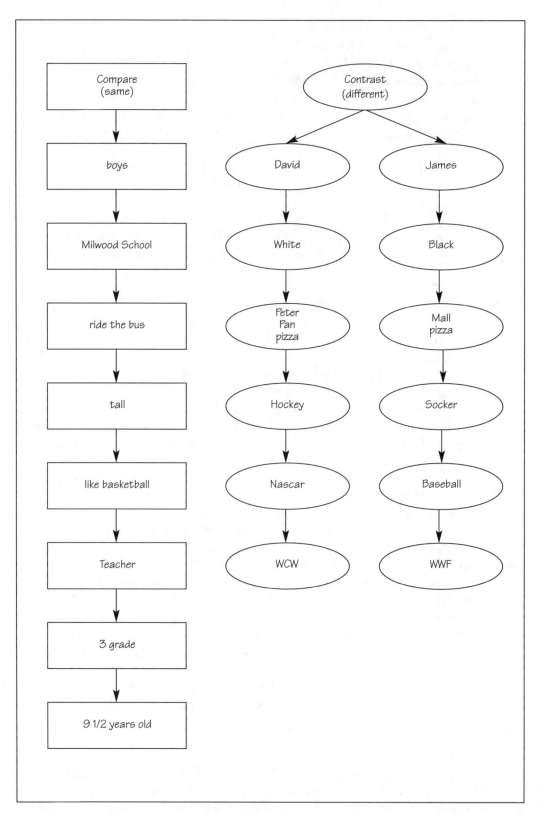

Figure 6.5. Compare–contrast organizer created by a peer dyad.

Scaffolding Other Discourse Genres

Beyond narrative and expository discourse, many other discourse possibilities exist. Each carries with it a set of enhanced language learning opportunities.

Scaffolding Friendly or Business Letters

Letter-writing projects present opportunities to make the authentic audience principle particularly salient. A framing scaffold for getting students started on letters to the school principal, for example, might be, "Pretend you saw Mrs. Clarkson in the hall. How would you start a conversation with her?" A letter to a local business to ask for information could begin by leading the class to brainstorm, "What do you think the people in the business would want to know about you?"

Scaffolding Poetry

Poetry projects are particularly suited to scaffolding students to use colorful language, interesting words, and language describing feelings. Scaffolds focused on how language sounds and its varied rhythms can be supported by reading poetry to students before getting them started on their own poems. Students who hear a variety of poems, some of which rhyme and some of which do not, have more choices for experimenting with the genre themselves. They can learn to write acrostic poems and haiku, which often are targeted in the general education curriculum, but they also can learn to create word pictures with their language in free verse. With free verse, students can decide where to break lines so that others will read the poem with their original intent for how the poem should sound. Focusing students on the "enter" or "return" feature on computer keyboards can make such line-break decisions more salient. Figure 4.2 includes an example of team planning related to taking advantage of the learning demands of poetry.

Summary of Scaffolding Other Discourse Genres

Part of the goal for teaching students to experiment with different discourse genres is to help them develop diverse ways of thinking and to develop cognitive structures they can draw on when faced with similar macrostructures in the general education curriculum. Another part of the goal is for students to be able to think dynamically about the best literate formats for communicating their ideas to others. One way to scaffold this manner of flexible thinking is to provide some free-writing opportunities in addition to structured class projects. During free writing, students should be allowed to select their discourse genre and topics and to control their writing schedules. One of our colleagues, a language arts specialist, devised a minilesson for helping students select a genre and plan specific goals for advancing their writing (see Figure 6.6). Opportunities for students to share their work, such as peer conferencing or author chair, are critical to keeping the authentic audience principle salient during such experiences. Instructors also can label discourse genres in their scaffolding comments (e.g., "Isn't it nice that Alicia chose to write a poem and Jesse chose to write a story? When authors choose different ways to share their work, they have different effects on their audience").

Scaffolding Other Discourse-Level Features

Beyond a focus on macrostructures, scaffolding at the discourse level can support students to improve such skills as sense of audience, use of cohesive devices, and syntactic transitions. The general approach is to help students attend to communicative purpose and effect.

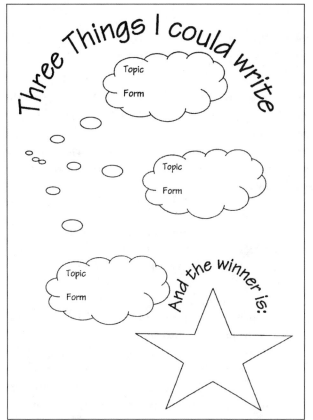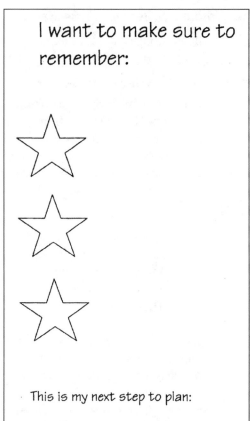

Figure 6.6. Anne Lape's minilesson for selecting discourse genres. ©2004 Anne Lape.

Sense of audience is a stylistic element that can be scaffolded across genres. In successful interactions, communicators provide information sufficient to meet partner needs without saying too much. In spoken conversations, adjustments are based on on-line feedback that is active and ongoing. In written discourse, authors must imagine their reading audience and decide what information to provide (Lund, 2000). The writing lab approach helps students acquire a sense of audience through peer feedback and adult scaffolding. When peers ask authentic questions about missing critical details, students begin to fine-tune their internalized sense of audience. Instructors also scaffold students to include appropriate levels of detail by asking strategic questions about missing information during drafting and revising processes.

Such techniques also can target linguistic cohesion and transition skills. These include strategies for making pronoun reference clear and unambiguous, for using logical or temporal connectors, and for making smooth transitions from one sentence to the next. For example, one third-grade student with language-learning risks wrote about her dog running away. She told how she discovered her dog tied up at a neighbor's house and how she went to get her mother. At that point, her draft read,

> When I first saw Lucky on a short rope and I ran back to my house and told her their was a dog on a rope and I had to bag her to come and then she got up When we got their my mom talked to her and she asked if the dog was for sale and she said yes so she paid her and then When we pet her for a few meanuts we let him out side When he got out side he just stude there.

In scaffolding this student, the instructor made some decisions about the child's emotional state and openness to revision possibilities. Two things stood out in this portion of the discourse: problems with pronoun reference and frequent (but not quite accurate) initiation of sentences with *when* introducing a subordinate clause. This second feature was recognized as a sign of growth for this student because her earlier stories had consisted almost exclusively of simple sentences, and now she was starting to indicate transitions and connect ideas with complex sentences. Therefore, at the moment, a choice was made to bring up only the pronoun reference issue so as not to overwhelm the student. Recommendations for scaffolding at this point, include the following:

1. Start the scaffolding interaction with a genuine compliment about a positive feature (e.g., "I love the details you are putting in your story. I can picture your dog on the short rope").

2. Frame the problem of pronoun reference (e.g., "But I do get confused in a couple of places").

3. Focus the student on the first *her* by pointing to it (e.g., "When you write *her* right here, I am not sure who you mean." Scaffold the student to change *her* to *my mom*).

4. Scaffold the student to use a rereading strategy to support revision (e.g., "Let's reread what you have now for that sentence." Read the sentence aloud. "It's sounding a lot clearer now, isn't it?").

5. Scaffold a higher degree of independence in repeating the new strategy (e.g., "Why don't you read the next sentence and see if all your characters are clear in that one, too?"). Try having the student read the next sentence. If necessary, use a feedback scaffold to convey uncertainty about which "*she*" said yes, and scaffold the student to recognize the need to indicate *the girl* for clarity.

6. Frame the problem with inconsistent pronoun gender reference to the dog (e.g., "I also wasn't sure if it was a girl dog or a boy dog. Why don't you read this sentence again and see if it says what you want." In this case, the student was able to detect the inconsistency and make the revision with minimal scaffolding.).

7. Unless the student is starting to show frustration, at this point the instructor could frame the problem of smooth transitions and gauge the student's response (e.g., "Is it okay if I show you one more thing?" If the student says no, the instructor must respect that, perhaps indicating, "I'll let you work on your story a while by yourself and come back in a little bit. It's really good, but I think you can make a few more improvements." If the student, indicates yes, the scaffolding can continue. "Here's what I want to know. After your mom paid and you got your dog back, did you go back home before you started petting the dog, or did you pet him at the neighbor's house and let him outside there?").

8. Encourage revisions to clarify the transition issue, perhaps in spoken language first, then helping the student to formulate the written discourse. A good idea is to walk away to encourage independence and to return later to check on progress. In this case, with minimal scaffolding, the student was able to revise the discourse orally to say, "We took him home. After we petted him for a few minutes, we let him outside." She was able to make those changes on her paper independently.)

As evident in this example, discourse transitions are thoroughly intertwined with syntax. In fact, students can be scaffolded to attempt a wider variety of discourse transition techniques through encouragement to experiment with syntactic alternatives. For example, Wong (2000) described the use of a "prompt card" to support high school students in thinking of transition phrases, referred to as "signal words," that they could use in their opinion essays. These prompt cards, which were available to the students while drafting, included (Wong, Butler, Ficzere, & Kuperis, 1996)

- Introductory phrases (e.g., *in my opinion, I disagree/agree with, from my point of view, I believe*)

- Countering phrases (e.g., *although, on the other hand, on the contrary, however*)

- Concluding phrases (e.g., *after considering both sides, even though, to sum up, in conclusion*)

- Supporting words and phrases (e.g., *first, second, finally, equally important, for instance, as well*)

Computer supports are particularly helpful for scaffolding more mature transitions because transitions make good targets during the revision process. Revising is less frustrating when computer tools can be used rather than recopying. Author groups and author chair audiences provide feedback that can be used to identify points in discourse where greater clarity or smoother cohesion is needed. Then, transitions can be improved while revising at the computer or while revising computer printouts in the classroom (with revisions to be made at the computer later).

Sentence-Level Targets and Scaffolds

Throughout this book, we recommend scaffolds aimed at achieving communicative purposes. In the previous section, we emphasized communicative roles played by sentence-level devices within larger discourse structures. Focusing scaffolds can be used to make such relationships apparent. The by-product will be the achievement of sentence-level goals, such as production of complete and correct sentences of advancing complexity. In writing lab contexts, such goals are not an end in themselves but a means to a more relevant and permanent set of effective literate language communication skills. General suggestions for scaffolding at the sentence level include the following recommendations:

1. Have students with relatively stronger spoken language skills read or tell a story and add spoken features to their written drafts.

2. Ask questions about sentence links that do not seem logical to get students to clarify relationships.

3. Use rereading focus and feedback scaffolding to help students notice errors in grammatical structure.

4. Model more complex syntax in discussions with students about their meanings.

Scaffolding students to higher levels of sentence-level ability requires instructional teams to increase goal expectations over time. Long before they come to school, young children acquire competence with basic sentence structures. By the time they enter school, most know how to produce and understand basic subject–predicate propositions; to elaborate noun and verb phrases by adding adjectives and adverbs; and to embed, combine, and subordinate phrases and clauses. The same may not be true for students with LLDs and other needs (see Chapter 3 and summaries in Nelson, 1998; Paul, 2001; Silliman et al., 2000).

Even children who develop conversational competence with simple and complex sentences in their preschool years may not have a firm sense of what a sentence is at the meta-level. Generally, experience with the literate forms of written sentences is necessary to gain such metalinguistic understandings. There is evidence to support modeling scaffolds in that children exposed to more complex syntactic structures in the discourse of others may begin to employ them in discourse of their own (Gummersall & Strong, 1999). As children learn to punctuate sentences, instructors can scaffold metalinguistic knowledge of sentence structures such as questions, statements, and exclamations.

Students with language limitations can learn to differentiate comments and questions on a metalinguistic level, as well, by using author chair experiences. When an author calls on two peers to make comments and two other peers to ask questions, students have an authentic reason to raise syntactic distinctions to a conscious level. For example, when one student with disabilities was called on to raise a question during an author chair activity, he demonstrated his growing metalinguistic skills for syntactic structures and functions by saying, "I liked the part . . . oh, that's a comment, I mean, was it a circus dog?" He realized that he was making a comment and corrected himself by asking a question.

The writing lab approach employs teacher and peer scaffolding to help children "hear" whether their drafted sentences make sense, are complete, and convey enough information for the reader. Ultimately, the test of a sentence's adequacy should rest not on its structure, but on the degree to which it achieves its communicative function. Similarly, the best scaffolds are those that help children identify communication breakdowns (Lund, 2000). In conference about their written work, students often can provide information that may be missing from the words on the page. They can develop sentence-level skills as they learn to express their ideas in more complex language through scaffolding aimed at repairing communication breakdowns. Students who demonstrate higher-level syntax in spoken and written language expression have more knowledge for spoken and written language comprehension as well.

Constructing one's own sentences on a computer screen offers unique opportunities for reflecting on sentence formulation and tinkering with it. Spoken sentences are gone once uttered, but sentences in a computer file have relative permanence, enhancing possibilities for later revision. The insert and cut-and-paste functions of computer software programs allow students to revise their own language forms. The possibility to insert words, such as conjunctions, or to use cut-and-paste features to revise syntax can contribute to metalinguistic concepts about sentence structure.

Word-Level Targets and Scaffolds

Word-level targets can be considered from the perspective of vocabulary fluency and specificity. They also can be considered from the perspective of phonological encoding and spelling. Both perspectives have important implications across spoken and written language domains.

Scaffolding Vocabulary Fluency and Specificity

General suggestions for scaffolding appropriately specific and descriptive words include

1. Frame the problem by helping the student set goals to use more interesting words.

2. Focus the student on selecting words that will help readers see the same picture the author sees.

3. Focus the student on any new vocabulary that is part of the instructions or curriculum content in curriculum-driven projects.

4. Feedback cues about omitted or substituted words by reading back the text exactly as written, or use a speech synthesis computer software feature to do the same.

5. Feedback cues about words used imprecisely or incorrectly by expressing confusion about meanings.

6. Guide the student to find words that fit the discourse context by asking strategic questions.

7. Guide the student to use computer editing features to make word changes during revising.

8. Celebrate new and unusual word choices to activate the student's attention to new vocabulary in the environment.

Scaffolding interesting word choices involves helping students think about word pictures they are drawing for their reading audience. As students experience success in using interesting words that others appreciate, they begin to soak up new words from the environment. A scaffolding technique for encouraging more mature word choices is to express delight when a student revises a paper by inserting a specifically chosen and communicative word to replace such all-purpose words as *thing* or *stuff* as nouns; *do, make,* or *go* as verbs; and *good, pretty,* and *big* as adjectives. The focus in these scaffolding events is on how some words communicate better than others to the reader. One third-grade teacher on our team urged her student to produce more interesting descriptions by saying, "I want to *see* what you and Tasha were wearing as you walked down the street. I want to *taste* the candy you were carrying in the bag. I want to *hear* the sound of the bag breaking open and the candy hitting the ground. I want to *feel* how you felt when it was all gone."

As children develop literacy skills, they use more interesting words to communicate more elaborate meanings. Vocabulary development, word storage, and retrieval are interactive developmental processes (German, 1994). As students write, some struggle to think of words they know but cannot retrieve at the moment. In such instances of word-finding difficulty, instructors should use dynamic assessment to identify cues that work best for particular students to scaffold better word retrieval. For example, depending on the situation and the student, instructors might try 1) initial phoneme cues (e.g., "Can you think of what sound the girl's name started with?"); 2) meaning cues (e.g., "Are you looking for words to tell how the man looked when he was angry?"); or 3) syntactic closure cues (e.g., "The candy scattered when the bag . . . ").

Scaffolding at the word level shares the goal of helping students acquire higher-level skills and strategies they can deploy independently. As they mature in their writing, students can learn to use computer software thesaurus tools to help them find more interesting word choices, as described in Chapter 9.

Scaffolding Spelling

Targeting spelling as word-level knowledge emphasizes the integration of sound-level and word-level language abilities. Ehri (2000) noted that there are at least three distinct ways to read and spell words: by memory, by invention, and by analogy.

Scott (2000) summarized recommendations for helping poor spellers in the context of authentic writing activities. To do so, instructional teams should 1) schedule many opportunities for authentic reading and writing, 2) capitalize on teachable moments for helping students learn individualized spelling rules, 3) use text-level bridging activities in sessions where they use word-level activities, and 4) use high-interest text, such as e-mail and the Internet, to build spelling vocabularies. Treiman and Bourassa (2000a) found advantages for working on spelling concepts in writing rather than orally. They compared children's written and oral spelling capabilities and found that "children, like adults, more accurately analyze the linguistic structure of a spoken item when they can represent the results in a lasting, visible form than when they cannot" (p. 183).

Students' invented spellings reflect their perceptions of the phonetic structure of words. Literacy learning requires that children first grasp the alphabetic principle— "the idea that written spellings represent spoken words," but that is not enough (Snow et al., 1998, p. 4). Poor spellers often rely on memory for letter position and visual matching because they have difficulty learning sound–letter association rules (Kamhi & Hinton, 2000). Scaffolding students to spell unfamiliar words can help them associate letters with the auditory and kinesthetic patterns of their own speech—and vice versa. Scaffolding aimed at phonemic awareness might involve showing students how to "stretch" their word productions by watching the instructor's mouth and attempting to feel speech sound production features in their own mouths as they say words slowly in imitation. Reciprocal benefits can be observed on speech production, perception, reading, and writing.

Effective scaffolding for spelling varies with the developmental stage of the students. Research supports early intervention for at-risk spellers that starts by training the alphabetic principle (connections between phonemes and one- and two-letter spelling units), but then combines whole word and onset–rime feedback (Berninger, 2000). Our suggestion is to use individualized assessment (see Chapter 15) to gather evidence about the developmental spelling stage that seems best to characterize a student's current level of performance, then use scaffolding to focus the student on cues at the next higher level.

Developmental spelling scales can be controversial (Treiman & Bourassa, 2000a, 2000b). They also vary in their design and focus (Ehri, 1986, 2000). In Chapter 15, we describe a system that works well for us, which we adapted from Ehri (1986) and Gentry (1982). It aims at supporting students as they advance through five roughly divided stages:

1. Prephonetic—scribbled, letterlike symbols

2. Semiphonetic—real letters representing words, syllables, or sounds (e.g., "N E" for *any*)

3. Phonetic—invented spellings reflecting children's concepts of how words sound (e.g., "chree" for *tree*; "laik" for *like*)

4. Transitional—a mixture of phonetic and orthographic strategies with more conventional spelling for some morphemes (e.g., "loshun" for *lotion*; "lagh" for *laugh*; "menbers" for *members*; "soulution" for *solution*)

5. Conventional—fewer misspellings and facility with both regular and irregular orthographic patterns

Scaffolding Prephonetic Spellers

It is never too early to include students with disabilities in authentic writing projects. If necessary, these students can dictate their ideas and use emerging skills to decode words that others, such as a peer or instructor, have written for them. Opportunities for prephonetic spellers to take the author chair may provide them with the motivation they need to persist through more structured instructional activities and to link their developing skills to sense-making and communication.

Scaffolding techniques can be used to encourage students to attempt invented spellings, leading them to grasp the alphabetic principle that letters represent sounds. Some students with disabilities, however, need more explicit and concentrated instruction to develop phonemic awareness and sound–symbol associations. In particular, students with dyslexia may require special interventions (Catts & Kamhi, 1999). A variety of structured multisensory approaches are available to target phonemic awareness and sound–symbol associations directly, if necessary. For example, the Lindamood Phoneme Sequencing Program for Reading, Spelling, and Speech (http://www.lindamoodbell.com), the Wilson Language Training approach (http://www.wilsonlanguage.com), and the Orton-Gillingham approach (http://www.orton-gillingham.com) are some of the most well known.

These approaches can be implemented separately in special education or speech-language therapy rooms. Students who need such interventions also should be included in writing lab activities to practice their new skills in meaningful contexts, as recommended by Scott (2000). This intervention can happen as child and instructor share a pencil or computer keyboard and the instructor focuses the student on the multisensory cues that are being learned in the related context.

Scaffolding Semiphonetic Spellers

As students begin to acquire sound–symbol knowledge, instructors can assist them to make more automatic connections for a wider repertoire of phonemes and letters. For students with phonological awareness problems, writing lab activities provide both a functional need for and strategies to recall sound and syllable patterns. Scott's (2000) recommendation for authentic writing projects and extensive practice to build spelling skill can occur within the writing lab approach. The speech synthesis feature that is included in many children's writing software programs can help to provide feedback to support this process of recursive spelling and checking.

Scaffolding Phonetic Spellers

Many children with phonological awareness difficulties have age-level articulation abilities that instructors can use to scaffold them to the phonetic level. Modeling can be used to show them how to produce words slowly. Then, focus scaffolds can be used to encourage students to hear and feel sequences of sounds in the mouth. An instructor might scaffold a child to spell the word *ship*, for example, by bridging from speech production to phonemic awareness.

"Let's say that word really slowly and listen for the sounds. You can feel them too. /sh-I-p/." [Make sure that the child watches the instructor's mouth and actually produces the word along with the model.]

"What's the first sound you hear?"

"What letters make the /sh/ sound?"

"Let's say *ship* again, and stretch the second sound." [Extend the /I/ sound in the co-production and isolate it for the student if necessary.]

"/I/, /I/, how do you spell /I/?"

[Continue the procedure as necessary through the final sound, but encourage greater independence. Revisit later without modeling until the student can employ the strategies independently. Perhaps add the new word to the student's personal dictionary section of the author notebook.]

Scaffolding Transitional Spellers

Fluent reading and writing also require children to grasp the orthographic principle, that is, "the ability to use a direct visual route without phonological mediation to access semantic memory and word meaning" (Kamhi & Catts, 1999b, p. 35). Morphemic-orthographic patterns are learned as students expand their invented spelling skills and read back words they have written. Students with special language and learning needs are less likely to recognize such repeatable patterns without explicit instruction. Their difficulties with automatic learning can be addressed through group minilessons to help all students "see" the patterns, followed by individual minilessons and extra practice for students with LLDs, supported by a special page in their author notebooks.

As students learn to associate syllables with patterns of letters, they recognize that such orthographic patterns as *lye, lie,* and *ligh* all are pronounced the same. This provides an important tool for decoding irregularly spelled words. Often, transitional spellers begin to experiment in their written work to achieve dictionary spellings independently. Also, when students develop orthographic stage recognition skills, they can begin to use computerized spelling-checker features more effectively. At this point, students can offer alternative spellings when words are highlighted as incorrect, and they can judge which alternative spelling offered by computer software represents the word they are seeking.

Research indicates that learning to decode words supports learning to spell them, and vice versa (Ehri, 2000). We have found that many students with wobbly phonological awareness skills spell both *in* and *and* as "in." This provides an opportunity to scaffold students' awareness of the two words' distinct meanings, pronunciations, and related spellings. The result is improved metalinguistic concepts that are critical to advancing to the level of conventional spelling. An instructor might say, for example, "I notice that you have the word *in* here in your story when you talk about "my dog in me." This is pretty tricky because sometimes that word does sound like *in* when we say it as, "my dog 'n me," but I think the word you mean is *and*. Let's say it together slowly. How would you spell that word?"

Other instructional opportunities for transitional learning arise in the context of helping students recognize spellings associated with common grammatical morphemes, such as, "There's that /-ing/ chunk again. Do you remember how to spell it?" If necessary, encourage students to turn to a section of their author notebooks, where spelling families are included. The goal is to scaffold students toward independent strategy use. The instructor could also say, "I see that you have heard the *-ed* ending in 'peekt.' You're right that it sounds like /t/, but we spell most of those *-ed* endings the same like this."

Next, the student can be taught to connect irregular but recognizable print patterns to spoken syllables of known words. For example, an instructor might say, "Let's look at that word *could.* You know some other words that sound like it—*would* and *should* are spelled the same way. How about if we put those into the word families section of your author notebook?"

Scaffolding Conventional Spellers

By definition, conventional spellers spell most words correctly. All spellers can continue to grow, however, and most adults—even strong spellers—have some spelling insecurities. Conventional spellers can use spelling-checker features with ease, so computer software can provide most of the scaffolding. Scaffolding could also focus conventional spellers on the morphological spelling conventions related to word etymology, such as those listed in Chapter 2. Bear, Inverness, Templeton, and Johnson (2000) related spelling and vocabulary development. This is one of the connections the writing lab approach is particularly able to support.

Scaffolding Writing Conventions

Scaffolds for writing conventions and speech clarity are parallel in that both focus on the surface features of communication rather than underlying meanings. Thus, timing is important to convey the sense that what students have to say is more important than how they say or write it. Although this basic value is established and continually reinforced, it is not frivolous to be concerned about elements of presentation (Graham, Berninger, Abbott, Abbott, & Whitaker, 1997).

A general rule of thumb is to scaffold writing conventions as aids to communication rather than treating them as features to be checked for errors. Writing conventions also deserve to be treated with respect in their own right. Errors of form not only can influence whether a message is actually received, but also whether it is received with a positive attitude and without distraction. Intervention teams, therefore, should focus scaffolding on the communicative value of such features and also communicative problems associated with their omission.

Writing conventions include capitalization, end punctuation, commas, quotation marks, and formatting. Formatting knowledge includes margins and paragraph indentation. Other formatting concerns are genre specific, such as line breaks in poetry and the address, salutation, and signature features in formal letters.

Using the keep it simple principle, instructional teams might limit their focus to a subset of writing conventions initially and add responsibilities for including new editorial conventions as students gain confidence. General curricular materials can be used to decide when and how to introduce minilessons on writing conventions and when to hold children responsible for independent application.

Instructors can use computer features to scaffold awareness of capitalization cues by guiding students to use the shift key. The motor act of capitalizing becomes more salient when students learn to hold the shift key down while typing the first letters of their names, main words in the titles of their stories, and first words in sentences. Thus, metalinguistic knowledge can be enhanced. This has helped some of our students move beyond the early stage of interspersing capital and lowercase letters in handwriting to strategic, language-based rules for capitalization.

Scaffolding for punctuation might start with guidance to insert end punctuation during editing processes at computers or desks. When one third-grade student with learning disabilities omitted all end punctuation, her classroom teacher provided good-natured feedback by telling the student she would read the story and take a breath when the punctuation told her to. Then, the teacher read on and on because there was, of course, no end punctuation. As the teacher became increasingly breathless, the student began to giggle. Then, she went back to her original draft, first with scaffolding, but then with increasing independence to add periods at sentence boundaries so her poor teacher would know when to breathe. This scaffolding helped the student make implicit knowledge of sentences explicit. Then, she learned to apply the newfound metalinguistic skill to using writing conventions.

The speech synthesis feature on children's writing software programs can be used similarly to scaffold this learning. For this to work, instructors must help students discover that the computer does not know where to end sentences unless the author uses punctuation to show it. They can only make the synthesized reading sound right if they punctuate correctly.

When children begin to include dialogue in their stories, they often are motivated to learn new punctuation, especially if an instructor expresses delight and appreciation for this emerging stylistic device. Sometimes, a student with disabilities is the first to experiment with dialogue. We have observed that some students are particularly fond of including dialogue in their stories, often preferring play writing and drama over narration. The appearance of dialogue in an authoring community sets the stage for minilessons on quotation marks, highlighting a particular student's contribution.

Scaffolds for writing conventions can be provided with any of the generic techniques described previously. A summary list includes

1. Read what the student wrote exactly as punctuated, or use the speech synthesis feature in children's software programs.

2. Scaffold the student to reread his or her own work, and note the value of punctuation for knowing where to pause.

3. Stress the value of writing conventions for making meanings clear and improving readability.

4. Emphasize editing for writing conventions in the editing stage for younger and less mature writers, using computer features to insert punctuation, change capital letters, and complete other age and ability appropriate edits.

5. Encourage more mature writers to develop their skills for monitoring the use of writing conventions as they write or type.

Scaffolding Spoken Communication Interactions

A full consideration of strategies for scaffolding children's spoken language development would require a book in itself. The fact that we devote less space to spoken language in describing the writing lab approach should not signal a lesser commitment to helping all children maximize their spoken as well as written language abilities. In fact, most of the writing lab contexts are designed to build on and contribute to students' spoken communication abilities explicitly.

Assessment guidelines and targets for spoken communication interactions, which are discussed in Chapter 15, include four areas of emphasis—listening comprehension, manner of speech production, topic maintenance, and linguistic skill. Spoken communication abilities are observed and scaffolded in contexts of peer editing and author groups, adult–child instructional scaffolding, and in author chair and formal presentations.

Listening comprehension targets include both social interaction and linguistic concerns. Social conventions include making eye contact with the speaker and listening without interrupting. Linguistic elements include direction following, as well as syntactic-pragmatic abilities for seeking clarification when needed.

Manner of speech production includes clear articulation and fluent speaking. Pragmatic features of appropriate eye gaze, proxemics (how close to stand), and vocal loudness can be targeted both in interpersonal and larger group interactions. When children have voice or fluency issues, practicing for formal presentations offers a powerful context for emphasizing other speech-language IEP goals.

Some students with communication issues struggle with topic maintenance. The writing lab offers many opportunities to observe whether students have conversation abilities that are appropriate to the situation in that they provide adequate information for their listeners, maintain the topic, and exhibit appropriate turn-taking skills. For example, in a peer editing session, an adult might scaffold students to take turns by beginning, "One suggestion is . . . " Students can practice asking relevant questions and sharing opinions in a sensitive manner during author groups and following author chair presentations. They can develop their topic maintenance skills in the context of discourse organization activities.

Treating behavior problems as communication and learning issues switches the focus from reward and punishment to learning new social skills. Students who are rejected by their peers can be engaged in setting goals related to peer interaction and to learning new skills that will enhance their acceptance. For example, they might learn about appropriate social distance and touching expectations, as in the case study presented in Chapter 13. Assessment might identify other factors at work when students are rarely asked to participate. When we observed one fifth-grade student who habitually was rejected by his peers, a part of the problem became apparent: a pattern of interruption and failing to listen to his peers. For him, things began to improve when he was taught to wait his turn and to be sensitive to cues that it was his turn to speak. In Randy's case, which was described in Box 6.2, behavioral problems subsided as he experienced positive feelings associated with helping a peer with special needs.

General suggestions for scaffolding spoken communication include

1. Encourage students to develop a public voice for group discussions and presentations.

2. Develop a routine for author group leadership and participation so that students can develop social communication and leadership skills.

3. Provide opportunities for students to practice for publishing party presentations using videotaped feedback, and provide chances for students to set personal goals.

4. Consider whether violations of social-pragmatic expectations might be a source of apparent behavior problems, and help students develop goals and new communication skills that will keep them from repeating well-practiced, negative routines that get them in trouble and isolate them from peers.

Summary of Scaffolding for Addressing Language Targets

The goals that result from language assessment activities can be used to plan scaffolding aimed at language targets at the discourse, sentence, and word levels. The word level includes word selection and retrieval targets, as well as spelling strategies. Developmental sequences are used when available to guide scaffolding decisions. Examples are provided for scaffolding students at next higher narrative and spelling levels. Language targets also include writing conventions and spoken communication. Scaffolding techniques are described for these as well.

SUMMARY

This chapter describes uses of scaffolding to support the development of higher-level writing processes and language targets. Scaffolding techniques are presented for the writing processes of planning, organizing, drafting, revising, editing, and presenting; for language targets at the level of discourse, sentences, and words (including syllables, morphemes, and phonemes for spelling); and for writing conventions and spoken communication.

Using Software Features to Support the Writing Process

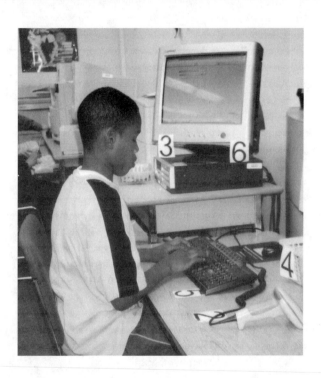

Personal computers are an integral component of nearly all aspects of life. New hardware and software applications are continually developed, produced, and marketed to meet a wide array of consumer needs. Although the proliferation of software ensures healthy competition in the market, the sheer volume of software choices can overwhelm consumers. Thousands of programs can be purchased from retail stores, ordered directly from publishers, or downloaded from the Internet. For education, software applications are available to support nearly all components of classroom instruction. They include drill-and-practice games, tutorials, electronic encyclopedias, grade book software, teacher utilities, student information systems, and multimedia authoring tools, to name just a few. For educators, identifying appropriate software to meet student needs is an enormous challenge.

One of the most popular uses of computers in education is word processing (Roblyer, Edwards, & Havriluk, 1997). Word processing can make the writing process more effi-

Planning and organizing		
	Idea generation tools	Organizational aids
Graphics-based	Stimulus pictures Clip art Scene creation tools Drawing and painting tools Multimedia authoring	Graphic organizers
Text-based	Brainstorming Mixed-up phrases Idea lists Story starters On-screen notepad	Outliners Prompted writing Text-based templates

Drafting
Picture symbols Word prediction and word banks Abbreviation expansion and macros Collaborative writing Speech recognition

Revising and editing
Standard editing tools Thesaurus and rhyming word tools Spelling checkers Homonym checkers Grammar checkers On-screen manuals Speech synthesis

Publishing	
Desktop publishing	Desktop presentation
Desktop publishing features Book formatting Alternative publishing formats	Multimedia options Electronic book formatting Publishing on the World Wide Web

Figure II.1 Taxonomy of software features.

cient, allow teachers and students to produce professional looking documents, and facilitate information sharing. It has been defined in a variety of ways:

- Using the computer to enter, store, manipulate, and print text in letters, reports, and books (Long, 1988)

- A computer application that enables the user to write, edit, format, print, store, and retrieve text (Mandell & Mandell, 1989)

- Computer software designed to facilitate the efficient collecting, revising, storing, and printing of text (Simonson & Thompson, 1997)

- A computer writing tool that replaces traditional writing tools, such as paper and pencil or typewriter (Maddux, Johnson, & Willis, 1997)

- Simply put, typing on a computer (Roblyer et al., 1997)

Many word processing programs are on the market. Choosing one can take considerable thought and time. For adults, the selection process is relatively simple. Although dozens of word processing programs are designed for adults, only a handful are widely adopted; thus, choices are fairly limited. The decision to choose an adult word processing program often is based simply on what colleagues or friends are using. Most adults prefer to use a word processor that is compatible with co-workers and others with whom they might share files.

The process of selecting word processing software for children, however, is considerably more complicated. Teachers and parents who have examined educational software catalogues know that there are dozens of word processing and creativity programs for children. Unfortunately, there is no standardization and little agreement about which programs are best, particularly for students who experience difficulties with the writing process.

Complicating the selection process, most children's word processing programs contain a limited set of features, and those features vary widely among titles. For example, some programs support the production of text and graphics and include clip art libraries or graphics production tools. Other programs emphasize the planning and organizing stage of the writing process and include features such as outliners and story starters. Others emphasize the revision process and include synthetic speech output enabling young writers to hear what they have written.

To facilitate the software selection process, we have developed a taxonomy of children's word processing features in Figure II.1. Recognizing that individual software titles come and go, the taxonomy focuses on software features rather than particular programs. The taxonomy represents our belief that word processing software can be used as more than just a typing tool. It is organized around the principal stages of the writing process—planning and organizing (prewriting), drafting, revising and editing, and publishing.

Although some features can support more than one stage of the writing process, we have categorized each feature according to its primary use. For example, speech synthesis, a feature found in talking word processors, can let young authors hear what they have written, thus providing feedback scaffolds for their revising and editing efforts. It also can be used as a publishing tool, allowing students to share their stories with peers by having the computer read aloud the text they have written. In the taxonomy, we chose to categorize speech synthesis as a feature that supports revising and editing because that is its primary scaffolding function. Readers should keep in mind, however, that a single feature might support more than one stage of the writing process.

Chapters 7–10 describe features in detail related to the writing process stages they support: planning and organizing (Chapter 7), drafting (Chapter 8), revising and editing (Chapter 9), and publishing (Chapter 10). These chapters also provide examples of word processing programs exemplifying each feature. The software examples should not be construed as recommendations or endorsements for particular products or publishers. Our intent is to provide a resource that educators can use to:

- Identify relevant software features that support the major stages of the writing process

- Quickly identify some children's writing programs that include those features

- Match software features to individual student needs

Chapter 11 describes specialized hardware and software adaptations for early stage readers and writers as well as students with various sensory, motor, and cognitive disabilities. This chapter also addresses keyboarding issues for young children. Chapter 12 describes how to make word processing selections for students by using the software features taxonomy and a related form we have designed to document software features. Chapter 12 also includes information about locating, evaluating, and selecting appropriate word processing tools to meet students' individualized writing needs.

A variety of word processing and related tools have features for supporting students through all stages of the writing process. Some of these are designed particularly for students with special needs, but many students can benefit from them. Computers are not just for publishing and certainly not just for playing educational games. Software should be selected deliberately for meeting instructional goals.

Software Features that Support Planning and Organizing

Faced with a blank piece of paper, students sometimes complain that they don't know what to write about, especially in the early stages of writing lab participation. The process of generating ideas and organizing them into a coherent story or report is difficult for many students, particularly those with special language and learning needs (MacArthur, 2000).

Computers and word processing software can scaffold students who struggle with the initial stage of the writing process, giving them confidence in their ability to generate worthwhile ideas about which to write. Many word processing programs designed for children include an array of prewriting tools and activities to scaffold students during this important first stage. Because there are so many planning and organizing features, we categorize them as idea generation tools and organizational aids and further subdivide them into graphics-based and text-based features (see Figure 7.1).

GRAPHICS-BASED IDEA GENERATION TOOLS

Children's word processing programs contain a variety of graphics-based features that can be used by students to stimulate ideas for writing. Some of these features are designed deliberately to support idea generation, such as stimulus pictures. Others are not necessarily intended to support the idea generation stage of writing, but can be used for that purpose. These include

- Stimulus pictures
- Clip art

225

Planning and organizing		
	Idea generation tools	Organizational aids
Graphics-based	Stimulus pictures Clip art Scene creation tools Drawing and painting tools Multimedia authoring	Graphic organizers
Text-based	Brainstorming Mixed-up phrases Idea lists Story starters On-screen notepad	Outliners Prompted writing Text-based templates

Figure 7.1. Taxonomy of software features that support prewriting.

- Scene creation tools
- Drawing and painting tools
- Multimedia authoring

Stimulus Pictures

Stimulus pictures are on-screen pictures that students can view to help them trigger ideas for writing. Usually, stimulus pictures depict characters engaging in some type of action (see Figure 7.2). These pictures may be in the form of line drawings, photographs, or even moving digital video images. Students can select a picture or pictures, then compose text to describe the characters, action, or scene contained in the image. Selected pictures typically can be embedded into students' writing documents as illustrations. *Creative Writer 2* (Microsoft) is a children's writing program that includes stimulus pictures.

Considerations for Use

Although some children may enjoy using stimulus pictures to spark ideas, others may find them too constraining. Many stimulus pictures depict ambiguous scenes that students may not fully understand. They often include cartoon-like images or fantasy characters that may be unfamiliar to students or unrelated to their cultural or background experiences. Although scanning through stimulus pictures may help some students think of ideas about which to write when they are particularly stymied, in our own experience, most children prefer to create their own characters and scenes and to write about events and activities that are personally meaningful to them.

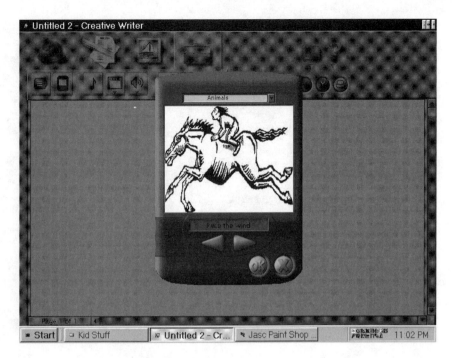

Figure 7.2.   Stimulus picture from *Creative Writer 2*.

Clip Art

Many word processing programs enable users to add clip art to their documents. Clip art refers to graphic images that have been created with a computer and stored as files on a disk or CD-ROM. They usually depict individual objects, such as a tree, dog, or toothbrush, isolated from any background, but also may depict complete scenes or decorative borders. Clip art images may be in black and white or in color. The programs often allow users to resize, crop, and edit clip art images that have been selected and pasted into writing documents. Some children's word processing programs include clip art libraries, that is, collections of clip art images, usually arranged in thematic categories (see Figure 7.3). Students simply 1) access the clip art library (by clicking on a menu bar command or icon), 2) select and "copy" the image they want, and 3) "paste" it into their writing document. Usually, they can move the image around, resize it, or in some programs, even recolor or redraw the image.

Some word processing programs that do not include a clip art library enable users to import clip art images from other applications. These word processors require users to obtain clip art images from a separate clip art disk or CD-ROM that can be purchased commercially. Many collections of clip art also are available as shareware and public domain software that is downloadable from web sites. Note, however, that not all clip art images work with all word processing programs. Clip art images are saved in various graphic file formats, and users must know which formats are compatible with their particular word processor.

Some children's word processors offer a variation on clip art, referred to as "stamps" or "stickers." Based on the idea of rubber stamps, stickers are small graphic images,

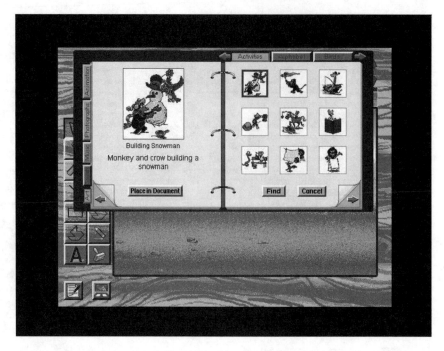

Figure 7.3. Clip art image from *Ultimate Writing & Creativity Center.* © 2003 Riverdeep Interactive Learning Limited, and its licensors.

either abstract designs or concrete objects that can be "stamped" on the computer screen with the click of a mouse. In some programs, students can select the color and size of the stamps, and in other programs, colors are predetermined and size may not be modifiable.

Although clip art and stamps or stickers are not designed specifically to stimulate ideas, they can be useful to students during the prewriting stage of the writing process. Students who cannot think of a story idea can scroll through clip art libraries or stamp collections, select an image that interests them, then compose text to accompany that picture. Students can even select multiple images, arrange them in a sequence or combine them to create a scene, then begin to write. This tactic was used by Andrea and is illustrated in Box 7.1.

Some programs that include clip art, stamp, or sticker options are

- *EasyBook Deluxe* (Sunburst)
- *Imagination Express* (Riverdeep/Edmark)
- *Kid Pix Deluxe 3* (Broderbund)
- *Kid Pix Studio Deluxe* (Broderbund)
- *Kid Works Deluxe* (Knowledge Adventure)
- *Student Writing Center* (Riverdeep/The Learning Company)
- *The Amazing Writing Machine* (Riverdeep/The Learning Company)
- *The Print Shop* (Broderbund)
- *Ultimate Writing & Creativity Center* (Riverdeep/The Learning Company)

Box 7.1.   Using Clip Art to Spark Story Ideas

In our computer-based writing lab, a fifth-grade student named Andrea used clip art as a scaffold during the idea generation stage. She spent the first several writing sessions browsing in clip art files in *The Writing Center* (Riverdeep/The Learning Company) software and choosing images that she liked. After selecting a cat, a dolphin, and a dog, Andrea arranged the images in a horizontal row across the top of her document, then wrote a story to accompany the pictures (see Figure 7.4). Several months later, while using *Creative Writer 2* (Microsoft), she employed the same strategy to generate story ideas, this time selecting pictures of a radio, a backpack, and a wrapped gift, again writing a corresponding story beneath the pictures (see Figure 7.5). Our research comparing the students' use of programs using these features showed that the presence of a greater number of graphic options could lead to less text productivity as students experimented with all of the options (Bahr, Nelson, Van Meter, & Yanna, 1996). That may be the explanation for Andrea's second story being shorter.

The cat and dog.

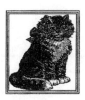 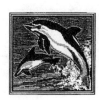 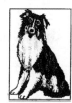

Once upon a time there was a dog named Buster and a cat named Charlie. They were best friends and one day Charlie ran a way. There owners were sad so they sent a search team to find him but it didn't help. So Buster went to find him. Then Buster got lost so they had to send a search team to find them, but that didn't help at all so Andrea B. the Gail that played with him was so sad she was crying like fire So she went to find them her self. So she snuck out during the nite and was gone. She went all over the state and finely found them in Tokyo Japan with there friends the Dolphins named Shamow and Kaite. Then all of them went to Paris and France They enjoyed French fries and milkshakes. Then they went to Florida and stayed with her Grandpa Jasick in a condo. Buy then Her parents were really worried so they called all there friends that had children but they said that Andrea was not there. So Andrea's mommy called Andrea's Grandpa but he said that she was not there because she told him not to her mommy and daddy that she was not there so she stayed there for ever and ever.

The End

Figure 7.4.   Andrea's *Writing Center* story with three images.

(continued)

Box 7.1.   *(continued)*

The Cool Stuff.

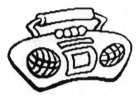 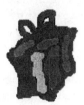

Once upon a time there was a girl named Jasmine she got every thing she wanted because she was a princess. The worst part of being a princess was that you had to marry a prince buy your 10th birthday. Jasmine was in love with Prince Ali of Bogwa. So she married him and they lived happaly after.

The End

Figure 7.5.   Andrea's *Creative Writer 2* story with three images.

Considerations for Use

Clip art is relatively easy to use and involves selecting, copying, and pasting images into a writing document. Most students enjoy browsing through clip art collections and finding images to spark story or report ideas. Some students, however, may "get lost" in clip art, spending so much time searching for images that they devote little time to writing text. Others find images quickly but spend considerable time editing those images (e.g., rotating, resizing, cropping, cutting, pasting) once the images are placed in their documents (Bahr, Nelson, Van Meter, & Yanna, 1996). Like stimulus pictures, clip art may actually constrain some students' creativity and idea generating skills if they cannot find familiar images. Teachers may need to watch as students use clip art and monitor the amount of time they spend browsing through clip art collections and manipulating clip art images in their documents.

Scene Creation Tools

Several word processing programs designed for children offer scene creation tools, a feature more elaborate than clip art. These programs allow students to create full scenes by selecting from a menu of premade backgrounds (e.g., a desert, forest, underwater image) and adding objects to the selected background (e.g., people, animals, vehicles). An example appears in Figure 7.6. Some programs even enable students to attach sound effects to selected objects or to the entire scene. Usually, objects placed on backgrounds can be resized, edited, rotated, and cropped like clip art images. Once a scene is created, students can add text, generally in a space reserved on the bottom of the page. Most programs that include scene creation tools allow users to create documents consisting of multiple pages, perhaps containing a different scene on each page.

Scene creation tools are quite useful to students who have difficulty generating ideas for stories. Selecting a background image can help students focus on a particular theme and setting. As students select and place individual objects on the background, they can begin to think about the characters and actions that could take place within a particular scene. An interesting way to encourage development of a cohesive plot is to have students copy a scene from one page to the next, changing the background or objects to reflect progression of the story. This was the approach taken by Chung when he constructed his time travel story (see Box 7.2).

Some scene creation tools also provide word generation and spelling assistance to students by labeling objects. *Storybook Weaver Deluxe* (Riverdeep/The Learning Company), for example, provides an on-screen list of object labels. Students click on the labels to display graphic objects one at a time, then select and drag the objects to place them in a scene. Box 7.3 describes how one fifth-grade student with emerging literacy abilities used scene creation tools to generate a personal word bank for his stories.

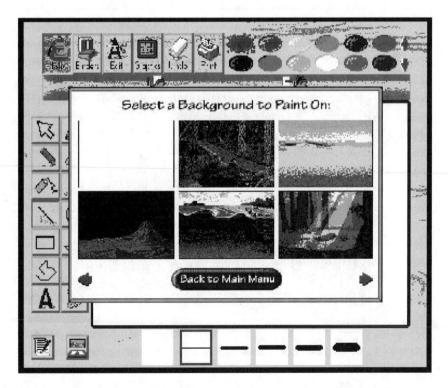

Figure 7.6. Scene creation tool from *Ultimate Writing & Creativity Center.* © 2003 Riverdeep Interactive Learning Limited, and its licensors.

Box 7.2. Using Scene Creation Tools to Develop a Story Sequence

In our computer-based writing lab, a young author named Chung used the scene creation feature in the *Once Upon a Time* (Compu-Teach) software to develop a story sequence. He started his story about a crew traveling in space by creating a scene depicting the inside of a spaceship looking out toward several planets (See Figure 7.7). Below the scene, he wrote a few story lines about the crew traveling toward an orange planet, then finding themselves in a different time period. On the next page, he created a medieval scene. He described the characters in the scene, then continued the time changing strategy for two more frames.

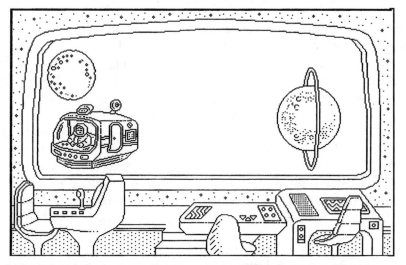

The crew was in space when they headed towards a weird plant. The color was orange.Then they started to spin around and around they went. Suddenly they were in a different time.

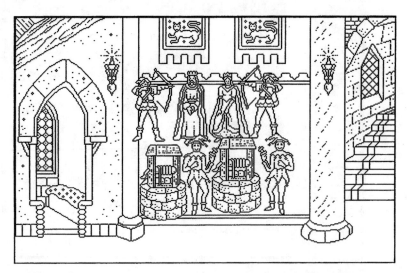

When they got to their new time ,it was midieval time. There were 2jesters, 2 archers, 2 wells, a king and a queen. The archers were aiming at there head. Then they changed times.

Figure 7.7. Chung's time travel story.

232

Box 7.3.　Using Graphic Object Labels as a Scaffold for Spelling Assistance

In our computer-based writing lab, a fourth-grade student with LLDs used the graphic object labels in *Once Upon a Time* (Compu-Teach) as a scaffold for spelling assistance. Although Manuel had limited ability to spell words independently, he developed a strategy for finding words using the graphics feature. He clicked the mouse on graphic object labels (e.g., *rhinoceros, hippopotamus, elephant*), listened to the pronunciation of each, copied the correct spelling of selected objects to a piece of paper, then used the paper as a guide while typing his story. Not surprisingly, most of the characters and objects Manuel wrote about could be found in the *Once Upon a Time* graphics collection.

Some programs that include scene creation tools are

- *EasyBook Deluxe* (Sunburst)
- *Imagination Express* (Riverdeep/Edmark)
- *Kid Pix Deluxe 3* (Broderbund)
- *Kid Works Deluxe* (Knowledge Adventure)
- *Once Upon a Time* (Compu-Teach)
- *Stanley's Sticker Stories* (Riverdeep/Edmark)
- *Storybook Weaver Deluxe* (Riverdeep/The Learning Company)
- *Ultimate Writing & Creativity Center* (Riverdeep/The Learning Company)

Considerations for Use

The same caveats apply to scene creation tools as to clip art. With limited backgrounds and objects from which to choose, some students may feel constrained by the graphics. Others may spend an inordinate amount of time creating and manipulating scenes, leaving little time to write. If problems occur, teachers may need to develop strategies to help students control their use of scene creation tools, perhaps limiting the introduction of graphics to certain points in the writing process.

Drawing and Painting Tools

Many students prefer to create their own artwork rather than using existing clip art, stamps, stickers, and scenes to spark ideas. For them, word processors that include drawing or painting tools are most appropriate. All drawing and painting tools produce graphic images made up of tiny dots called pixels. Although drawing and painting are often thought to be the same, they really are two distinct processes that produce two different kinds of graphics—vector-drawn graphics or bit-mapped graphics.

Drawing programs produce *vector-drawn graphics*. As the user draws, the computer remembers the steps involved in drawing a particular graphic image. Each piece

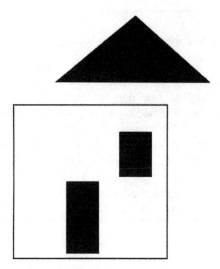

Figure 7.8. Image created with drawing tools.

of the graphic, produced by a different step, is considered a separate object and must be edited separately. For example, in Figure 7.8, the house consists of four objects: a square, a triangle for the roof, and two rectangles depicting the door and window. To change the roof, a student would select the triangle (by clicking the mouse on it), then edit its size, color, rotation, or position on the screen. Each command entered will affect the entire triangle, or roof.

Painting programs produce *bit-mapped graphics.* In this case, each pixel corresponds to a specific spot on the computer screen. Thus, bit-mapped graphics can be edited pixel by pixel, meaning that students can select, change, or move any piece of a bit-mapped graphic, even a single pixel. To change the roof of the bit-mapped house in Figure 7.9, a student would select any portion of the image (by using a selection tool and dragging the mouse around an area), change the color of the pixels in the selected area, or move the selected area to another place on the screen. Changes would affect only the selected pixels, not the entire roof.

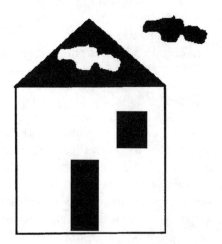

Figure 7.9. Image created with painting tools.

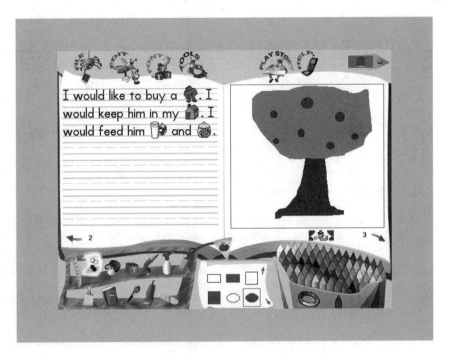

Figure 7.10. Painting tools in *Kid Works Deluxe*.

Most children's word processing programs with graphics creation features use painting tools rather than drawing tools. Many types of painting tools are available, and a word processing program may include just a few or several. Usually, painting tools are represented and selected by icons that resemble tools a real artist would use. They may even generate realistic sound effects when activated. An erasing tool, for example, might be represented by a pencil eraser icon and make a scratchy sound when used. A color filling tool, used to fill color into selected closed spaces, might be represented by a paint bucket icon and make a dripping sound when used (see Figure 7.10).

The advantage of painting programs is that they enable students to create very detailed images. Unlike drawn objects, however, it is more difficult to change painted images once they have been created. For example, if students paint a circle, then decide to get rid of it, they must use an eraser tool to delete the circle but also may inadvertently erase other objects near the circle. With a drawing program, they simply could click the mouse to select the circle (an independent object), and then press the delete key to erase it without affecting any other object in the scene.

Some programs that include drawing or painting tools are

- *Creative Writer 2* (Microsoft)

- *EasyBook Deluxe* (Sunburst)

- *Kid Pix Studio Deluxe* (Broderbund)

- *Kids Media Magic* (Sunburst)

- *Kid Works Deluxe* (Knowledge Adventure)

- *The Amazing Writing Machine* (Riverdeep/The Learning Company)

- *Ultimate Writing & Creativity Center* (Riverdeep/The Learning Company)

> **Teaching Tip 7.1** Using a Drawing or Painting Program to Stimulate Writing
>
> Drawing and painting tools are particularly good for introducing kindergarten and first-grade students to the constructive process of creating an original work, as well as to the mechanical aspects of using a mouse to make selections and to draw images. In a computer lab, an instructor could model the tools first, then take the children through a series of steps in unison, such as drawing a house.
>
> We worked with one first-grade teacher who used *Kid Pix* (Broderbund) as a tool for generating expository text about natural phenomena (e.g., insects, clouds). He made available a series of simply written books, which the students used for conducting their library research. They also conducted their own scientific observations. To produce their reports, a group of students worked on the same topic. First, each created a picture related to their topic. Then, they added sentence descriptions to accompany their pictures. When the reports were complete, the class compiled the related pages and produced several class books, all of which had different authors for each page. Students with special needs produced pages (with SLP scaffolding) that looked similar to their peers' pages.

Stand-alone painting programs designed for children, such as *Kid Pix Deluxe 3* (Broderbund), also are available. These offer a more comprehensive collection of painting tools than can be found in most children's word processing programs. Students can use stand-alone painting software to create elaborate graphics and then import their images into compatible word processing programs that allow images to be imported. Or, for limited text, they can use the painting software instead of a word processor, simply typing their stories on top of their graphic pictures using the text or alphabet tool (a standard tool in most painting programs).

Considerations for Use

Some students experience difficulty generating story or report ideas when faced with unfamiliar clip art pictures or scenes. They may lack background information about the pictures or sufficient vocabulary to describe what they see. These students may have greater success generating ideas if they can work through the process of creating their own original illustrations using drawing or painting tools. Because drawing and painting tools work differently, it is important that students know what tools are available and how to use them. When new software is introduced, teachers may need to spend several sessions demonstrating features and helping students master new tools.

Multimedia Authoring

Some software products enable users to create multimedia documents, that is, documents that include not only text and still-image graphics, but also video and sound. These multimedia authoring programs are not word processors per se, but they include text generation capabilities; thus, they can be used by students to write stories en-

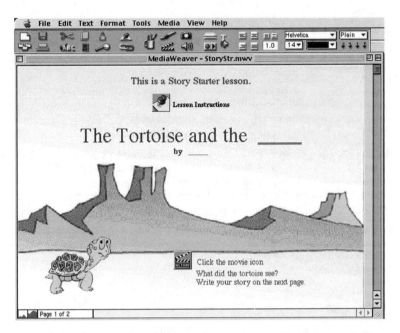

Figure 7.11. Screen from *Media Weaver*.

hanced by graphics, video, and sound. Typically, the resulting multimedia document is presented on a computer (desktop presentation) rather than printed on paper (desktop publication).

MediaWeaver (Sunburst) is an example of a multimedia-authoring tool designed for children (see Figure 7.11). In addition to a word processor, the program includes interactive media buttons. Students can create text with the word processor, then illustrate their work with the built-in paint tools or choose from hundreds of graphic, sound, movie, and photo clips.

Students can use multimedia-authoring programs as a means of generating story ideas or to help them think about relationships among their ideas and facilitate story organization. They also can engage in multimedia composing; taking or scanning pictures; shooting video; and recording sounds about people, places, and things in their own lives as a means of creating a context for writing (Daiute, 1992). Table 7.1 lists some additional hardware and software accessories that can enhance the multimedia composing process. Box 7.4 provides an example of how one student used sound effects to stimulate ideas and organize his stories.

Some multimedia authoring programs are

- *HyperStudio 4* (Knowledge Adventure)

- *Kid Pix Deluxe 3* (Broderbund)

- *Kid Pix Studio Deluxe* (Broderbund)

- *Leonardo's Multimedia Toolbox* (Riverdeep/The Learning Company)

- *MediaWeaver* (Sunburst)

- *MP Express* (Bytes of Learning)

- *mPOWER* (Multimedia Design Corporation)

Table 7.1.   Hardware and software accessories for multimedia composing

Accessory	Function in multimedia composing
Graphics scanner	Scanning images (pictures, drawings, paintings) into the computer; converting paper-based images to digital format
Photo scanner	Scanning photographs only into the computer; converting paper-based photographs to digital format
Microphone	Recording live voice, music, sounds
Digital video camera	Recording video images in digital format
Digital still camera	Taking still pictures in digital format (images would already be in compatible format and would not have to be scanned into computer)
Video digitizer	Board inside computer to transfer images from video cassette recorder or videodisc to digital computer-compatible format
Image editing software	Software to manipulate digital images (recolor, crop, rotate)
Sound editing software	Software to manipulate sound files (record, play, cut, paste, change pitch, frequency)

Considerations for Use

Teachers should be aware that multimedia elements, which serve as a powerful scaffold for some students, might not be as useful to others. It is best to provide students with a wealth of resources and to let them use the ones that are most meaningful to them. Multimedia authoring can be highly motivating to students who are reluctant to write (Daiute & Morse, 1994), but the process of creating a multimedia document including text, graphics, video, and sound is time consuming. Teams should be aware that students may produce less written text when they are focused on incorporating other media (Bahr, Nelson, & Van Meter, 1996).

TEXT-BASED IDEA GENERATION TOOLS

As an alternative to graphics-based tools, many text-based features can scaffold students to generate initial ideas for stories or reports. These text-based idea generators include

- Brainstorming
- Mixed-up phrases
- Idea lists
- Story starters
- On-screen notepads

Brainstorming

The brainstorming feature allows students to record their ideas as they come to mind without worrying about spelling, punctuation, or grammar. Students typically start with a topic, then type concepts or ideas related to the topic as quickly as they can think of them. For example, *Inspiration* (Inspiration Software) is a graphic organizer

---

Box 7.4. Using Sounds to Spark Story Ideas

A young author named Carl demonstrated the power of multimedia for scaffolding idea generation. Carl generated story ideas by searching the sound library in *My Words* (Hartley). He created a story about a trip to Florida by incorporating three of the sound clips available in the software: a laugh, a cough, and a "halleluiah!" (see Figure 7.12). A few months later, when introduced to another word processor that included clip art, but no sounds, Carl expressed extreme disappointment and had great difficulty generating new story ideas. He had enjoyed using the audio sounds as a scaffold for idea generation and simply was not inspired by pictures.

> *A trip to Florida*
>
> *Once apon a time*
> *   Autumn and Carl went to*
> *Florida. The first thing they did was*
> *funny laugh* 🍎 *. When they got there,*
> *Carl said, "I am having fun*
> *already!" "Yeah, so am I!" said Mom.*
> *The next thing they did was go on*
> *the Rollercoaster ride.   Mom said, "*
> *This is fun. Oh no, here comes a*
> *funny laugh* 🍎 *! Carl said, "I can't*
> *stop laughing* 🍎 *!" Then Carl said, "I*
> *can't go" said Carl. "Why?" said*
> *Mom. "Because I am sick* 🍎 🍎 *!" The*
> *last thing they did was go to the*
> *movies they saw Mrs. Doubt Fire. And*
> *in the movie they sang, "Halleiujah* 🍎 *!"*
> *Finally, they got home. Carl said,*
> *"There's no place like home." Mom*
> *said, "Home sweet home."*

Figure 7.12.   Carl's story incorporating sounds.

that includes a feature called RapidFire. It allows students to enter brainstorming ideas quickly into a concept map or web just by pressing the return key on the keyboard.

Considerations for Use

In our computer-based writing labs, we encourage students to use this feature to brainstorm ideas without worrying about spelling or writing conventions while brainstorming. Intense focus on spelling during the early stages of writing can inhibit the

---

Teaching Tip 7.2.   Exploring Options and Sharing Multimedia Products

After presenting guided minilessons on software use, allow students time to explore freely some of the multimedia features such as graphics, animations, sounds, and music options.

This is a good time for students to share what they are learning about the features with each other as well. Preteaching some features to children with special needs can elevate their status by preparing them to demonstrate such features for their classmates without disabilities.

Because of the time multimedia requires for authoring, to maximize writing time it may be better to use a multimedia-authoring program a few times per year for special occasions, such as the end of a thematic unit or for writing about an upcoming holiday or event, rather than as the daily writing tool.

Documents created with multimedia authoring tools must be presented on a computer rather than printed on paper to retain all of their features. Desktop presentation enables the audience not only to hear the text, but also to hear sounds or music embedded in the document and to see moving animations or video clips on the screen. One strategy we have used for desktop presentation is to have pairs of students take turns presenting their documents on the computer screen to one another or to their parents at a publishing party.

---

idea generation process among students who lack confidence in their spelling skills. Students who are fearful of making errors often avoid typing ideas that they think they cannot spell correctly. The quick action of the brainstorm feature may help such students overcome this tendency.

Mixed-Up Phrases

Another text-based idea generation tool is mixed-up phrases. With this feature, unrelated words and phrases are randomly linked to create unusual sentences. Students can use these resulting sentences to spark ideas. Different programs offer variations on the mixed-up phrases feature. For example, *Creative Writer 2* (Microsoft) has a "Splot Machine" option that students can use to create silly sentences (see Figure 7.14). With the push of a button (mouse click), words and phrases scroll briskly across three windows. The top window contains subject phrases; the middle window contains predicates; and the bottom window contains prepositional phrases. When the machine comes to a stop, it shows three phrases comprising a complete sentence, such as:

The energetic short-order cook
stayed up late
in the garbage dump.

Students can save the resulting sentence in an electronic notebook, paste it into a writing document and begin writing with it, click on the button again to get a new sentence, or change just one of the three sentence parts.

Teaching Tip 7.3. Using the RapidFire Tool in *Inspiration*

Try demonstrating the RapidFire tool in a group brainstorming session first. This could involve, for example, modeling how to brainstorm multiple ideas in two or three categories for personal narratives, such as for a pet story or cooking mishap story. The minilesson instructor might start by modeling self-talk about his or her own ideas, then solicit ideas from the students about other possibilities.

As an example, we used the RapidFire tool to introduce a class of third graders to the genre of debate, having them brainstorm points for and against a "Lunch and Learn" program their school had introduced to replace the traditional lunchroom and recess program. Figures 7.13a and 7.13b show examples of a RapidFire brainstorm for a class of third-grade students divided into two subgroups. One generated pro ideas, and the other, con ideas. Each was led by an instructor who typed in the students' ideas using the RapidFire feature. Later, the two groups lined up across from each other and took turns making points from printouts of their side's arguments. The activity ended with each student taking a stand about his or her position.

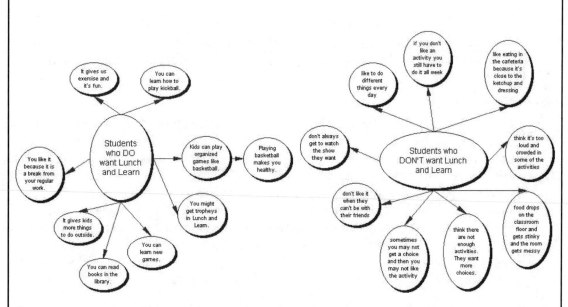

Figure 7.13a. Pro arguments brainstormed with RapidFire tool in *Inspiration*.

Figure 7.13b. Con arguments brainstormed with RapidFire tool in *Inspiration*.

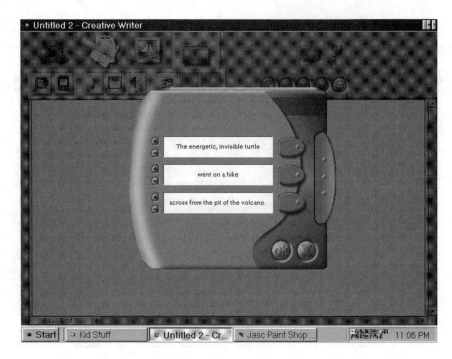

Figure 7.14. Splot machine in *Creative Writer 2*.

Some programs that include the mixed-up phrases tool are *Creative Writer 2* (Microsoft) and *The Amazing Writing Machine* (Riverdeep/The Learning Company).

Considerations for Use

The mixed-up phrases tool may give students ideas for unusual characters or settings, but it may not be the best way to generate a true narrative. Some sentences that result from combining unrelated phrases may be so far removed from children's own fields of knowledge that they are not particularly useful. Furthermore, students who use the mixed-up phrases tool must be able to understand the language incorporated in the resulting sentence. Most important, the use of mixed-up phrases seems to violate the value of authors engaging in an authentic communication act—starting with meaning and then formulating the language to express it. In our experience, we found that students were generally amused by the mixed-up phrases feature and played with it, but they did not often use the results as a basis for their stories.

Idea Lists

Another prewriting tool that helps students generate story ideas is an idea list. An idea list may contain items such as little known facts, famous quotations, potential story titles, or open-ended questions to help spark ideas for a narrative. Students can scroll through the idea list until they find a topic in which they are interested, then use it as a basis for their writing.

Imagination Express (Riverdeep/Edmark) provides an idea list feature that presents digitized video clips of children suggesting story topics. When students press the story idea button, a short, randomly selected video clip is displayed. For example, one clip shows a girl who says, "Interviews make great stories. Ask your mom about things she did when she was your age. You'll probably be surprised." Another says, "Shhh . . . don't tell anyone, but I like making up stories about my secret powers."

Some programs that include idea lists are

- *Imagination Express* (Riverdeep/Edmark)

- *The Amazing Writing Machine* (Riverdeep/The Learning Company)

- *Ultimate Writing & Creativity Center* (Riverdeep/The Learning Company)

Considerations for Use

Idea lists are helpful for some students, providing them an array of topics and suggestions about which to write. Teachers should be aware, however, that different idea lists might stimulate different types of discourse. There may be problems if the teacher requests one type of discourse (e.g., narrative) and the idea list scaffolds another (e.g., expository).

Story Starters

Many educators use story starters to help students generate ideas for writing. Story starters usually consist of a phrase or a few sentences designed to serve as the beginning of a writing document. Students complete the story starter and continue writing. For example, when a user clicks the mouse on a picture of a turtle in the *Ultimate Writing & Creativity Center* (Riverdeep/The Learning Company), the software provides the following story starter, "Once there was a sea turtle who felt ugly, so it carried a beautiful sea anemone on its back. 'Now I'm beautiful,' thought the turtle, but . . . "

The student can copy the story starter, then paste it into a writing document, and continue typing a story.

Some programs that include story starters are

- *Kid Works Deluxe* (Knowledge Adventure)

- *Sunbuddy Writer* (Sunburst)

- *Storybook Weaver Deluxe* (Riverdeep/The Learning Company)

- *The Amazing Writing Machine* (Riverdeep/The Learning Company)

- *Ultimate Writing & Creativity Center* (Riverdeep/The Learning Company)

Considerations for Use

Story starters provide more structure than simple idea lists because they typically present a few prewritten sentences to get students started. They may be useful for students who tend to write about the same thing over and over, showing reluctance to take risks in their writing, or for students who have well-developed spoken language skills but struggle to put words on paper. However, for some students, story starters prohibit their natural flow of ideas and confine them to writing about topics in which they have little interest.

In our experience, we have found that most children prefer to write about their own ideas, and some may even rebel against the constraints of story starters. For example, when a second-grade teacher gave his students a story starter about a big yellow bus, one student who was disappointed about the prescribed topic changed the bus to blue and made it crash. Story starters are probably best used occasionally rather than routinely in most classrooms or as one of several choices including students' own ideas.

On-Screen Notepads

As students accumulate writing ideas, through graphics or text-based idea generation tools, they need to keep track of those ideas in some way. Of course, students can keep paper and pencils next to their computers so that they can jot down ideas as they occur to them. Some word processing programs eliminate the need for extra notetaking materials, however, by including an on-screen notepad, also called a journal or a diary. Students can click on a notepad button that brings up a floating window on top of their writing document (see Figure 7.15). They can type notes in the window, then select, copy, and paste these notes from the notepad window directly into their writing document, or they can cut and paste material from other open windows.

Some programs that include an on-screen notepad are *Draft: Builder* (Don Johnston), *Student Writing Center* (Riverdeep/The Learning Company), and *Ultimate Writing & Creativity Center* (Riverdeep/The Learning Company).

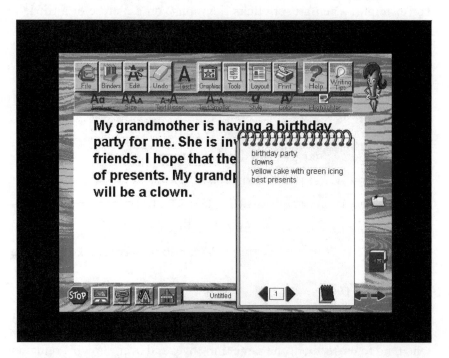

Figure 7.15. On-screen notepad in *Ultimate Writing & Creativity Center*. © 2003 Riverdeep Interactive Learning Limited, and its licensors.

Teaching Tip 7.4.　Using Graphic Organizers

- Introduce graphic organizers by modeling how the instructor might use the feature to plan and organize his or her work, such as story or report writing.
- Give students teacher-generated organizers to fill in story or report information on the computer or hard-copy print out.
- Allow students to explore features of graphic organizer software to create their own structures about topics that interest them.
- Use graphic organizers to categorize concepts in subject areas such as science and social studies. Show students how to see relationships between elements, such as superordinate and subordinate, compare and contrast, and sequences.
- Use graphic organizers to teach discourse structures, such as stories, science reports, reviews, and persuasive essays.
- Use graphic organizers to outline prewriting ideas.

Considerations for Use

The on-screen notepad feature is particularly useful for expository writing tasks. If students use electronic resource materials such as an encyclopedia CD-ROM, they can copy text from the CD-ROM and paste it directly into an open notepad window. Then, after they have accumulated sufficient information, they can choose the notes they want to keep and selectively paste those into their writing documents. The notepad feature allows students to collect a large number of ideas without actually putting all of them into their writing document. That way, they do not have to delete unused ideas later. Although the notepad feature can be useful during the idea generation stage, students who lack proficient keyboarding skills may find it easier and faster to record their ideas with paper and pencil rather than to type them into the notepad window, unless they can use an electronic cut and paste. Teachers can help students decide whether the notepad feature will save them time and effort in the writing process.

GRAPHICS-BASED ORGANIZATIONAL AIDS

Once students have selected a topic and generated some ideas for writing, they must organize those ideas to produce a coherent story or report. Educators use an array of paper-and-pencil based tools to help students make connections, such as note cards, outlines, and story maps. Many word processors provide similar organizational aids that can scaffold this stage of the writing process. We refer to these organizational tools as graphic organizers.

Graphic Organizers

Graphic organizers are graphical representations of ideas and their relationships to one another. Various terms are used to describe different types of graphic organizers, such as *story webs, story maps, semantic webs, concept maps,* and *frames,* to name just a few. They usually consist of on-screen geometric shapes containing text and sometimes pictures, linked with lines. The lines depict how the various ideas are related conceptually or temporally to one another. Educators can provide blank graphic organizer printouts for students to fill on paper, or students can create their own organizational structures. Some educators use graphic organizers to help students generate ideas and vocabulary for narratives or expository pieces. Others use them to help students plan the sequence of their stories, create relationships among characters and events, or organize main ideas and details.

Several computer programs are designed to support production of graphic organizers. For example, *Inspiration* and *Kidspiration* (Inspiration Software) allow students to create many types of graphic organizers, such as concept maps, idea maps, webs, and storyboards. Figure 7.16a presents a graphic organizer concept map, and Figure 7.16b shows the same information altered to appear in outline view. Students can toggle between the visual diagram view of their graphic organizer and the text-based outline view by clicking an icon on the tool bar. Changes made in the diagram are automatically updated in the outline, and vice versa. Students can print their graphic organizers on paper (provided a printer is connected to the computer) and use them as guides for writing text, or they can convert them to outlines on the computer, then expand the outlines by typing full sentences and paragraphs to create complete narratives or reports.

If projected on a large monitor or video projector, graphic organizer software also can be used to facilitate large group planning for writing. Students can work collaboratively to generate ideas and create links depicting relationships among them. Then, they can break into small groups or work individually to draft stories or reports using ideas generated by the class. Most children's word processing programs do not include

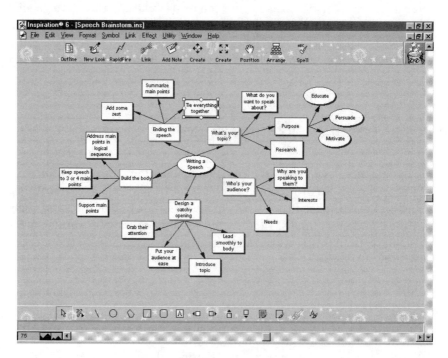

Figure 7.16a. Concept map produced with *Inspiration.*

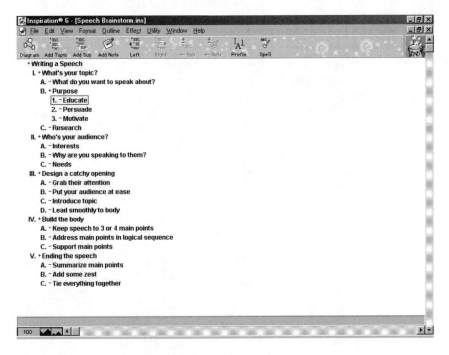

Figure 7.16b. Outline produced with *Inspiration*.

built-in graphic organizer features; however, programs marketed as graphic organizers usually include some word processing capabilities or the option of exporting text to an external word processor.

Some graphic organizer programs or programs that include a graphic organizer are

- *CREATE Together* (Bytes of Learning)

- *Draft: Builder* (Don Johnston)

- *Inspiration* (Inspiration Software)

- *Kidspiration* (Inspiration Software)

Considerations for Use

Graphic organizers can be quite useful to students during the organizational stage of the writing process. The ability to convert graphic plans to text-based outlines with the click of a mouse is a special benefit of planning on a computer. Some children, however, need significant teacher support while using graphic organizers. They may link their ideas randomly or rely on a "what next" strategy to make connections. Most elementary and middle school students require specific instruction in the use of graphic organizer software before they can effectively use it as an organizational tool (Sturm & Koppenhaver, 2000). With scaffolding, however, most students can learn to use graphic organizers, with noticeable benefits to their general cognitive organization and self-organization skills. Sturm and Rankin-Erickson (2002) found that middle school students with learning disabilities produced descriptive essays with more words, more T-units, and higher holistic scores after planning with hand-mapping or computer-

Teaching Tip 7.5. Using Graphic Organizer Templates

Inspiration includes a list of preestablished planning templates for various genres. Writing lab teams can use these to stimulate discussions of the features they want to see in their students' writing for a particular genre at a particular grade level. The software permits modification of these templates or the creation of new ones, which then can be saved as templates for student use. An example of a narrative-planning template appears in Figure 7.17a, and a compare-contrast planning template appears in Figure 7.17b.

When customizing a template, put it on a floppy disk and open and save it on each of the computers in a computer lab. When students open the template, scaffold them to save immediately under a new name if you want to preserve the original graphic template.

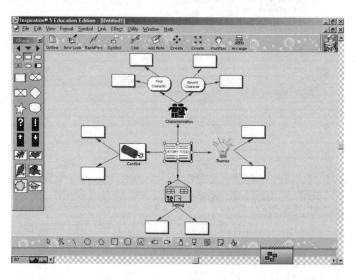

Figure 7.17a. Narrative planning graphic organizer template in *Inspiration*.

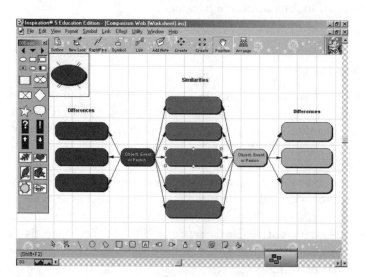

Figure 7.17b. Compare-contrast graphic organizer template in *Inspiration*.

mapping (compared to baseline) than in a no-mapping condition. They also found that students' attitudes toward writing were more positive in the computer-mapping condition than the hand-mapping or no-mapping conditions.

TEXT-BASED ORGANIZATIONAL AIDS

Some children's word processors include text-based organizational aids, activities that use words rather than graphics to help students organize their ideas. On a continuum of providing least to most support, these include

- Outliners
- Prompted writing
- Text-based templates

Each of these tools might be more useful to some students than to others; therefore, educators must determine which organizational aids will best support their students.

Outliners

A common way to organize ideas is to develop a written outline encompassing main and subordinate ideas. Most popular adult word processing programs and some children's word processors include outlining capabilities. Generally, users can turn the outlining feature on or off while writing, and they can choose among various numbering styles. Later, when the outline is edited, it is automatically renumbered to reflect changes that have been made. If the outline feature is part of a graphic organizer program (e.g., *Inspiration*), the outline can be converted to a concept map or web with the click of a button.

Some programs that include outliners are

- *Draft:Builder* (Don Johnston)
- *Inspiration* (Inspiration Software)
- *Kidspiration* (Inspiration Software)
- *The Amazing Writing Machine* (Riverdeep/The Learning Company)

Considerations for Use

In order to use outliners effectively, students must be familiar with the parts of an outline, various numbering systems, and the notion of main and subordinate, or supporting, ideas. In addition, outliners are most useful for planning and organizing expository text rather than creative narratives.

Prompted Writing

Another text-based organizational aid is prompted writing. Prompted writing refers to a series of on-screen prompts that assist students to organize their ideas. Typically, prompts consist of questions requiring students to elaborate on a particular topic or idea. Some programs provide prompts that guide students through each step of the writing process according to a particular genre. *Writing Process Workshop* (Educational Activities Software/Siboney Learning Group), for example, offers four different titles: *Persuasive Writing, Report of Information/Observation, Autobiographical Incident,* and *Evaluation.* The software guides students step by step with prompted instructions through the stages of readiness, brainstorming, prewriting, drafting, revising, editing, and proofreading.

Another program, *Author's Toolkit* (Sunburst), prompts students to begin by selecting the purpose for their writing: imaginative, personal, or functional. Then, they proceed to the *NoteTaker* tool, which prompts them to begin prewriting by gathering information. After using the *NoteTaker* tool, students access the *StructureMaker* tool that helps them to organize their notes in a logical order. Using *DraftMaker,* students add to their notes to create sentences and paragraphs. Finally, students transfer their work to the built-in word processor that allows them to check spelling, import graphics, and format the document for printing.

Some programs that include prompted writing are

- *Author's Toolkit* (Sunburst)

- *Intellitalk II* (Intellitools)

- *Paragraph Power* (Gamco/Siboney Learning Group)

- *Writing Process Workshop* (Educational Activities Software/Siboney Learning Group)

Considerations for Use

For students who are learning about story grammar (see Chapter 16) or who have difficulty organizing their many ideas into a coherent story or report, prompted writing can help to scaffold their planning and organizing processes (Bahr, Nelson, & Van Meter, 1996). Of course, the quality of the scaffolding depends on the nature of the prompts provided. Students must be able to read the prompts and understand their meaning. The prompts must be sufficiently open-ended so as not to constrain students' ideas.

Text-Based Templates

A text-based template is a preformatted document with some of the words already filled in. These also may be called *framed paragraphs.* Some word processors include premade templates corresponding to different writing genres, such as lab reports, memos, letters, field notes, résumés, book reports, and stories. Students select the appropriate genre, open a template (sometimes there are several options for each genre), and then fill in their own content in the spaces provided.

Some programs allow users to create and save their own custom template files. When the saved template is opened, a new untitled document appears, allowing the user to save the new document under a new name without changing the original template. Of course, even without a template saving feature, students or instructional teams can use any word processor to create documents, then save and use them as templates for future documents. However, they must be careful to change the filename for the new document so that it does not replace the original template document.

Teaching Tip 7.6.　Using Text-Based Prompted Writing

To set up a text-based prompted writing template, start by analyzing the genre the instructional team intends the students to produce. Then, create sections with prompt questions to correspond with the macrostructure of the genre.

A set of prompts for story writing might ask students to think about 1) the setting (characters, time, and place), 2) the problem the characters are facing, 3) the things they decide to do to attempt to solve the problem, 4) the results or what happens, and 5) an ending that brings it all together.

A set of prompts for an opinion essay might prompt students to enter 1) an introduction with a clear statement of their position, 2) at least three paragraphs with supporting statements and details, and 3) a concluding paragraph that summarizes their position and draws the essay to a close.

The Amazing Writing Machine (Riverdeep/The Learning Company) offers a unique variation on templates for writers who may need more support than a blank template offers or who may not know how to change a prewritten template story. This program offers "spin" stories, prewritten stories that include buttons, scattered throughout the text, for changing individual words and phrases. When students click the mouse on a word or phrase button, a list of appropriate alternative words or phrases is displayed. Students can scroll through the list of alternatives and select a different word or phrase to replace the original in the story or type their own original replacement in the space provided.

For younger students, *Bailey's Book House* (Riverdeep/Edmark) offers text-based templates along with pictures (see Figure 7.18). When the student clicks on an object choice, the corresponding word fills the slot in the sentence (e.g., This is a story about *Sammy*). Then, the program shows a new frame using information from the first (e.g., Sammy is taking a trip in a _____). The student makes another choice, and the story continues to build. This feature provides the greatest degree of scaffolding for students who have difficulty generating story ideas and organizing those ideas in a coherent way.

Some programs that include premade templates or a template saving option are

- *Student Writing Center* (Riverdeep/The Learning Company)
- *The Amazing Writing Machine* (Riverdeep/The Learning Company)
- *Bailey's Book House* (Riverdeep/Edmark)

Considerations for Use

Because text-based templates are relatively restrictive, they probably are best reserved for the most reluctant writers who do not believe they have the ability to write creative narratives or expository pieces. A template can provide a textual framework from which to start, giving students something other than a blank screen with which to work right from the beginning; however, educators should pay careful attention to the

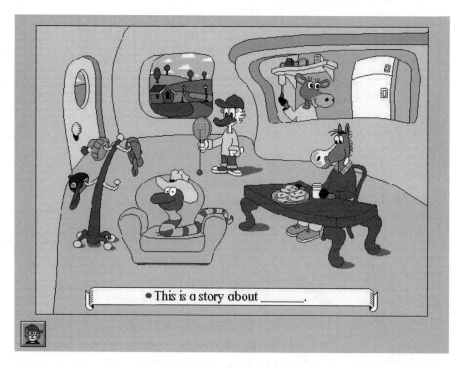

Figure 7.18.   Story template feature in *Bailey's Book House.* © 2003 Riverdeep Interactive Learning Limited, and its licensors.

syntax used in the template to ensure that students can understand it. Students who need this relatively intense level of scaffolding support may also benefit from speech synthesis to hear the template text read aloud. This was the case with one first-grade student with autism who used *Bailey's Book House* (Riverdeep/Edmark) while his classmates used more open-ended word processing programs.

SUMMARY

For students who are stymied by a blank screen or who write over and over again about the same topics, word processors offer several features that can scaffold them during the idea generating process. Students can scroll through stimulus pictures designed to spark ideas; browse clip art, stamps, and stickers; or create story scenes by combining premade backgrounds and clip art objects. For students who prefer to draw their own pictures as a stimulus for writing ideas, some word processors include drawing or painting tools. Although these drawing and painting tools require that students generate ideas themselves, many students prefer to write about their original artwork than to write about characters and objects with which they are unfamiliar. In addition, multimedia authoring tools can be used to combine text, still images, video, and sounds. Students can browse through multimedia resource files or, with additional hardware and software accessories, generate their own resources to create a familiar context for writing.

Beyond graphics-based features, some children's word processors include text-based idea generation tools, such as brainstorming activities, mixed-up phrases, idea

---

Teaching Tip 7.7. Using Text-Based Templates

One strategy for helping students who have difficulty organizing their ideas in a logical sequence is to create partially written stories or reports and save them as templates. For example, try scaffolding a reluctant student to tell a story or report orally, and then enter the student's main ideas as the first line of each of several paragraphs. The student can use the template as a starting point, filling in the supporting sentences in each paragraph.

In an inclusive setting, even though some lower-functioning students with developmental disabilities might need the maximum support provided by text-based templates, if possible, produce the template using the same software the student's classmates are using. This will yield a final product that looks similar. A footnote could be added to the printout to make it clear which parts of the story were produced directly by the student.

---

lists, and sentence- and story starters. Students can interact with idea generation activities, then use their responses as a springboard for writing.

Many students can think of topics and ideas but require assistance to arrange those ideas into a coherent story sequence or report structure. They may benefit from organizational aids provided by word processors. Some children's word processors provide graphic organizers, enabling students to arrange their ideas spatially before beginning to draft.

Several word processors also provide text-based prewriting activities to scaffold organizational skills. Depending on the level of support needed, students can use outliners, prompted writing, or text-based templates. Students who have an understanding of story grammar and sequence can benefit from the process of creating an outline prior to writing. But, for students who are less familiar with the organization of a narrative story or an expository report, educators can create prompts to assist them with the various parts. Some programs even provide templates for various writing genre, including narrative stories, reports, and letters. For students just beginning to learn how to organize their ideas, or for those who have great difficulty generating text, prewritten templates can provide the most support for getting started and feeling successful with the writing process.

Idea generation tools and organizational aids provided by word processors can provide support for students during the prewriting stage of the writing process. While many of these prewriting activities could be done on paper, the word processor enables prewriting products to be embedded directly into writing documents, saving time and effort during the drafting stage. Even proficient writers can benefit from the use of prewriting tools, such as outliners and graphic organizers, during the important first step of the writing process.

Software Features
that Support Drafting

8

Drafting text on a computer requires diverse skills, such as word retrieval, spelling, sentence construction, and keyboarding proficiency. Several software features can be used to scaffold students during this stage of the writing process. Figure 8.1 lists software features that help students to select appropriate vocabulary, spell words, and type them.

PICTURE SYMBOLS

Picture symbols are small graphic icons that represent words (similar to Rebus symbols). Some word processors include picture symbols that students can select instead of typing words. While writing, students can switch to a picture symbol library, find a symbol they want, select it (by clicking the mouse), and place it directly into a sentence in their writing document. Later, they can click the mouse on a conversion button to change all picture symbols to words or vice versa. Picture symbols might be organized alphabetically as a whole or arranged alphabetically within thematic categories, such as those found in *Kid Works Deluxe* (Knowledge Adventure) (see Figure 8.2).

Picture symbols are especially useful to very young students or any students at emergent literacy levels who may not know how to spell the words they want to use. Instead of trying to type a word, they can select a corresponding picture symbol and then use the conversion button to change the symbol to a word. This feature provides a quick way for students who are not proficient spellers to generate correctly spelled words. Picture symbols also may be useful to students who demonstrate limited written vocabulary. Students can scroll through the picture symbol library and select words (symbols) for their stories that they otherwise might not have considered.

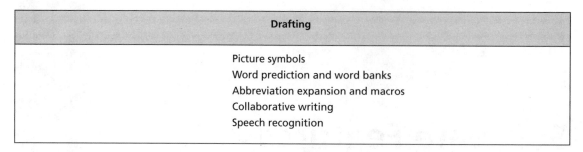

Figure 8.1. Taxonomy of software features that support drafting.

Some software programs that include picture symbols are

- *Clicker* (Crick Software)

- *Intellitalk II* (Intellitools)

- *Kid Works Deluxe* (Knowledge Adventure)

- *Kids Media Magic* (Sunburst)

- *PixWriter* (Slater Software)

- *Sunbuddy Writer* (Sunburst)

- *The Amazing Writing Machine* (Riverdeep/The Learning Company)

- *Writing with Symbols 2000* (Widget Software Ltd.)

Considerations for Use

One limitation of picture symbols is that symbol libraries generally are limited to several hundred or fewer words, and most of those are concrete words that can be depicted easily. Thus, they are not particularly useful to older students with higher cognitive functioning who have developed more extensive vocabularies incorporating abstract concepts, and they may be frustrating to any child who generates unique ideas. Some picture symbols require that students operate at a metalinguistic level. A child who can only function at a literal level and who cannot treat words as abstract objects may not be able to select the picture of a tin can, for example, to represent the auxiliary verb *can* in a sentence, or the picture of a bumblebee to represent the verb *be.*

WORD PREDICTION AND WORD BANKS

Many students (and adults) have not developed sufficient keyboarding skills to type accurately and efficiently. Chapter 11 describes keyboarding requirements and instructional methods that educators can use to help students develop proficient keyboarding skills; however, word prediction can provide assistance during the drafting stage for students who have not yet mastered typing, those who have difficulty with spelling, or those who struggle with the physical demands of accessing and pressing keys.

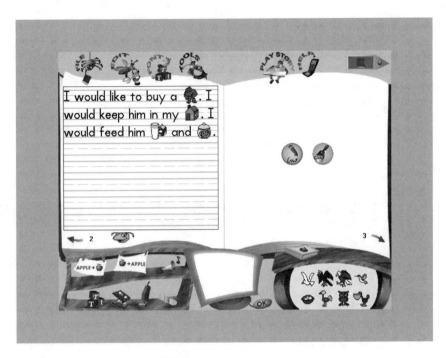

Figure 8.2. Picture symbols in *Kid Works Deluxe.*

Word prediction reduces the number of keystrokes required while typing. With word prediction, a short numbered list of words is displayed on the screen as the student types. The word prediction list changes as each character is entered, with the most likely words displayed at the top of the list. When the desired word appears in the word prediction list, students select and enter it into their writing documents by typing its corresponding number (see Figure 8.3).

Word prediction was developed originally to assist individuals with motor impairments and restricted typing speed, but it has become popular for students who require spelling assistance. If students can identify the initial sounds of a word and type the first letter or two, they often can locate the desired word in the prediction list and simply type its corresponding number to enter it into their writing document. They do not have to know how to spell the entire word, but they must be able to recognize and select it from a short list.

Some programs that include word prediction are

- *Co:Writer 4000* (Don Johnston)
- *Clicker* (Crick Software)
- *Read & Write* (textHELP! Systems Ltd.)
- *Type & Talk* (textHELP! Systems Ltd.)

A related activity to support drafting is to create a personal word bank of key vocabulary for a particular composition or project. A personal word bank may be developed by taking dictation from an oral story and making the words available to the student while drafting through an on-screen notepad or word bank. A program called *My*

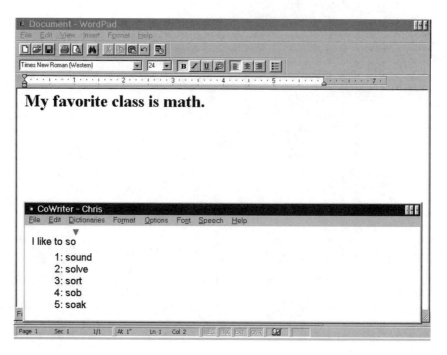

Figure 8.3. Word prediction window in *Co:Writer 4000*.

Words (Hartley) provided this feature, but it is no longer available for purchase (although it could be available in an existing computer lab). In Chapter 7, the notepad feature was discussed, and Figure 7.15 shows an example of an on-screen notepad. This feature can be adapted easily to serve as a personal word bank with a small set of words customized for a particular student and project.

Some programs that include an on-screen notepad are *Student Writing Center* (Riverdeep/The Learning Company) and *Ultimate Writing & Creativity Center* (Riverdeep/The Learning Company). A program that includes a word bank feature is *Intellitalk II* (Intellitools).

Considerations for Use

The word prediction feature varies across software programs. After reviewing research on word prediction, MacArthur concluded, "Design issues, such as the size of the vocabulary, its match to the writing task, and the complexity of the interface, clearly make a difference in the impact" (2000, p. 95).

Some word prediction programs allow users to determine the number of words in the prediction window, the size of the window, and its location on the screen. Some allow users to create and retrieve word lists relating to a specific topic, thus reducing the number of irrelevant words that may appear in the word prediction window. Vocabulary control seems to be an important feature for students with LLDs. MacArthur (1998) found a dramatic effect on the legibility and spelling of students' writing when the word prediction vocabulary for interacting in dialogue journals with teachers closely matched the task. Newell, Booth, Arnott, and Beattie (1992) also reported positive effects of using a word prediction program. They described increased spelling accuracy, writing productivity, and motivation to write in a series of case studies on 17 students with diverse disabilities. Only one student did not like to use the word prediction software because it was too slow.

Most word prediction programs allow users to add suffixes or other modifications to words in the list with a single keystroke. Some more complex word prediction programs "learn" over time, automatically updating the predicted word list vocabulary on the basis of factors such as frequency and recent use of words, common word associations, or grammatical patterns. Finally, some word prediction programs include additional support features such as abbreviation expansion (explained in next section) and speech synthesis (explained in Chapter 9, with revising and editing tools).

When word prediction algorithms grow in complexity, however, some evidence suggests that children with learning disabilities may have more difficulty using the feature. MacArthur (1999) found limited benefits for three students with learning disabilities who used a program with a large vocabulary and prediction that altered word choices based on syntax and frequency of use. Two students, in particular, had difficulty finding the correct word in the predicted word list. Speech synthesis is a feature that might overcome this limitation by having the computer read aloud the words in the prediction list, making it easier for students with reading problems to recognize the words (MacArthur, 2000).

Word prediction is designed to save keystrokes, but it is not particularly useful to students who know how to spell and can type more than 20 words per minute. For students who type less than 20 words per minute, including students with physical disabilities or hunt-and-peck typists, word prediction can accelerate the drafting process. For proficient typists, the additional cognitive tasks of scanning the prediction list, reading the options, selecting the desired word, and translating its number to a keystroke may only serve to slow down the writing process. For students who are reluctant writers because of limited spelling skills, word prediction can provide scaffolding they need to take risks in their writing, particularly if the vocabulary is controlled and speech synthesis is available to help them identify intended words from the list. Personalized word banks offer another way to achieve this function.

ABBREVIATION EXPANSION AND MACROS

Abbreviation expansion and macros are two other features designed to reduce keystrokes. With abbreviation expansion, writers can type short (typically one-, two-, or three-character) abbreviations that will be converted to longer words, phrases, or sentences on the screen. This feature is especially useful to individuals who have physical limitations that reduce their typing speed. Abbreviation expansion, however, requires that users remember the abbreviations available to them and what they stand for.

A macro is a series of commands saved as a file that can be replayed with a few keystrokes or a mouse click. To assign a series of commands or keystrokes to a macro file, students must turn on the macro feature; enter the text, commands, or menu selections they want to record; then save the file. To replay the macro file, they must locate the file and play the macro. Some programs that offer the macro feature allow users to store frequently used macro files on a macro button bar, enabling users simply to click the mouse on the button bar to play the macro they select. Macros can be used to store long strings of text, such as words, phrases, sentences, paragraphs, or frequently used command series. For example, a student could record a macro to select a particular font, apply a bold style, center text, and type his or her name, school, grade, and teacher's name. Then, the student could assign the whole series of keystrokes to a macro called *header*. When the header macro is played, the following text would appear in the writing document:

Billy Smith

Johnson School

Grade 4

Miss Lang

Macros are most useful for setting up text formatting options, creating headers and title pages, or recording text that will be repeated many times. They can assist students to do complex tasks and reduce the amount of time it takes students to enter text that they use regularly. Macros are found in many full-featured adult word processing programs and a few programs designed for children.

Some programs that include abbreviation expansion or macros are

- *Co:Writer 4000* (Don Johnston)

- *Read & Write* (textHELP Systems Ltd.)

- *Word* (Microsoft)

Considerations for Use

Abbreviation expansion and macros can save students many keystrokes; however, students must remember which commands are stored under each abbreviation or macro file. It may be helpful for teachers (or students themselves) to create and post lists of abbreviations and macros they have defined near the computer.

COLLABORATIVE WRITING

Another way to scaffold students during the drafting stage of the writing process is to allow them to write collaboratively with a partner (see Box 8.1). Two students seated at the same computer may be able to generate text better than one student working alone. They can help each other think of words, spell, and locate characters on the keyboard; however, it is difficult for both students to reach the keyboard or to type at the same time. Collaborative writing programs have been developed to enable two or more writers to work together on the same writing document at the same time while seated at two different networked computers. Some programs also provide a chat window, allowing students to send comments back and forth to each other while they write.

Some programs designed to support collaborative writing are

- *CollaborEdit* (PaperFly Corporation)

- *CREATE Together* (Bytes of Learning)

- *Storyspace* (Eastgate Systems)

In addition to programs designed specifically for collaborative writing, there are general use electronic conferencing programs that enable two or more users to exchange audio and/or video with each other. Electronic conferencing systems support real-time communication, allowing users who are separated by geographic space, (e.g., across a building, a city, or the world) but connected via a network (e.g., cable, satellite) to talk back and forth with each other and, with some systems, to see each other while communicating. They range from the relatively simple and inexpensive (costing a few hundred dollars) to highly sophisticated and expensive systems (costing several thousand dollars), depending on the quality and speed of the audio and video exchange.

Many electronic conferencing systems also include a shared "whiteboard," which is a window that allows conference users to view and mark up shared text and/or graphic images. For example, a group of users engaged in an electronic conference could talk back and forth with each other about their plans for an upcoming event, then each bring up the shared whiteboard window and collaboratively view and mark up a flyer that one of them has posted.

Although many school systems do not yet have electronic conferencing equipment, the technology is rapidly becoming more affordable and reliable. One day, it may be commonplace for students to engage in real-time collaborative writing with co-authors around the world.

Considerations for Use

Although the research on collaborative writing is limited (nonexistent in the case of collaborative writing programs), there is some evidence to suggest that students with disabilities can benefit from working together in a computer-supported writing environment (MacArthur, 2000). Daiute and Dalton (1993) found that posttest stories written by low achieving third-grade students incorporated more story elements and reflected earlier discussions between the students when they had worked in pairs at their computers. Other researchers (Cosden, Goldman, & Hine, 1990; Hine, Goldman, & Cosden, 1990), who compared solo and paired performance for students with mild educational disabilities in a computer-supported writing summer program, found no advantage for the collaborative condition. In his review, MacArthur (2000) suggested, however, that this result might have stemmed from the fact that the pairs were given no guidance in how to interact constructively. Research is also needed on heterogeneous pairs, in which students with or without disabilities work together in an inclusive writing lab. Our experience in inclusive writing labs has taught us that such collaborative relationships can be beneficial. We observed some success among a group of students with written language disabilities using specialized software in an after-school project.

SPEECH RECOGNITION

Speech recognition technology has the potential to revolutionize the way people interact with computers and the way authors compose text. This promising tool can assist struggling writers whose spoken communication is relatively better than their written communication. The technology, also referred to as *voice input* technology,

Box 8.1. Individual Preferences for Collaborative Writing Software

In our work with collaborative writing software in an after-school writing lab, we found that some students with written language disabilities enjoyed the experience of working with a partner while others felt limited by the requirement to work with another student. For example, two students decided to write a story about cats. However, one student wrote about her two cats, and the other wrote about his cat. Only after significant scaffolding by teachers did the two students collaborate to add a section to the end of their story describing how all three cats got lost and then found.

Two other students, however, collaborated readily to write a mystery about some missing dinosaur and alien eggs. They worked together to develop the characters and plot and even inserted the idea of teamwork into the storyline. Figure 8.4 shows their work in progress before final editing.

We also found that students differed in their use of the chat window. Some pairs used the chat window to exchange relevant ideas about the story they were writing. Others used the chat window to send comments about the class or jokes to each other. Students with less developed social skills sometimes sent unintelligible strings of characters back and forth, a less sophisticated form of interaction, but interaction nevertheless.

The Mysterey Of the Missing Eggs

     In the middle of downtown Detroit an alien floo to earth on a spaceship. Then the kind scientist found out how to bring a dinosaur back to life. They had mixed different kinds of animal's blood to gather.

     The dinosaur and the alien were missing there eggs. Then they were fiting because they thought they had took each other's eggs. They had not known what they had been doing when they were fighting.

     The alien throo the dinosaur agenst the tower. Wen the dinosaur landed he saw a man with thare eggs.

"stop!" he sed. " Let's go get them!"

     They figured out who stole their eggs. They became a team to get there eggs back.

     The dinosaur and the alien got ther eggs back wen thay fond thare eggs in som ones house. Then the eggs did not hatch becaus the eggs war too colde . then the dinosaur and alien got married.   the end

Figure 8.4. Leann and Aaron's story.

Teaching Tip 8.1. Scaffolding Peer Interactions in Collaborative Writing

A critical variable in collaborative writing is selection of writing partners. In our work, depending on immediate objectives, we have assigned partners on the basis of writing strengths and weaknesses, shared interests, and compatible personalities. A few pairs consisted of one boy and one girl. In some cases, pairs worked well initially; in others, heavy intervention was required to encourage the collaboration. Students almost always prefer to select their own writing partners, and we recommend that they be allowed to do so, at least occasionally (McAlister et al., 1999). At other times, it may be worth the extra scaffolding effort to support students to work together who otherwise would not. It can provide a unique opportunity to teach new social interaction skills or tolerance for interpersonal differences.

Scaffolding of peer interactions is a consistent theme of this book. Effective inclusion of students with disabilities almost always requires scaffolding. In cases in which the team consists of one partner who is more capable, a private conversation about the importance of the role of this student can set the stage for a more positive interaction.

Any collaborative writing pair attempting to write simultaneously in the same document can benefit from assistance in structuring the collaboration. When investigating collaborative writing software, we used a series of text-based story grammar prompts (as explained in Chapter 7) to assist students to select which part of the story one of them would work on at any point in time. For example, one might work on a paragraph that tells about setting while another is drafting the paragraph in which the problem is explained. They might use the chat box to discuss how to end their story and who will take responsibility for producing the first draft of the conclusion. These structural supports, coupled with instructor scaffolding, make it possible for some students to work with peers who previously avoided such interactions.

allows a user to speak into a microphone attached to the computer rather than to type characters on a keyboard. Spoken words then appear as printed text in the writing document.

Speech recognition programs vary along several dimensions. First, some programs are dictation systems and others are command and control systems. Dictation systems place spoken words in a dictation window on the screen. After dictation, the user can copy and paste the contents of the dictation window into an open word processing document. Command and control systems, however, are not designed for text entry, but rather for controlling various operations and functions of the computer. They are most useful for people with physical disabilities that prohibit use of the keyboard.

Some speech recognition programs are discrete speech recognition systems, and others recognize continuous speech. Discrete speech recognition programs require the user to speak one word at a time, with a slight pause between words. Continuous speech programs allow the user to speak in normal conversational phrases, and the programs recognize longer strings of words. In fact, continuous speech recognition programs recognize longer phrases more accurately than discrete words.

Speech recognition systems also vary along training dimensions. Some systems are referred to as *speaker independent* and generally display high recognition rates with little or no speaker training required. Other systems are *speaker dependent*. They cannot be used at all unless they have been trained to recognize an individual speaker's voice. Speech recognition programs vary in the size of their dictionaries as well. Programs with smaller dictionaries have more difficulty recognizing unique words and require more individual user training than systems with more extensive dictionaries. Future research should shed light on best ways to use this feature.

Some speech recognition programs are

- *Dragon Dictate* (ScanSoft)

- *Dragon NaturallySpeaking* (ScanSoft)

- *ViaVoice* (IBM)

Considerations for Use

Research on speech recognition software is limited, but in one study, Higgins and Raskind (1995) found that college students with learning disabilities produced higher-rated essays in a computer-supported speech recognition condition compared with an unassisted condition. Although not directly attributable to speech recognition software, research also has shown that dictation to a human transcriber can help students with learning disabilities circumvent problems with mechanics and produce papers that are longer and higher in quality (Graham, 1990; MacArthur & Graham, 1987).

Speech recognition technology has great promise, but it also has problems. In the past, speech recognition software was extremely expensive and unreliable. Despite technological advances that have made it more affordable and accurate, some serious limitations remain. These include added cognitive burdens (e.g., remembering to dictate punctuation and formatting commands, demands on abilities to recognize and correct mistakes) and continuing accuracy problems, particularly for individuals with nonstandard pronunciation or language disorders (MacArthur, 2000).

When addressing the cognitive burden issue, instructors should review the ways that spoken communication differs from printed text (see Chapter 2). Whereas people often use partial sentences and phrases when they speak, relying on tone of voice and expression to clarify meaning, a different set of standards operates when writing. In written language, words alone must convey the meaning, necessitating a shift in register as well as modality, during dictation. On a more basic level, students need concepts of word boundaries to use a discrete word recognition system, the use of which, however, might provide opportunities to scaffold that understanding reciprocally.

In addition, although speech recognition eliminates the need to type, it requires students to monitor the screen continuously to ensure that the words or phrases they dictated are indeed the word or phrases that the computer has recognized and printed on the screen. This constant monitoring may tax some students, particularly those with limited spelling skills who cannot read what the computer displays. Such students may need a word processor with speech synthesis to hear what has been printed on the screen.

Cognitive demands also are associated with the training phase. Because speech recognition programs generally are separate applications, rather than an integrated feature of a word processor, they must be used in conjunction with one's selected word processor. Because these programs are not built-in to word processors, they have an add-on set of commands, icons, and menu bars that students must learn, which requires a focused effort, generally involving repeated readings of standard text—another skill likely to be impaired for students with LLDs.

The limited research that is available on speech recognition programs provides some evidence that discrete speech recognition programs are easier for students with LLDs to use than continuous speech recognition systems (Follansbee, 1999). Continuous speech systems require the user to think in complete phrases and sentences before dictating and to enunciate words clearly and consistently within a stream of continuous speech, meanwhile reflecting on and modifying performance while dictating and avoiding extraneous vocalizations (MacArthur, 2000). Discrete speech recognition systems slow down the dictation process so that language processing, pronunciation, and monitoring are more manageable for inexperienced writers. Problems remain, however, related to cognitive demands for sustained attention and adequate working memory, as well as environmental demands for quiet environments. In general, when working with younger students and students with special language and learning needs, we recommend starting with dictation to a human who can scaffold intentionally, then moving to a discrete speech recognition program.

Another caveat for using speech recognition software is that the software may not be accurate enough to save time and effort during the writing process, particularly if students have nonstandard or disordered pronunciation. Students must learn how to "speak" to the computer to optimize recognition, and any extraneous noise will affect the accuracy. If the software does not accurately recognize the student's speech and print the correct words, the student may spend too much time correcting speech recognition errors instead of writing. Teachers may need to monitor students' error rates for several weeks to determine whether the software makes the drafting process easier or more difficult and time consuming. The bottom line is that although speech recognition software has the potential to support some students to write independently who otherwise would be unable to do so, it is not a panacea for solving the varied transcription problems for all students with written language difficulties.

SUMMARY

During the drafting stage, students may require scaffolding for word retrieval, spelling, and typing tasks. Students who are unable to spell or generate any written text can select picture symbols instead of words and then convert the symbols to text with the click of a mouse. Another option for students who need spelling assistance during the drafting stage is word prediction or a word bank feature. With word prediction, students can select words from a constantly changing numbered list of predicted options and simply enter a corresponding number rather than typing a complete word. Customized word banks (or notepads) provide a lower technology alternative to word prediction by making words available on the screen as a model to support the student while drafting. Abbreviation expansion and macros also provide assistance to students during the drafting stage. For text that must be entered over and over again, such as a header or title page, students can type short abbreviations that will expand to longer strings of text, or they can access macro files to activate a series of saved commands and keystrokes. Collaborative writing can also help students during the drafting stage by enabling two or more students to work together on a shared document. Finally, although it adds cognitive demands in some areas, speech recognition technology can allow students to bypass the keyboard altogether and dictate text instead.

Software Features that Support Revising and Editing

9

Most educators appreciate the benefits of using word processors for revising and editing. Rather than erasing, crossing out, and rewriting on paper, students can use a variety of editing tools to revise and edit text on screen. Just providing the technology is not enough, however. "Word processing does not directly help students learn how to evaluate their writing, diagnose problems, or fix those problems" (MacArthur, 2000).

Revising and editing often are thought of as synonymous, but actually they are two different, but related, processes. Revising refers to changing the organization or content of a document to enhance its clarity or meaning. For example, after rereading a piece of work for content and clarity, a student might seek to improve it by reordering paragraphs, adding or deleting sentences, changing vocabulary, or revising the macrostructure. Editing, on the other hand, involves careful proofreading of surface-level details to identify whether changes are needed related to mechanics. Examples include fixing spelling errors, adding punctuation, capitalizing letters, or changing verb tenses. Editing enhances the accuracy of a document but does not necessarily alter its meaning.

Typically, when students write stories, they engage in a repetitive process of drafting, revising, and redrafting, but they do most of their editing just prior to printing or publishing. Figure 9.1 lists word processing features that can scaffold students during both the revising and editing stages.

STANDARD EDITING TOOLS

Nearly all word processors, whether designed for adults or children, include basic, standard editing tools such as cut, copy, and paste. Most word processors allow users to highlight (by dragging the mouse) a letter, word, or string of text; copy it to the com-

Revising and editing
Standard editing tools
Thesaurus and rhyming word tools
Spelling checkers
Homonym checkers
Grammar checkers
On-screen manuals
Speech synthesis

Figure 9.1. Taxonomy of software features that support revising and editing.

puter's memory; and duplicate it (i.e., paste it) somewhere else in the document or in another document. Likewise, most word processors allow users to cut highlighted text and then paste it in another location in the same document or in another document. These standard features make it easy for students to move whole words, sentences, or even paragraphs around as they revise their stories and reports.

Many word processors also include editing tools that allow users to search for particular words they have typed, then edit or replace those words (see Figure 9.2). For example, a student who wanted to change the word *dog* to *Dalmatian* every time it occurred in a story could select the replace tool, enter the word *dog* for "find what" and the word *Dalmatian* for "replace with," then click "find next" to begin the search and replace process.

The find-and-replace function requires the user to specify appropriate replacement words. For some students who have difficulty generating alternative words for ones they have already typed, a tool that provides recommendations, such as a thesaurus (described in the next section), may be more useful.

Some children's word processors that include standard editing tools are

- *Creative Writer 2* (Microsoft)

- *Student Writing Center* (Riverdeep/The Learning Company)

- *Ultimate Writing & Creativity Center* (Riverdeep/The Learning Company)

Considerations for Use

The biggest direct challenge when using revising and editing tools in children's word processors is figuring out and remembering which icons represent which tasks. Unlike adult word processors that use a relatively standard set of icons to depict such actions as cut, copy, and paste, some children's tools use different sets of metaphoric images. For example, in *Creative Writer* (Microsoft), students must select an icon depicting a chicken and cracked egg to undo the previous action, whereas in most adult word processors, selecting "edit/undo" performs this process. A toaster serves as the icon for the printer, with a metaphoric meaning that escapes even most adults. For some programs,

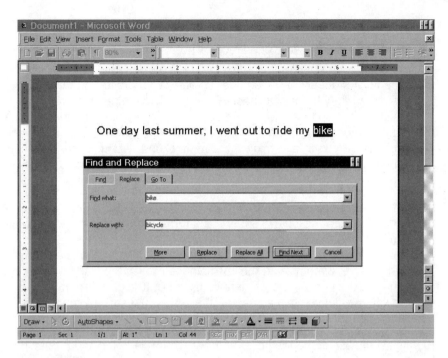

Figure 9.2. Replace tool in *Word*.

especially those that use a unique set of icons such as these, teachers may need to instruct students directly about symbols (perhaps leading a discussion about choosing symbols that would be less abstract). The instructional team also could create and post a command reference sheet near the computer.

The most significant indirect challenge when teaching students to use revising and editing tools is the need to help them acquire the metacognitive and metalinguistic skills for evaluating work critically and deciding when and how to make changes. One study found that simple access to word processing does not change the amount or quality of revisions made by students with learning disabilities (MacArthur & Graham, 1987). Learning revising tools can help to make the possibilities for change more salient, however, if combined with instruction in revision. MacArthur and his associates found that such instruction improved students' revising and overall writing produced with word processors (Graham & MacArthur, 1988; MacArthur et al., 1991a).

THESAURUS AND RHYMING WORD TOOLS

Many word processing programs offer features that can help students generate alternative words for ones they have typed. The most common example of this word replacement feature is a thesaurus. An on-screen thesaurus contains synonyms, and sometimes antonyms, for selected words. Students highlight a word they have typed, select the thesaurus tool from the menu bar, scroll through a list of synonyms for the target word, then click again to replace the target word in their document with the selected

---

Teaching Tip 9.1.   Teaching Students to Use Standard Editing Tools

When first introducing students to standard word processing features, be aware of the opportunity for new vocabulary learning and the need to provide explicit instruction to introduce it (e.g., *keyboard, shift key, space bar, mouse, click and hold, left click, right click, double click, highlight, drag, cut and paste*). Remember that students with disabilities might need more exposure and concrete experience to learn key vocabulary, but expect them to be highly motivated in the computer-use context, and expect them to learn along with their classmates.

Often, the opportunity to teach revising software features (and to check on knowledge of related vocabulary) arises in the form of teachable moments while working with students at their computers. The scaffolding instructor might ask, "Do you want me to show you a cool way to move those words to where you want them?" If the answer is affirmative, the instructor can coach the student to use the highlight-and-drag or cut-and-paste features. If not, the instructor might say, "Okay, let me know when you're ready, and I can show you what this cut-and-paste thing is all about."

Relate the use of the tool to what the student is learning about the writing process. For example, if a student is learning to connect sentences with transition words or conjunctions other than *and then,* scaffolding might focus on deleting excessive examples of *and.* Then, the student could be scaffolded to have the computer reread the selection and to reflect on whether the text sounds okay without *and,* or if there could be a better way to say it. When a deleted *and* is determined to be necessary after all, the opportunity may be right to teach the "undo" feature.

Early in this process, students should be taught that if they highlight a block of text and type anything, even a single letter, what they type would replace the text they have highlighted. This is a good thing to model in a minilesson introducing the editing features, along with the "undo" feature.

---

word from the thesaurus (see Figure 9.3). Most full-featured adult word processors include a thesaurus as a standard feature.

Several children's programs also incorporate this feature:

- *EasyBook Deluxe* (Sunburst)

- *Student Writing Center* (Riverdeep/The Learning Company)

- *The Amazing Writing Machine* (Riverdeep/The Learning Company)

- *Ultimate Writing & Creativity Center* (Riverdeep/The Learning Company)

Another word replacement feature found in some programs is a rhyming word tool. Similar to a thesaurus that provides synonyms and antonyms, this feature provides a list of words that rhyme with the target word.

A children's word processor that includes a rhyming word feature is *The Amazing Writing Machine* (Riverdeep/The Learning Company).

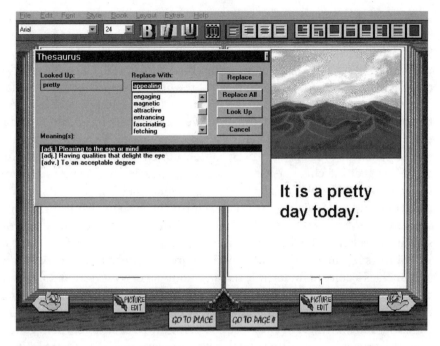

Figure 9.3. Thesaurus in *EasyBook Deluxe.*

Considerations for Use

Although we have not directly studied the use of an on-screen thesaurus with students who have writing difficulties, we have observed some students using the feature on their own. Students must have fairly good decoding skills to read the alternative words that are presented on the screen. If not, teams might look for thesaurus tools that can accommodate users with poor reading skills by including speech synthesis, enabling the computer to read the word list aloud. Also, students must understand various parts of speech and have a rich inner vocabulary to avoid choosing inappropriate words from the list of alternatives.

The rhyming word option might be especially helpful when students compose poetry. Word replacement features such as a thesaurus or a rhyming word tool are used most often during the revising and editing stage after students have already produced some text. Students with word finding problems, however, might use such tools to scaffold themselves during the planning and organizing or drafting stages.

SPELLING CHECKERS

Most word processors designed for adults, and many designed for children, include spelling checkers. Spelling checkers perform two basic functions—identifying misspelled words and suggesting correct spellings (MacArthur, Graham, Haynes, & DeLaPaz, 1996). Typically, students enter and revise text, then invoke the spelling checker when they are ready to edit. The spelling checker searches the writing document for words that are not contained in its spelling checker dictionary. When it finds a spelling error (i.e., a word not in its dictionary), the program highlights the word and suggests several alternative correct spellings. Users can select one of the correctly spelled words, type in a different attempt, or skip the word altogether. They also might have the option of adding a new replacement word to the spelling checker dictionary so that the "error" is not highlighted again (see Figure 9.4). We strongly advise refraining from introducing this option to students, however, and if they have discovered it, prohibiting them from using it independently. This step is essential to prevent the software spelling dictionary from becoming contaminated with incorrectly spelled words.

Most spelling checkers require author activation after text has been entered. Typically, students should be encouraged to invoke spelling checkers after they have finished drafting and revising, during the editing phase, and just prior to publishing. Some students, however, prefer to check their spelling more frequently and may access the spelling checker while drafting and revising, using it as a scaffold for text generation.

Some spelling checkers alert writers immediately to misspellings by providing a cue, such as a colored underline, flash, or sound. For some students, this feature is helpful, enabling them to check and correct their spelling as they write. For others, particularly those who make frequent errors, this feature may interfere with planning, organizing, and drafting. For these students, it may be best to let them generate and revise text, then access the spelling checker only when they are ready to edit. Instructors are advised to observe and talk with students about their individual spelling checker preferences and to look for a program with selection options.

Spelling checkers use either typographic or phonetic algorithms (rules) for matching errors to possible correct words. An algorithm based on typographic principles chooses

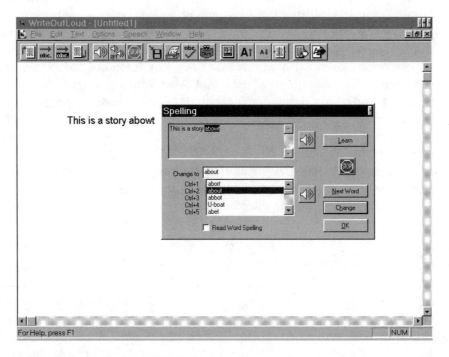

Figure 9.4. Spelling checker in *Write: Outloud.*

alternative words based on how closely the letters match the "misspelled" word. This type of spelling checker, typically found in adult word processors, is designed for relatively competent spellers who occasionally make a typographical error. Spelling checkers that use a phonetic algorithm display words that are phonetically similar to the misspelled word. These are generally more useful for children who are poor spellers who may spell words like they sound. Unfortunately, software catalogs do not identify the type of algorithm used in spelling checkers. Educators must try out various spelling checkers to learn their features.

Some children's word processors that include spelling checkers are

- *Co:Writer 4000* (Don Johnston)

- *Draft:Builder* (Don Johnston)

- *Dr. Peet's Talk/Writer* (Interest-Driven Learning)

- *EasyBook Deluxe* (Sunburst)

- *Intellitalk II* (Intellitools)

- *Student Writing Center* (Riverdeep/The Learning Company)

- *The Amazing Writing Machine* (Riverdeep/The Learning Company)

- *Type & Talk* (textHELP! Systems Ltd.)

- *Ultimate Writing & Creativity Center* (Riverdeep/The Learning Company)

- *Write:Outloud* (Don Johnston)

Considerations for Use

The handful of studies that have been conducted on spelling checkers support the effectiveness of using them. MacArthur and his colleagues (1996) investigated the use of spelling checkers with middle school students with learning disabilities and moderate to severe spelling problems, who misspelled 4%–35% of their words at baseline. The students were able to correct 37% of the errors with a computerized spelling checker, compared with correcting 9% of errors unaided. McNaughton, Hughes, and Clark (1997) studied proofreading and editing processes among college students with learning disabilities. They compared assistance provided by a handheld spelling checker or a dictionary with use of spelling checkers integrated into word processing software. Neither the handheld tool nor the dictionary assisted the students to detect spelling errors (although they did assist the students to correct errors), but with the integrated spelling checker, students were able to detect and correct about 60% of their spelling errors.

Although spelling checkers can be useful during editing, there are limitations. Spelling checkers may not find 100% of spelling errors in a document, as they are not able to identify misspellings that match the correct spellings of other words, such as homonyms. In their research, MacArthur and colleagues (1996) found that 37% of students' misspellings were not detected because the words were homonyms. Spelling checkers also may be unable to suggest correct spellings for words that are dramatically misspelled. The spelling checker in the study by MacArthur and colleagues (1996) failed to present a correct choice for 42% of students' misspellings. Even if the cor-

Teaching Tip 9.2. Teaching Students to Use Spelling Checkers

If the software program your students are using has a spelling checker feature, wait to introduce it until the students have had some experience entering text. Then, teach the feature by modeling it in a minilesson by using a spelling checker on a composition of your own in which you have planted numerous spelling errors to demonstrate the features of the program. Model by thinking aloud through the process, asking students for suggestions to activate their constructive problem solving when a correct word does not appear in the list, or in the case of homonyms, showing them how important careful proofreading is. After the minilesson, provide additional scaffolding to individual students who need it. As a rule, suggest that students wait to check for spelling until the editing phase of their writing.

When a spelling checker identifies a misspelled word, encourage students to generate their own alternative before consulting the spelling checker list. The spelling checker in the program *Ultimate Writing & Creativity Center* (Riverdeep/The Learning Company), for example, opens a window that allows children the option of typing in a corrected spelling before choosing to see the list. One of the third-grade teachers with whom we worked required her students to try at least one alternative spelling on their own before checking the list.

Help children understand that spelling checkers often do not recognize the correct spellings of their proper names, but if at all possible, prevent them from using the feature to add a word to the software spelling dictionary. Once students learn this feature, there is a risk that they will add words indiscriminately, with the result that the program will begin to treat a number of added misspelled words as if they were spelled correctly. This contaminates the feature for them and others who use the same computer.

rectly spelled word does appear, students with disabilities may have difficulty identifying and selecting the correct alternative if their reading decoding skills are inadequate or the list is too long. To assist students, some spelling checkers provide speech synthesis to pronounce alternative words aloud, making it easier for students with special needs to recognize and select their intended word from the list. Students also can benefit from instruction in how to generate additional suggestions if the list does not include the intended word (McNaughton, Hughes, & Ofiesh, 1997).

HOMONYM CHECKERS

In addition to checking spelling, a few word processing programs check for homonyms (e.g., *there, their; two, to, too; here, hear*). These programs highlight homonyms found in the writing document and provide students with on-screen definitions. After reviewing the definitions, students are expected to select the appropriate word to use or to go on to the next homonym.

Some programs that include homonym checkers are *Type & Talk* (textHELP! Systems Ltd.) and *Write:Outloud* (Don Johnston)

Considerations for Use

To use a homonym checker effectively, students must understand the concept of homonyms, and they must be able to read the definitions offered by the computer. Most young authors need instruction and scaffolding to learn how to use this feature; however, a homonym checker could serve as a technological scaffold to frame those cues for a student, supported by instructor scaffolding to interpret and respond to them.

GRAMMAR CHECKERS

In addition to spelling, many students struggle with sentence structure and syntax. Some word processors offer grammar checkers to assist students with editing for punctuation, word usage, and grammatical errors. These programs highlight possible problems, such as missing words or punctuation, possessive errors, noun–verb agreement errors, or double negatives, and then offer advice about how to fix the problem(s). For example, if a student types the phrase, *the boy gived the dog a bone,* a grammar checker might highlight the word *gived* and recommend that the student use the correct past tense form of the verb *to give.* A word processor that includes a grammar checker is *Word* (Microsoft).

Considerations for Use

To use a grammar checker successfully, the tool must highlight errors appropriately, and students must be able to understand the advice given by the tool in order to make corrections. Thus, grammar-checking tools are likely to be more useful for older students and those with greater language competence, who can understand the feedback that is provided.

Research on this feature suggests that further development is needed before it will be really useful (MacArthur, 2000). In perhaps the only experimental study of a grammar checker by students with disabilities, Lewis, Ashton, Haapa, Kieley, and Fielden (1999) studied a software program designed specifically for students with disabilities and found that it 1) identified fewer than half of students' grammatical errors, 2) provided feedback that was confusing to the students, and 3) did not result in any reduction in grammatical errors in the students' compositions. At this point, it appears that instructor- or peer scaffolding might be necessary to assist students to identify grammatical errors and reformulate them. Speech synthesis provides an alternative for scaffolding students to identify missing or inappropriate words or phrasing more independently and to focus them on the need for edits.

ON-SCREEN MANUALS

Some word processing programs include on-screen manuals whereby students can look up grammar, punctuation, or writing tips, much like they might do with a reference book. These on-screen manuals look like books and allow students to search the contents for information about topics in which they are interested. For example, *Student Writing Center* (Riverdeep/The Learning Company) includes a feature called "Tips." Students can click on the Tips button, then select report, newsletter, journal, letter, sign, writing, or grammar tips. Once they are in a particular section, students can search for tips on a specific topic, such as commas, and read general information about that topic (see Figure 9.5). The advantage of an on-screen manual versus a hard copy of the same is that it can be searched quickly and does not clutter one's writing space.

Examples of word processors that include an on-screen manual are *Student Writing Center* (Riverdeep/The Learning Company) and *Ultimate Writing & Creativity Center* (Riverdeep/The Learning Company).

Considerations for Use

Use of on-screen manuals requires relatively well-developed decoding and comprehension skills. Students must be able to determine the topic about which they need more information, find the appropriate section of the manual, read the information, and then apply the information to their own writing. For students with severe reading difficulties, the process of accessing and using on-screen manuals may not be feasible.

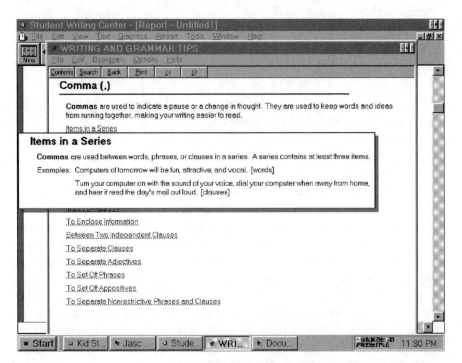

Figure 9.5. Tips about comma use in *Student Writing Center.* © 2003 Riverdeep Interactive Learning Limited, and its licensors.

SPEECH SYNTHESIS

In our experience, one of the most useful features for students across all stages of the writing process is speech synthesis, also known as *text-to-speech* capability. As noted throughout Section II, speech synthesis can facilitate access to other tools for students with limited word decoding abilities. Word processors equipped with full speech synthesis capabilities can be used to pronounce individual letters, words, sentences, paragraphs, or whole documents aloud, enabling young authors to hear what they have written.

Auditory feedback provided by speech synthesis can help students detect spelling or typing errors, alert them to missing or incorrect words, and help them to determine whether or not their stories are clearly written. Most word processors that include speech synthesis allow writers to choose a voice for the speech synthesis, to select the level of speech desired (e.g., letters, words, or sentences), and to turn the feature on or off at any time. For example, students might turn on speech synthesis during drafting, or only activate it when they are ready to revise and edit. In the early learning stages, listening to the computer read one's work might be more a novelty than an intentional aid to revising, but as students become more sophisticated, they are more likely to activate the feature to conduct a conscious review of their work.

In a computer-supported writing lab, some educators prefer students to listen to their documents with the speech synthesizer before requesting teacher assistance. To minimize excessive noise, headphones can be attached to student computers.

Some word processors that include text-to-speech capabilities are

- *Clicker* (Crick Software)
- *Dr. Peet's Talk/Writer* (Interest-Driven Learning)
- *EasyBook Deluxe* (Sunburst)
- *Intellitalk II* (Intellitools)
- *Kids Media Magic* (Sunburst)
- *Storybook Weaver Deluxe* (Riverdeep/The Learning Company)
- *The Amazing Writing Machine* (Riverdeep/The Learning Company)
- *Type & Talk* (textHELP! Systems Ltd.)
- *Ultimate Writing & Creativity Center* (Riverdeep/The Learning Company)
- *Write:Outloud* (Don Johnston)

Considerations for Use

Because speech synthesizers use complex algorithms to convert text to speech, they may occasionally mispronounce correctly spelled words. This may confuse some students, making them think they have made an error when they have not. Most programs that include speech synthesis allow teachers or students to edit pronunciations by entering phonetic spellings of words into a speech dictionary. This process takes time,

---

Teaching Tip 9.3.   Using the Scaffolding Support of Speech Synthesis

Students with limited word decoding skills should be acquainted with opportunities to use speech synthesis to support their use of other software tools (e.g., spelling checkers, word prediction). For all students, speech synthesis is particularly good at providing feedback without evaluation or judgment. This makes it easier for students to use the feedback independently to reflect on their work and to implement revising and editing processes.

Encourage the use of speech synthesis feedback to aid editing processes, as well as revising. For example, punctuation omission at the ends of sentences would lead the computer to read a selection without a pause. This cue might be brought to the student's attention with scaffolding about sentence boundaries. One third-grade student, who had spelled "Mr." without the period, complained to his instructor, "That thing reads my story wrong. It says 'M' 'R' instead of 'mister.'" The instructor responded with a scaffolding question, "Is there anything you could do to make the computer read it right?" Immediately, the student observed, "Oh, I need to add a period." In such ways, computer-based scaffolds and human scaffolds support each other.

---

however, and time is always at a premium in a busy writing lab. We have found that most students learn to make allowances for bad pronunciation of proper nouns, in particular, and that they may become more conscious of the distinction between proper and common nouns in the process.

In our own work with speech synthesis, we found that some students relied on speech synthesis throughout the writing process, even using it to check their spelling after every two or three words. Other students rarely invoked the speech synthesizer, choosing instead to read their stories silently. For such students, speech synthesis with personal headphones would afford support with privacy. Headphones offer a way to hold down the cacophony in a computer writing lab but they may interfere with instructor scaffolding.

The experimental research on speech synthesis is extremely limited at this point and inconclusive. MacArthur concluded, "More research is needed before conclusions can be reached about the value of speech synthesis as a support for revising" (2000, p. 93). Anecdotally, however, our experience has been that it is a useful feature across all stages of the writing process.

SUMMARY

Word processors provide several tools that can scaffold students during the revising and editing stage, often the most difficult process for young writers to master. Most word processors include standard editing tools that allow students to copy or move blocks of text around easily within or between documents.

Students who have difficulty thinking of the precise words they want to use or who struggle with using a variety of vocabulary words in their writing pieces may benefit from word replacement tools, such as a thesaurus or a rhyming word option. They can draft words with which they are familiar and then find alternative words with similar or opposite meanings during the revising stage. A few programs include a rhyming word option, providing lists of words that rhyme with target words selected by students.

Many word processing programs provide features that help students find and fix spelling, homonyms, or grammatical errors. Several word processors include a speech synthesis feature, enabling young writers to hear what they have written. Others provide on-screen manuals that students can search for general information about punctuation, grammar, or writing tips. Through careful consideration of the revising and editing tools available, teams can select programs that best meet the needs of their students during this important phase of the writing process.

Software Features that Support Publishing

A critical feature of the writing lab approach is publishing for an authentic audience. During the writing process, printing student work on paper generally is referred to as *desktop publishing.* Students also can publish their final work in electronic format on a computer screen. Stories presented on screen can include not only static text and graphics but also animation, video, and sound. Electronic publishing generally is referred to as *desktop presentation.* Word processors offer students many features to support printing their work on paper or presenting it on a computer screen (see Figure 10.1).

DESKTOP PUBLISHING

Even before students start the writing process, it is important for them to know the purpose of their writing, who their audience will be, and how their work will be published—whether on paper or on a computer screen. If the goal is to produce text that will be printed on paper, it is helpful to use a word processing program that provides desktop publishing support. Such word processors may include

- Desktop publishing features
- Book formatting features
- Alternative publishing format features

Desktop Publishing Features

Nearly all word processors, even the simplest, include what can now be called standard desktop publishing features. These include options to change the text font, size, and

Publishing	
Desktop publishing	Desktop presentation
Desktop publishing features Book formatting Alternative publishing formats	Multimedia options Electronic book formatting Publishing on the World Wide Web

Figure 10.1. Taxonomy of software features that support publishing.

style. A *font* is a typeface. Typically, word processors offer several different fonts from which to choose and enable writers to mix various fonts in a single document. For example, this text is typed in Arial font and this text is typed in Times New Roman font. In a process approach to writing, students choose the fonts they want to use in their stories, with encouragement to select fonts that are most readable for their intended audiences.

In addition to changing fonts, most word processors allow users to determine the size of the text. Text size is measured in units called points with one point equivalent to approximately $1/72$ of an inch. Thus, larger numbers indicate larger text size.

This is 12-point text.

This is 14-point text.

This is 18-point text.

Some word processors include just a few fonts and text sizes from which to choose. Others provide "scalable" fonts, that is, fonts that can be sized as large or small as the user specifies, without losing any print quality.

Various styles also can be applied to printed text. Most word processors designed for children include at least two or three basic style options such as **bold,** *italics,* and <u>underline</u>. Others, particularly those designed for adults, offer additional style options such as <u>double underline</u>, ~~strikethrough~~, and shadow, to name a few. *Creative Writer 2* (Microsoft) even offers animated style options that are visible on the computer screen but not when printed on paper, such as shimmering text, sparkling text, text that fades in and out, blinking text, and marching ants (a moving border around text).

In addition to text font, size, and style, some word processors offer other desktop publishing features to help writers format their text for the printed page. These features vary from program to program and may include tools enabling users to

- Merge text and graphics together on the same page
- Use drawing and painting tools to illustrate their works
- Add borders
- Change text and background colors
- Create text shapes
- Justify text (left, center, right, or full justification)
- Set margin width

- Set line spacing
- Create tables
- Print text in columns
- Create headers and footers
- Number pages
- Use bullets
- Select alternative paper size
- Print vertically (portrait mode) or horizontally (landscape mode)

Considerations for Use

Most children's word processors provide a subset of the desktop publishing features found in programs designed for adults, but programs vary widely and few include exactly the same set of tools as adult programs. Typically, programs designed for younger children include fewer desktop publishing features than those designed for older students and adults. Programs with limited desktop publishing features may prohibit students from formatting their final printed work exactly the way they want it to look.

Modifying fonts and other features can be fun, but it also can take attention away from writing and can lead students to produce shorter texts (Bahr, Nelson, Van Meter, & Yanna, 1996). As students become more proficient in using special features and more confident in their writing, however, they can generally achieve a balance in how they approach the task. Teaching Tip 10.1 also provides some suggestions about scaffolding the use of presentation features.

Desktop publishing is a great leveler. As one collaborating teacher commented (see Chapter 13), students' products "can look similar as far as the overall appearance of the product that gets printed out," although, "if you look at the details, you might see differences in the vocabulary usage or the spelling." In this way, desktop publishing is a major contributor to the inclusion of students with special needs with their peers.

Book Formatting

In a process-writing classroom, one of the most common ways for children to publish their writing is in book form. Typically, books are created as paperback books (construction paper covers over paper) or as hardcover books (cardboard and cloth). Several word processing programs designed for children facilitate the creation of books by formatting students' writing as book pages. Rather than presenting a blank screen that students fill with text, and then format afterwards, these programs present a preformatted book page layout on the computer screen (see Figure 10.2). The on-screen page layout usually includes separate areas for entering graphics and text. Sometimes, the author can determine the size and position of these areas. After authors fill in the preformatted areas with text and graphics, they can print the pages and bind them together

Teaching Tip 10.1. Using Desktop Publishing Features

When introducing new features, it is wise to give students some time to explore and share with one another as they learn about the features. As soon as possible, however, it is important to teach them to connect the idea of using particular features deliberately, with the intention of achieving particular effects in their audience. Chapter 13 describes case examples that illustrate the power of giving students with disabilities the opportunities to be the knowledgeable ones at times, engaging them to demonstrate new features for peers.

To encourage reluctant writers, plan an early project that has only a small amount of text and that offers opportunities to try out interesting desktop publishing features. For example, About the Author pieces are appropriate across a wide range of grade levels. They allow students to write about things they know, using words, such as family names, that they are more likely to know how to spell. Author photos may be taken with a digital camera and imported into documents. Then, students can explore various formatting options, such as borders, font variations, and clip art.

If necessary, instructional teams can set limits as to when and how much time students should spend using desktop publishing features, perhaps reserving formatting for the final stages, after editing. Keep in mind, though, that it is the application of such features that may be the initial hook for some reluctant writers (see Chapter 5). We do not think it is wise to punish students who have difficulty generating text by prohibiting them from working on the visual aspects of their work, an area in which they may have greater strengths. Rather, scaffolding might consist of helping students control their own decisions, suggesting, for example, "Let's see if we can finish this paragraph. I am sure you will want to have some time to make your work look really nice." Even if their early works are shorter than peers', it is important for them to have a finished product that looks good.

Adding illustrations and other features works better after a minilesson on how to choose appropriate images to augment the content of the piece. This is a good opportunity to model the decision-making process, starting with consideration of some inappropriate choices and leading the students in a discussion of why such choices would not make sense and would not achieve the author's purpose as well as others.

Working on a collaborative project, such as producing a newspaper or an activity book, can provide opportunities to try out many different features and to create a product that incorporates the work of a whole class of students, including those with disabilities.

into a book. Typically, book-formatting programs also provide an initial screen that prompts students to create a book cover page, including a title, author, and graphics. Most also provide an automatic page numbering option.

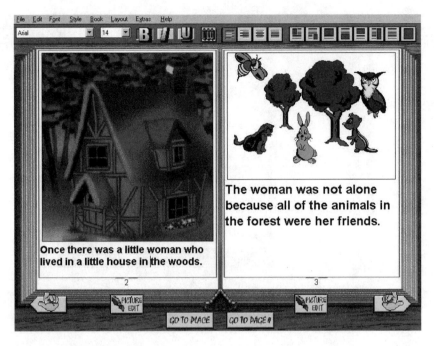

Figure 10.2. On-screen page layout from *EasyBook Deluxe*.

In addition to facilitating publication of standard size books on 8.5″ x 11″ paper, a few programs offer options to create "big books." These programs typically enable students to print their stories in several different sizes. *EasyBook Deluxe* (Sunburst), for example, allows users to create four sizes of books: mini-books, half-page size, full-page size, and poster books (see Figure 10.3). The pages can be printed on standard size paper, then folded or taped together, as directed by the program.

Some children's word processors that provide features to support book publishing are

- *EasyBook Deluxe* (Sunburst)

- *Kid Works Deluxe* (Knowledge Adventure)

- *Storybook Weaver Deluxe* (Riverdeep/The Learning Company)

- *The Amazing Writing Machine* (Riverdeep/The Learning Company)

Considerations for Use

Some book-formatting software does not allow text to wrap from one page to the next when new language is inserted during the revision process. This became a problem when we were attempting to use *EasyBook Deluxe* with third graders. Although the students liked being able to choose whether to put text or illustrations on each page, they found it frustrating to attempt to add text in the middle of a full page. Adult assistance was required to cut and paste text from one page to the next after one became full.

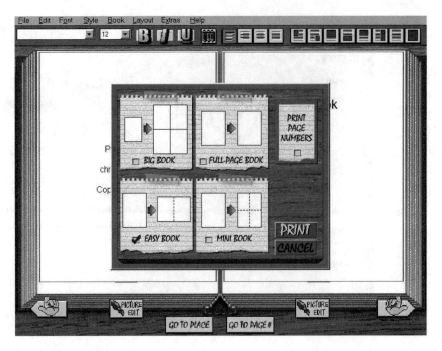

Figure 10.3. Book format from *EasyBook Deluxe*.

Publishing a hardback book of their own is extremely motivating to students. In one school, we literally cut and pasted pages produced with a word processor into blank books that already had been bound. The students' original illustrations were particularly wonderful, and the students were so proud of their books that the effort was worth it.

Alternative Publishing Formats

In a writing lab approach classroom, students frequently publish their stories in book form, but also benefit from opportunities to publish other kinds of written documents, such as newspapers, signs, and greeting cards. Some word processing tools provide specific support for alternative publishing formats. *The Print Shop* (Broderbund) family of products, for example, prompts users first to select a publishing format and then guides users through the process of creating the selected product. The program helps students create banners, signs, certificates, posters, bookmarks, stationery, calendars, labels, greeting cards, and other printed products. It includes thousands of graphics, ready-made design layouts, scalable fonts, and text effects (or text styles).

Some programs that support alternative publishing formats are

- *The Print Shop* (Broderbund)

- *Ultimate Writing & Creativity Center* (Riverdeep/The Learning Company)

- *Creative Writer 2* (Microsoft)

Considerations for Use

When the goal is to increase written language skill, it is best to engage students in projects that involve planning and writing extended discourse texts. Alternative publishing formats, however, provide opportunities for students to explore different features and prepare products to achieve particular purposes.

DESKTOP AND WEB PRESENTATION

In addition to supporting the traditional method of publishing text on paper, some writing programs allow students to publish, or *present,* their work on a computer screen. Desktop presentation programs enable printed work to come alive with animation and sound. Instead of printing their work on paper, students play their stories on a computer screen. Desktop presentation features include

- Tools that provide multimedia options

- Features that support electronic book formatting

- Tools that facilitate publishing on the web

Multimedia Options

As discussed in Chapter 7, some word processing programs provide multimedia options, allowing students to enhance their text with graphics, sounds, and video images. Programs that provide multimedia options are most useful for desktop presentation of student work. While writing, students are not limited to production of text and still graphic images. They can embed sound effects, animated text styles, and video images in their stories. Usually, multimedia programs allow students to import graphic, sound, and video resources from other programs, or they provide built-in tools enabling students to create their own resources. For example, to promote ownership of their work and a real sense of authorship, students can record themselves reading their own stories or reports aloud, save the recordings, then embed them into their writing documents. When such multimedia-enhanced documents are presented on a computer screen, an audience can hear young authors read their own work.

Several software programs that provide multimedia options to facilitate desktop presentation are

- *CREATE Together* (Bytes of Learning)

- *HyperStudio* (Knowledge Adventure)

- *Kid Pix Deluxe 3* (Broderbund)

- *Kid Pix Studio Deluxe* (Broderbund)

- *Kid Works Deluxe* (Knowledge Adventure)

- *Kids Media Magic* (Sunburst)

- *MediaWeaver* (Sunburst)
- *mPOWER4* (Multimedia Design Corporation)
- *MP Express* (Bytes of Learning)
- *Ultimate Writing & Creativity Center* (Riverdeep/The Learning Company)

Considerations for Use

Qualitative research has supported the intuitive expectation that multimedia authoring can be highly motivating to students (Daiute & Morse, 1994), although quantitative research suggests that the time spent formatting and inserting unique features may mean less time writing (Bahr, Nelson, Van Meter, & Yanna, 1996). Students whose strengths lie in areas of graphic design and spoken language rather than in written language production particularly may be able to shine in the production of multimedia presentations. The result may be that increased self-esteem creates a willingness to risk trying new things in other areas of learning.

Electronic Book Formatting

Electronic book formatting refers to the presentation of a book on a computer screen. Programs that include electronic book formatting capabilities combine two features: book formatting (discussed in Desktop Publishing) and multimedia options. In other words, electronic book programs present a preformatted book on the computer screen and allow students to enter text, graphics, sounds, or video images. Typically, readers turn pages by clicking forward or backward arrows or icons located at the top or bottom of each page. As pages turn, sounds or video images may play automatically, or readers may need to click on particular words, graphics, or buttons to hear associated sound effects or see moving video images.

Several programs that support electronic book formatting are

- *EasyBook Deluxe* (Sunburst)
- *Imagination Express* (Riverdeep/Edmark)
- *Stanley's Sticker Stories* (Riverdeep/Edmark)
- *The Amazing Writing Machine* (Riverdeep/The Learning Company)

Considerations for Use

The problem with presenting a book on the computer screen is that it limits the size of audience who can appreciate a work, and it restricts the opportunity for sharing across time and space. Most electronically formatted books can be printed as well, however, making it possible to share the work in more than one way.

Publishing on the Web

Until recently, most student writers were limited to sharing their work with local audiences, such as teachers, parents, or peers, via handmade books. With the introduction of multimedia software, computer-based presentations could be run on desktop com-

Teaching Tip 10.2.   Presenting on the Desktop or Web

When publishing on the desktop in a school's computer lab, students can enjoy the special effects of their own works-in-progress and also can share their works with their immediate neighbors. Holding peer conferences at the computer during drafting and revising processes can provide opportunities for scaffolding social interactions. Students also can practice giving and receiving praise and constructive criticism as they try out and reflect on interesting features in their work.

As a publication date approaches, it helps to bring a sense of closure to the project by planning a date for bringing in a new audience of other students and adults who have not yet seen the presentation. This can be as simple as sharing with another class of students who have been working on similar projects so that two students share a computer and take turns presenting their work to each other. A more elaborate celebration could also be scheduled, bringing in caregivers and siblings for a publishing party in which students might participate in planning an agenda and refreshments. This experience is especially meaningful for parents and grandparents of students with disabilities, who previously might not have been included in such general education performances.

The opportunity to experience *being* the audience, as well as *having* an audience helps students develop a metacognitive framework for considering deliberately how others will perceive their work. Presenting on the desktop or the web offers ways to enhance the audience experience. Teams might start the process of web publishing by introducing students to web sites where students of similar ages are publishing. Consider setting up a minilesson in which students work in pairs or small groups to talk about features in the text that appeal to them, as well as multimedia features of the presentation mode. Later, make sure the students know how to upload their work and to access it themselves to share with others.

puters, but the audience had to be present in the room. Advances in telecommunications technology now enable students to share their writing with audiences around the world, even with people they will never meet face to face. The simplest way to share work with a global audience is to publish it on the web. The web is a multimedia component of the Internet that allows users to send and receive text, graphics, video, and sounds. When students publish their work on the web, anyone with a computer, Internet access, and a web browser (e.g., Netscape, Internet Explorer) can read their work and, if properly configured, can even send comments back to the authors.

There are two ways to publish student writing on the web. Many schools and districts have set up their own web servers (i.e., computers connected to the Internet that store and manage text, graphics, video, and sound files). If a school or district maintains such a web server, students can upload and store their work on that computer. If students do not have access to a local web server, they can send their work to other servers around the world designed for publication of student writing, such as the KidPub site at http://www.kidpub.com (see Figure 10.4). Table 10.1 lists several examples of web sites that accept and publish original writing by students.

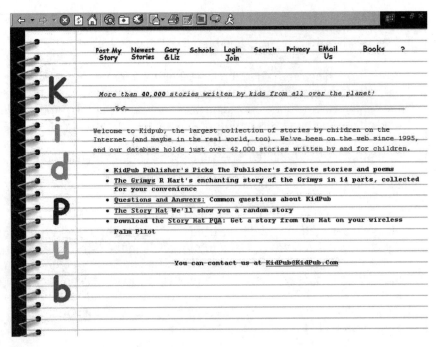

Figure 10.4. Opening screen from KidPub.

In order to publish one's work on the web, files must be formatted in a special language called *HyperText Markup Language,* or *HTML.* HTML is essentially a coding system that embeds formatting tags into documents. These tags specify how documents will appear when they are viewed on the web. It is not necessary for students to learn HTML coding, as several word processors offer built-in HTML editing features or HTML conversion utilities. One of the options on the opening screen of *Creative Writer 2* (Microsoft), for example, is to create a web page. The program automatically saves student work in HTML format, then guides students through the process of uploading their documents to a web server (see Figure 10.5).

Several programs that facilitate web publishing by simplifying HTML formatting are

- *Clicker* (Crick Software)

- *CREATE Together* (Bytes of Learning)

- *Creative Writer 2* (Microsoft)

- *Leonardo's Multimedia Toolbox* (Riverdeep/The Learning Company)

- *mPOWER* (Multimedia Design Corporation)

- *Storybook Weaver Deluxe* (Riverdeep/The Learning Company)

- *The Print Shop* (Broderbund)

- *Web Workshop* (Sunburst)

Table 10.1. Web publishing sites for children

Site name	Web site	Description
KidAuthors	http://www.kidauthors.com	Accepts stories and poems from children ages 6–18
		Includes monthly writing contests
KidNews	http://kidnews.com	Publishes writing from students of all ages
		Accepts poetry, fiction, reviews, sports articles, and autobiographical pieces from individuals or whole classrooms
		Includes areas for kids and adults to exchange information, ask questions, and share ideas
KidPub	http://www.kidpub.com	Accepts stories submitted by children
		Allows children to read works written by other children
		Includes a section called "KidPub Schools" where classes can publish their writing
		Allows students to add to a collaborative, never-ending story
KidsBookshelf	http://www.kidsbookshelf.com	Accepts book reviews, poems, and short stories from children
		Publishes teachers' and parents' original writing
MidLink Magazine	http://www.cs.ucf.edu/~MidLink	Is an electronic magazine created by kids specifically for kids in the middle grades, ages 10 to 15
		Publishes four times a year
The Young Writers Club	http://www.cs.bilkent.edu.tr/~david/derya/ywc.html	Is a club for young writers to read peers' work, send in their own, and participate in contests and activities
		Publishes *Global Wave*, a monthly electronic magazine for kids and teens
Writers' Window	http://english.unitechnology.ac.nz/writers/home.html	Publishes writing from children ages 5–18
		Includes continuous stories, a discussion board, and a writer's workshop guide

Considerations for Use

It is, of course, essential to obtain parental permission before publishing students' works on the web. Although doing so can be highly motivating to students, it should be a personal choice, and students who decline should have their wishes honored.

SUMMARY

Publishing is the last, but very important, stage of the writing process. Students can publish their work on paper or present it on a computer. Children's word processors offer various options to facilitate the publishing process. Most offer some basic desktop publishing features; others provide a more extensive array of options. Some programs are designed specifically to support book formatting and may allow students to

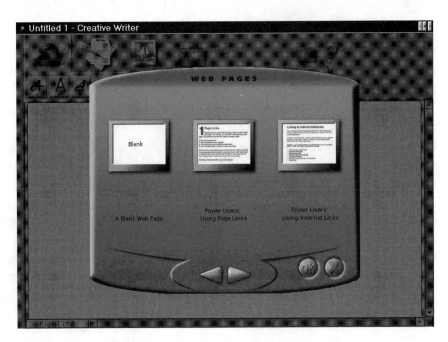

Figure 10.5. Save document as web page option in *Creative Writer 2*.

print books in several different sizes. Other programs provide support for alternative publishing formats, such as greeting cards, calendars, and posters.

Students who prefer to present their work on a computer screen are not limited to static text and graphics but may embed sounds and video images into their writing documents. Desktop presentation programs that combine multimedia capabilities with book formatting features support production of electronic books that can be displayed on a computer screen. Finally, advances in telecommunications open up vast new audiences for student work. The web, in particular, offers tremendous opportunities for students to share their work with audiences around the world. Several writing programs offer HTML formatting features that facilitate the process of publishing documents on the web.

11

Specialized Access and Keyboarding

Previous chapters in Section II describe how computers and software features can support students with and without disabilities to complete all stages of the writing process. Students may have difficulty accessing such computer supports, however, if disabilities make it impossible for them to use standard computers in typical ways. For example, students with physical impairments may not be able to manipulate a standard keyboard or mouse. Students with visual impairments may be unable to see the text on a computer monitor. Students with cognitive impairments may have difficulty discriminating all 128 keys on a standard keyboard or understanding the relationship between mouse movements on a mouse pad and cursor movements on the screen.

Students with specialized access needs such as these may require adaptive hardware or software to enable them to use computers for writing processes. Adaptive computing solutions range from simple adaptations, such as propping up the keyboard, to more complex and expensive solutions, such as using an alternative keyboard or a single switch to scan and select characters from an on-screen keyboard. Access decisions require input of interdisciplinary team members. For example, an occupational therapist can make important contributions to a team's decisions about these and other positioning and technology adaptations.

This chapter describes specialized solutions for supporting students with physical, visual, or cognitive impairments to access computers for the writing process. It also provides information about keyboarding for all students. Resources for further information appear in Table 11.1.

Dr. Janet Sturm reviewed and provided input for this chapter.

Table 11.1. Selected assistive technology resources

Assistive technology databases

ABLEDATA—http://www.abledata.com

Assistivetech.net—http://www.assistivetech.net

Assistive technology organizations

The Alliance for Technology Access (ATA)—http://www.ataccess.org

Center for Applied Special Technology (CAST)—http://cast.org

Closing the Gap—http://www.closingthegap.com

Council for Exceptional Children (CEC), Technology and Media Division (TAM)—http://www.tamcec.org

International Society for Technology in Education (ISTE), Special Education Technology SIG—
http://www.iste.org/setsig

Rehabilitation Engineering and Assistive Technology Society of North America (RESNA)—
http://www.resna.org

Assistive technology training

Research Institute for Assistive and Training Technologies (RIATT) with The National Association of State
Directors of Special Education (NASDSE)—http://www.nasdse.com

Selected keyboarding software for children

All the Right Type (Ingenuity Works, Inc.)

Disney's Adventures in Typing with Timon and Pumbaa (Disney Interactive)

Jump Start Typing (Knowledge Adventure)

KidKeys (Knowledge Adventure)

Mavis Beacon Teaches Typing (Riverdeep/The Learning Company)

Stickybear Typing (Optimum Resource)

Type to Learn (Sunburst)

Type to Learn Jr. (Sunburst)

Typing Tutor 10 (Knowledge Adventure)

Typing Workshop (Optimum Resource)

UltraKey (Bytes of Learning)

ACCESS SOLUTIONS FOR STUDENTS WITH PHYSICAL IMPAIRMENTS

Students with physical impairments, such as cerebral palsy or other motor impairments, may have difficulty using a standard keyboard or mouse. They may experience various limitations such as inability to extend their arms far enough to reach a standard keyboard, difficulty grasping and moving a mouse, inadvertently striking keys other than those intended, uncontrollable finger bouncing on selected keys, or inability to release keys quickly enough to prevent repeated activation.

When considering adaptations to assist such students, it is best to try the simplest and least intrusive options first. If simple solutions do not work, then more complex and expensive options, such as alternative keyboards or input methods, may be appropriate. The access solutions described in this section are presented in the general order in which they should be considered for students with physical limitations.

KEYBOARD MODIFICATIONS

To assist students with physical impairments to use a standard keyboard, the simplest solution may be some type of hardware or software keyboard modification. Keyboard modifications maintain the standard keyboard, but modify it in some way. For example, for a student who has difficulty reaching the keyboard, moving the keyboard to a different location, such as on the student's wheelchair lap tray, or propping it up at an angle may be a simple modification that would enable the student to use a standard keyboard. For students who have difficulty controlling their arm movements, clamping the keyboard to a table or lap tray may provide the stability required for the student to use the standard keyboard.

For students who rest their hands on the keyboard or accidentally press keys they do not want, a keyguard may be helpful. A keyguard is a piece of metal or plexiglass with holes drilled in it matching the keys on a keyboard. The keyguard attaches to the sides of the keyboard and rests on top. It requires students to press their fingers down deliberately into the holes to strike the keys. Although a keyguard slows typing speed, it prevents students with limited fine motor control from accidentally pressing keys they do not intend to activate. Keyguards are available to fit a variety of different keyboards. They generally cost from $50 to $100.

For students who drool, a moisture guard can protect the keyboard. A moisture guard is a piece of transparent, flexible material that fits the profile on top of the keyboard. It prevents moisture or debris from falling between the keys and can be removed easily for cleaning.

Many keyboard modifications are software-based and cost nothing. For people who use PCs running a version of the Microsoft operating system *Windows* (e.g., *Windows 3.x, Windows 95, Windows 98, Windows 2000, Windows XP*), accessibility features are built into the operating system itself. Accessibility utilities can be located through the Start menu or under the Accessibility Options icon in the Control Panel. Accessibility Options can be turned on or off by the user, or they can be set up to activate automatically when the computer starts. Although the availability of specific utilities depends on the version of *Windows* installed on a particular computer, most versions include the following utilities:

- StickyKeys—This utility latches the Control, Shift, and Alt keys, which ordinarily require simultaneous activation, so that the user can press two or three keys in sequence rather than simultaneously and have them function correctly. This feature is helpful for students who cannot hold down more than one key at a time because they use a single finger, mouthstick, or headpointer to type.

- FilterKeys—This utility instructs applications to ignore repeated keystrokes or to adjust the repeat rate. It is helpful for students who accidentally hold down keys too long or press them more than once.

- MouseKeys—This utility allows users to control cursor movements using the arrows on the numeric keypad instead of a mouse. It is helpful for students who cannot manipulate a mouse but can use a keyboard.

In addition to Accessibility Options, users can modify the operation of the mouse by accessing the Mouse button in the Control Panel. Using Mouse Properties, one can reconfigure the mouse to be left-handed instead of right-handed. The double-click speed also can be adjusted to accommodate a user's double-click rate. The mouse pointer can be changed to a different image such as a three-dimensional pointer or to a larger *Windows* standard pointer. In addition, the pointer speed can be adjusted and a tail can be added to assist in visually tracking the pointer on the screen. Users running

Windows 95 or later also can adjust the keyboard repeat rate or delay by accessing the Keyboard Properties button in the Control Panel. Microsoft provides extensive on-line support to assist users in learning about and using the built-in Accessibility Options (http://www.Microsoft.com/enable).

Apple Computer also includes built-in accessibility features in its Macintosh operating system, beginning with *System 7.x.* The *Easy Access* system software, included with the operating system, provides three utilities:

- StickyKeys—This utility operates like the *Windows* version. It latches two or more keys and is especially useful for one-finger typists or those who use a mouthstick or headpointer to type.

- SlowKeys—This utility is the software equivalent of a keyguard. It enables the user to change the length of time it takes for a keystroke to be registered on the screen. It is useful for students who accidentally tap other keys while trying to strike the target key.

- MouseKeys—This utility operates like the *Windows* version. It allows users to control all mouse movements by typing on the numeric keypad.

In addition, the key-repeat function can be disabled so that multiple key presses are not recognized. Apple Computer provides detailed operating instructions for each of the built-in utilities on its web site (http://www.apple.com/disability/easyaccess.html).

Alternative Keyboards

If simple modifications do not make it possible for students to use a standard keyboard, it may be necessary to provide an alternative keyboard. Unlike built-in accessibility options that cost nothing extra, alternative keyboards carry additional cost. The prices depend on the sophistication and capabilities of the particular keyboard selected. Alternative keyboards may be smaller or larger than standard keyboards; they may have a membrane overlay instead of raised keys; or they may be part of an augmentative communication device.

A popular alternative keyboard used in many schools is the *Intellikeys* keyboard (Intellitools). *Intellikeys* is a programmable, alternative keyboard that works with any Macintosh or Windows computer. It comes in two versions, *Intellikeys Classic* and *Intellikeys USB*, and costs approximately $400. The USB model is compatible with *Windows 2000*. *Intellikeys* also offers Overlay Maker (for creating adapted overlays) and Click It (for on-screen scanning).

The *Intellikeys* keyboard is a flat panel that can be changed by sliding in different overlays. The keyboard ships with six standard overlays, but educators and parents can create custom-designed overlays (using Overlay Maker) to meet students' specific needs. Overlays can include letters, numbers, pictures, or even three-dimensional objects glued to the overlay. *Intellikeys* is especially useful for students who have physical impairments that make it difficult for them to press the small keys on a standard keyboard. A special setup overlay also allows users to customize keyboard settings such as the response rate and the repeat rate for students who press unwanted keys or who rest their finger on a key too long. Intellitools provides keyboard demonstrations and further product information on its web site (http://www.intellitools.com).

Other alternative keyboards are available, as well, ranging in price from approximately $200 to $1,000. *Discover:Board* (Madentec), like *Intellikeys,* comes with several overlays and allows users to modify, create, and print customized overlays to meet students' specific needs. The *BigKeys Keyboard* (Greystone Digital) is a standard size keyboard with very large keys. It comes with black, white, or colored letters configured in ABC or QWERTY order. The *King Keyboard* (Tash International) is an oversized alternative keyboard with recessed keys that provide both tactile and auditory feedback when pressed. In Mouse Mode, a user can control the mouse by pressing keyboard keys. Alternatively, the *Mini Keyboard* (Tash International) is a tiny keyboard that can be used by students with limited range of motion in their hands and arms. The keys are small and closely spaced, requiring minimal arm and wrist movement to access.

If a student already uses an augmentative and alternative communication (AAC) device, the keyboard on the AAC device may be used as an alternative keyboard for the student's computer. The Windows operating system has a built-in utility called *Serial Keys* that allows an AAC device keyboard to take the place of the computer keyboard. This is helpful for students with communication impairments as it enables them to use the same keyboard for speaking and writing.

Alternative Mouse Access

For students who have difficulty manipulating a standard mouse, many mouse alternatives are available. They include various types of rollerballs, joysticks, and head-controlled mouse devices. A rollerball, also called a trackball, is best described as an upside-down mouse. It consists of a stationary unit with a ball mounted in the middle. Students can roll their hands across the top of the ball to control movement of the cursor on the screen. Most devices have separate buttons on the side for click, double-click, and drag controls.

Joysticks, similar to those used with electronic games, can control the computer cursor. They come in a variety of sizes and shapes. Most include separate buttons or jacks for switches to control the click, double-click, and drag functions.

Other alternatives are head-mounted devices, such as the *Headmouse* (Origins), the *Penny and Giles Headway* (Don Johnston), or the *Tracker 2000* (Madentec). These allow users to control cursor movements by moving their heads up, down, left, or right. The head movements are converted to cursor control signals and sent through an infrared transmitter to the computer.

When selecting an alternative keyboard or mouse device, educators must first identify the specific reason that an alternative device is required, then, if possible, try out different models with the student before making a final decision.

Alternative Input Methods

If simple keyboard modifications or alternative keyboard and mouse devices (including the student's AAC device) cannot solve the accessibility problem, an alternative input method might be necessary to bypass the keyboard and mouse altogether. Two major types of alternative input methods are 1) speech recognition and 2) scanning with a switch and on-screen keyboard. If a standard, modified, or alternative keyboard does not work, it might be tempting to consider one of these two methods right away, but both are relatively complex and difficult to master. Thus, they should be considered for students only after simpler and less intrusive options have been eliminated.

Speech-recognition technology requires both hardware and software modifications. With an added microphone- and speech-recognition software installed, a user can speak words, phrases, or sentences into a microphone, and the computer will carry out a command or print what is said on the monitor. Speech-recognition software can be used to control the basic operations of the computer, such as opening and closing files, saving, and copying; composing text in a word processor; or interacting with other application software, such as drawing tools and spreadsheets.

As described in Chapter 8, there are two major types of speech recognition software—discrete speech and continuous speech. Discrete speech systems represent older speech-recognition technology. They require users to speak discrete words, one at a time, with brief pauses between each word. In contrast, the newer technology, continuous speech recognition, allows users to dictate by speaking at a normal rate of speech. For users without disabilities, continuous speech recognition systems are more efficient than discrete systems. However, some research suggests that students with learning disabilities, who are also emergent writers, or those with articulation difficulties, may find discrete speech systems easier to operate and control (Higgins & Raskind, 2000). Follansbee (2001) noted that by slowing down the dictation process, discrete speech makes it easier for inexperienced writers to deal with difficulties in language processing, pronunciation, and monitoring. In addition, the word-by-word style of discrete dictation reflects the text creation style of beginning writers more closely and makes error correction more comprehensible.

While it may appear easier to speak to a computer than to type, use of speech-recognition technology requires extensive training and constant monitoring for accuracy. Speech-recognition programs require an individual user to train the software to recognize the user's voice and speech pattern. This process of creating a voice file may take several hours or days for students to complete. After training, users must carefully monitor the software for words recognized incorrectly or other software operation problems. Students must correct such errors as they occur, or the speech recognition program will "learn" the errors, and recognition accuracy will gradually decrease. Students with poor spelling skills or general cognitive deficits may be unable to monitor the software for corrections while simultaneously generating words for their writing. Thus, although speech-recognition technology eliminates the need to use a keyboard or mouse, it introduces an additional set of cognitive demands that make it difficult for many students to master.

In addition, speech-recognition technology must be used in a location where background noise is not excessive and students can dictate without disturbing others. This generally is not possible in school settings, and it is contraindicated when a goal has been established to include students with disabilities with their typically learning peers, as it is in the writing lab approach. Yet, if it is the only method through which text can be entered independently, it may be worth the time, effort, and temporary separation.

Another alternative for students who cannot use keyboard input involves scanning with an on-screen keyboard and switch. An on-screen keyboard is a virtual representation of a keyboard contained in a separate window that floats in front of the open application, such as a standard word processing program. *Windows 2000* and later versions of the operating system include an On-Screen Keyboard utility. *Intellikeys* offers Click It for on-screen scanning. Other public domain software, shareware, and commercial on-screen keyboard programs also are available.

To select keys from the on-screen keyboard using single-switch scanning, the user first has to activate a switch to initiate the scanning process. A scanning pattern is generally programmed for an individual user and may vary by function. In row and column scanning, for example, activating the switch starts the scanning process by highlighting rows one at a time. When the desired row is indicated, the user activates the switch again to scan across columns until an intended key is highlighted. At that point, the user activates the switch at least one more time to stop on the desired key and to choose the desired item. Both the timing and the switch itself must be highly individualized to meet students' particular needs. For example, one student might be able to manage rapid scanning rates and a small button-type switch, whereas another may need slower scanning rates and a large flat panel switch. Another student might need a mercury switch that activates when moved to a vertical position or a pneumatic switch that requires sipping or puffing through a strawlike device.

As this description suggests, scanning is a slow and complex process, even for the most proficient users. Depending on the speed of the scanning and the dexterity of the user, it might require significantly more time and attention than typing on a keyboard. Thus, it should generally be considered only as a last resort when all other input options have been eliminated. When keyboard scanning is deemed necessary, rate of input may be enhanced by adding software with word prediction capabilities (described in Chapter 8).

ACCESS SOLUTIONS FOR STUDENTS WITH VISUAL IMPAIRMENTS

Similar to students with physical impairments, students with visual impairments may require specialized access solutions in order to use computers for writing. Fortunately, many hardware and software solutions are available to make computers accessible to students with low vision or blindness.

Low Vision

Many students with low vision benefit from enlarged text. Although it is easy enough to enlarge the font size in a word processing document, students with low vision also may require enlargement of the icons and menus on the screen. Fortunately, both Windows and Macintosh operating systems have built-in screen enlargement utilities.

Windows 2000 and later versions include a utility called *Magnifier*. This utility creates a separate window that displays a magnified portion of the screen. *Magnifier* allows users to adjust the magnification level of text and images in the magnification window; change the size, location, and position of the window; invert the screen colors; or use a high-contrast setting.

The Macintosh operating system includes a similar program called *CloseView*. It allows users to magnify screen images up to 16 times the normal size in a magnification window. It also includes an option to display black-on-white or white-on-black characters on the screen. Other public domain software, shareware, and more powerful commercial screen magnification programs are available if the built-in options are not sufficient.

Students with low vision also may need enlarged keyboard labels to make identifiers on keys more visible. Adhesive keyboard labels are available in various colors such as white on black, black on beige, or color-coded. These also can be used to enhance the visibility of selected keys, such as vowels, numbers, or keyboard functions.

Blindness

Students who are blind generally use speech-output devices or Braille to access print-based information. To use a computer for writing, they must either hear the words on the screen read aloud or feel the displayed text converted to Braille.

To assist users who are blind, *Windows 2000* includes a utility called *Narrator*. This text-to-speech utility reads what is displayed on the screen, including the contents of the active window, menu options, or text that has been typed. Users can adjust the speed, volume, and pitch of the voice.

Similarly, the Macintosh operating system includes a utility called *Text-to-Speech* as part of the Easy Access program. *Text-to-Speech* enables the computer to speak the alert messages that appear on the screen. In some application programs, the computer also can read aloud text that is contained in the documents. Users can select from 26 different voices.

Although *Narrator* and *Text-to-Speech* are included free with the Windows and Macintosh operating systems, respectively, users may want to purchase a more powerful commercial screen reader program. Commercial screen readers, such as *Jaws for Windows* (Freedom Scientific), *ZoomText* (Ai Squared) and *outSPOKEN* (ALVA Access Group), provide many additional options for customizing and controlling software.

For blind users who read Braille, refreshable Braille displays can be used instead of or in addition to a computer monitor. The *ALVA Satellite* (ALVA Access Group), for example, is a device that converts characters on a computer monitor to Braille pins. The device sits under a standard keyboard just below the space bar. When text is displayed on the monitor, the pins on the *ALVA Satellite* raise and lower in the configuration of Braille characters as the cursor scans across the letters. Users run their fingers over the moving Braille pins to read the text.

ACCESS SOLUTIONS FOR STUDENTS WITH COGNITIVE IMPAIRMENTS

Students with cognitive impairments may be overwhelmed by the complexity of a standard keyboard with 128 keys. A simple solution for some is to cover the keys that are not needed with a cardboard mask. Various masks can be made for individual programs and the masks can be fastened with Velcro to the keyboard and changed or removed, as needed. Another way to simplify the keyboard is to color code important keys or to apply adhesive labels with capital or lowercase letters to the keys. For students who need picture cues instead of letters and numbers, a team might try using custom overlays with picture symbols instead of letters and an alternative membrane keyboard, such as the *Intellikeys* (Intellitools). Emergent writers might use *Writing with Symbols 2000* (Widgit Software Ltd.), or they might benefit from a Word Bank, such as *Intellitalk II* (Intellitools) (see Chapter 8 for a discussion of Word Bank features).

For students who cannot grasp the relationship between keyboard commands or mouse movements and the control of text on the screen, a touchscreen may be helpful. A touchscreen attaches to the front of the monitor and allows students to touch the screen to enter information. With a touchscreen and on-screen keyboard program, a student can point to letters desired on the screen rather than type them on a keyboard. Educators should keep in mind, however, that extensive use of a touchscreen can cause fatigue to a student's shoulder and arm.

KEYBOARDING CONSIDERATIONS

Most educators agree that students must demonstrate some level of keyboarding proficiency to use computers effectively for writing. Significant questions remain, however, about how and when to teach keyboarding. In this section, we review the arguments and summarize the limited research literature. We also report on our own experiences with keyboarding instruction and make some preliminary recommendations based on that experience and the broader language and literacy learning goals of the writing lab approach.

Questions About Keyboarding

The ongoing debate about how and when to teach keyboarding centers around four issues: 1) whether keyboarding should be taught, 2) the best age to begin formal keyboarding instruction, 3) the most effective instructional strategies to use, and 4) levels of proficiency required before students can reap the benefits of computer-supported writing.

Should Keyboarding Be Taught?

Children and adults of all ages use personal computers extensively at school and at home for education, business, communication, and entertainment. Bartholome (2002) reported that 50% of the workforce uses computers on the job and 75% of 8- to 12-year-olds spend time on personal computers. Although it is possible to operate a computer without knowing how to touch type, people who rely on hunt-and-peck methods of typing often are frustrated by the effort required to enter information into the computer. Although the computer can process information with lightning speed, its efficiency is limited ultimately by the rate at which a user can operate the keyboard.

Touch-typing, that is, typing quickly and smoothly without looking at the keyboard, can greatly enhance a writer's ability to use a computer. Touch-typing is a psychomotor skill, similar to playing a musical instrument or performing athletically. It does not develop incidentally, but requires systematic instruction and significant practice to master. Some users, particularly adults, can learn to touch-type by reading self-instructional print-based manuals and practicing sequenced lessons on their own. Some can learn by interacting with sequenced, self-instructional, tutorial typing programs on the computer. Others require the direct instruction, guidance, feedback, and support provided by a face-to-face teacher. To learn proper keyboarding techniques and to develop speed and accuracy, users must devote time and effort to some type of systematic instruction.

At What Age Should Formal Keyboarding Instruction Begin?

Although keyboarding skills are important for children to acquire, developmental milestones may limit what children can do at early ages. Typically, children do not possess the dexterity and hand size to manipulate keys efficiently until third grade. Therefore, most educators suggest that formal keyboarding instruction should begin around age 10–12 years (Hopkins, 1998; Jackson & Berg, 1986; National Business Education Association, 1992). Prior to that age, however, students (even as young as preschool) can be introduced to the keyboard, learning where the letter and number keys are located and how to use high-frequency keys, such as *enter, backspace, shift,* and *space-bar*. They also may be encouraged to position their hands in the center of the keyboard and to use both their right and left hands to strike the keys (Starr, 2001). Young children generally should not be expected to use the proper fingers for touch-typing or to type without looking at the keys. Hunt-and-peck typing is the appropriate mode for students at this young age. Of course, drafting text on a computer is a slow process in such cases, but students are rewarded by the ease of revision and the polished look of the finished product. Also, children are bothered less by the slowness than adults.

An additional benefit of keyboard instruction is that children's metalinguistic understandings can be enhanced as they are scaffolded to use the keyboard to represent linguistic choices. For example, they can be scaffolded to make explicit letter choices to represent sounds in words they are attempting to spell, to use the space bar to define boundaries between words, and to use the shift key to capitalize certain letters based on linguistic factors.

Generally by third or fourth grade, at around age 9 or 10, students are developmentally ready to begin formal keyboarding instruction (Jackson & Berg, 1986). At this age, students can be given initial structured keyboarding instruction, followed by guided practice and consistent reinforcement. Through formal instruction, students learn how to position their hands and use the proper fingers for keying. They also learn to type by feel without looking at the keyboard.

Some states have mandated keyboarding classes at particular grade levels and have established standards for instructional time, as well as for students' speed and accuracy. It is generally agreed that keyboarding instruction should not be limited to a single grade, but reinforced in subsequent grades after initial instruction. When first learning to touch type, students need about 30 hours of formal keyboarding instruction to learn the correct fingers (McLean, 1994). After initial instruction, they require regular, short practice sessions, typically 15–20 minutes at a time, to maintain and improve their skill.

What Methods and Materials Should Be Used to Teach Keyboarding?

Educators generally agree that keyboarding instruction should be conducted by a knowledgeable teacher. This may be an elementary school teacher who has taken a keyboarding methods class or a business teacher who has knowledge of elementary learning methods. In many elementary schools, keyboarding instruction is provided by a designated "computer teacher" or a computer lab coordinator, who may be a licensed teacher or a teaching assistant.

Tutorial keyboarding software can play a role in the development of keyboarding skills. Although tutorial software cannot take the place of a qualified teacher, it can provide additional opportunities for students to practice their skills independently and to develop speed and accuracy. Keyboarding programs are on the market for students of all ages. Well-designed programs include developmentally sequenced lessons, automatic record-keeping functions, and incentives (e.g., arcade-style games, printable charts, certificates) for recording and rewarding mastery of speed and accuracy targets.

What Level of Keyboarding Proficiency Is Required to Use Computers for Writing?

Some educators argue that students should receive formal keyboarding instruction before they ever begin to use a computer for writing. Most (including the authors) agree, however, that students who have not received formal instruction and students as young as preschool age still can use a computer for some writing activities. It is generally accepted that when students can type about as fast as they can handwrite, they can use computers effectively and efficiently for substantive writing, such as composing sentences and paragraphs (Balajthy, 1988; Daiute, 1985; Wetzel, 1985). The payoff is that those who develop automatic motor patterns for writing with a pencil or typing on a keyboard are able to devote more attention to higher-level activities associated with writing processes. The less effort students must devote to conscious focus on the mechanical aspects of writing or typing, the more cognitive capacity they can devote to content, organization of ideas, and word choice. Thus, the faster students can handwrite or type accurately, the better. Cost-benefit decisions, however, must be weighed regarding whether extra keyboarding practice justifies withdrawing time from more substantive writing process instruction.

How fast do students handwrite? Pisha (1989) found that older elementary students could copy manually from a model at speeds between 8 and 17 words per minute, with an average of 11 words per minute. This rate does not hold for conditions when students must compose their own thoughts rather than copy printed text. Such rates could be expected to vary across students. A general rule of thumb, however, is that students should be able to type at least 10 words per minute to reap the benefits of computer use (Wetzel, 1985). Typing as few as 10 words per minute is equivalent to handwriting speed for many children in middle- to upper-elementary grades. Typing slower than that may indicate that students are devoting more cognitive energy to typing than they would to handwriting (depending on their personal rates and skills); thus, they may have less capacity to focus on the content of their writing. Over time, with consistent practice and frequent opportunities to use word processors, high school students may attain typing speeds of 40–50 words per minute.

Recommendations Based on Our Experiences

As we emphasize throughout this book, the computer can serve as much more than an expensive typewriter. Children as young as first grade can make effective use of computer supports for planning, entering, and revising text, as well as for illustrating and publishing their work, especially when children's word processing programs are available. When instructors sit side-by-side at computers with children who are at risk for language-learning difficulties, scaffolding can encompass using computer features to support language learning at multiple levels. We believe that these goals and possibilities justify exposing young children and children with disabilities to the uses of computers for supporting writing processes long before they can be expected to become touch-typists.

In our own writing lab experiences, we have used tutorial keyboarding software with several groups of students. In our most extensive implementation, we used keyboarding software-guided practice in a twice per week after-school university writing lab for students with disabilities from third- through eighth grade. The students used a keyboarding program during the first 10–15 minutes of each 75-minute lab session as a transition activity as they arrived at the computer lab and got settled. Students had varying keyboarding abilities, and the tutorial software included audio instruction via headphones. Therefore, the lessons were practiced independently and without adult scaffolding, except for encouraging students to stay on task. Students simply came to class each day and started their keyboarding program at whatever lesson they had not completed the day before. Instructors monitored student performance and provided occasional assistance, but students were able to work independently most of the time.

After 10–15 minutes at this task, all students were asked to come to a stopping point so we could begin the writing lesson for the day. The regular and systematic practice delivered via a series of short, structured sessions served as a consistent orientation and transition activity for the class. It helped this group of older elementary and secondary students improve their keyboarding accuracy and speed. They also charted their progress, which helped them develop a greater sense of ownership for their goals and accomplishments, as well as giving them an authentic reason to chart and understand data.

In subsequent experiences, we used tutorial keyboarding software less extensively, mostly due to time constraints of working in inclusive elementary school settings. We did use keyboarding software in one elementary school with two classes of third graders. The school employed a computer lab teacher who assisted in setting up the computers so that the students could use their computers for a full hour on the 1 day per week they were scheduled to use the computer lab. On the other 2 days, writing lab sessions were held in the students' classrooms, during which they wrote by hand when planning or drafting, or when editing print-outs of stories produced on their computer lab day. On classroom days, students also participated in such spoken language communication events as peer editing or author chair.

Our observation was that it would be impossible to fit 10–15 minutes of keyboarding practice into computer lab sessions shorter than 1 hour, and it is hard to give up any computer lab time to keyboarding when only 1 hour per week can be scheduled in the computer lab. We did observe that many children benefited from the computer-supported keyboarding instruction and practice; however, some students, particularly those with disabilities, became frustrated when they could not complete a full lesson in the limited time allotted because the software required them to start over on lessons they had not fully completed. Some teachers we have worked with have found ways to incorporate keyboarding practice at other points in their school day using videotapes and practice keyboards.

In implementing the writing lab approach with first- through fifth-grade students, we have found that most students can use computers effectively to write and revise their work even with only rudimentary keyboarding skills. In some instances, instructors share the keyboard with students to enter text, just as they sometimes share pencils with emergent writers to help them get their words on paper. If time is tight for meeting a publishing schedule, instructors might do more of the typing, but they still can scaffold students to make decisions about word choices, syntax, spelling, punctuation, and the like.

Learning features of keyboards can be valuable even without typing instruction. In addition, minilessons about basic keyboard functions can be used to instruct students about language. Keyboard vocabulary and related concepts give students authentic reasons to learn such words as *space, spacebar, capital, capitalize, shift, insert, delete, backspace, cursor, tab, arrow keys, alignment, center,* and *margin.* Vocabulary instruction in computer lab contexts also conveys the value of people sharing common language so they can replace such vague communication as, "Move that thingie over there," with more specific wording. Instructors also can take advantage of such language-learning opportunities to highlight morphological features of complex words. For example, when teaching the border feature in *Ultimate Writing and Creativity Center* (Riverdeep/The Learning Company), we might ask students whether they can recognize any part of words such as *format* or *alignment,* which appear on the relevant pull-down menus. This provides one more opportunity to help students think about how complex words often are constructed from smaller, more easily recognizable parts.

SUMMARY

Numerous assistive technologies are available to support the specialized access needs of students with physical, visual, or cognitive impairments. Students who have difficulty using standard keyboard and mouse technology can still participate in computer-supported writing if appropriate access solutions are identified. The many options for modifying standard keyboards and mouse controls to make them more accessible include activating the accessibility options built into Windows and Macintosh operating systems. If keyboard modifications are not sufficient, some students may benefit from use of an alternative keyboard or mouse device. Finally, if keyboard modifications and alternative keyboards and mouse devices do not help, speech recognition or scanning with a switch could be considered. Most specialized access solutions are relatively simple and inexpensive, yet they can make an enormous difference to the user. Some are more complex and carry heavy learning demands, yet they may provide the only path to greater independence.

A summary of views on keyboarding instruction suggests that it should begin early and continue throughout students' school years. Educators can systematically introduce young students to keyboard features (and related concepts) and show them how to operate the keys, encouraging them to use both hands and to learn specific vocabulary for talking about keys and functions. Formal touch-typing instruction might be introduced at around age 9 or 10 and can be supplemented in subsequent years with short practice sessions. Interacting with well-designed tutorial keyboarding software can help students increase their accuracy and speed, working independently at odd times throughout the day. Even if time cannot be allotted to formal keyboard instruction, students of all ages can benefit from performing some of their writing processes with computers.

12

Software Selection Processes

The writing lab approach requires systematic, step-by-step planning (see Chapter 4). Relatively early in the effort, teams need to select the optimal text-processing software for supporting students as they embark on the computer-supported writing process. This step, although complex, can be quite rewarding. As described in Chapters 7–11, the market is full of interesting writing tools for children, and new products are always emerging. The challenge for teachers and clinicians is to find appropriate tools to match the individualized learning needs of students who have undergone formal and informal assessment, while supporting all students to meet general curricular goals.

The software selection process involves three primary activities: 1) locating text-processing software, 2) evaluating potential software to determine the presence of critical design features, and 3) matching software features to student needs. In addition, educators must take into account factors such as hardware requirements, operating systems, networking capabilities, and costs. This chapter provides detailed information about the software selection process and offers tools to guide teams through the decision-making process.

LOCATING TEXT-PROCESSING SOFTWARE

When personal computers were first introduced in the early 1980s, little software was available, and most users had to program the machines themselves in order to accomplish various tasks. During those early years, schools placed significant emphasis on development of programming skills for both teachers and students. Since the 1980s, however, the situation has changed dramatically. Thousands of software programs are available to conduct virtually any task imaginable. Most computer users are not pro-

Table 12.1. Software types

Software type	Description
Commercial	Sold to users by commercial software publisher or distributor
	1976 U.S. Copyright Act and 1980 amendments permit owner to make back-up copy to use if original disk fails
	Back-up copies cannot be used on second computer at same time original is in use
	Consumers must read and understand licensing agreements for programs they purchase and use
Shareware	Also called freeware
	Can be freely copied, shared, and used on trial basis for limited time or number of uses
	Users required to send fee, usually $5–$20, to developer to pay for continued, long-term use
	Can be acquired at professional conferences, downloaded from Internet, or obtained from other users
Public domain	Noncommercial software that can be freely copied, shared, and used
	May be nominal charge for cost of disk and/or shipping and handling
	Can be acquired at professional conferences, downloaded from Internet, or obtained from other users

grammers; they rely instead on three types of software—commercial, shareware, and public domain—to meet their computing needs (see Table 12.1).

The first step in the selection process is to locate text-processing software. Although the software market changes daily, there are many ways to find out what is available and to stay abreast of revisions and additions. The primary places to find software include retail stores, software publishers, and the Internet.

Retail Stores

Most people find it hard to believe that finding commercial software for children used to be difficult except in specialty computer stores. Considerable growth in the computer industry has spurred the software market, and software is now available in many types of retail stores. Most large department and discount stores that sell computers also carry selected children's programs. Electronics stores generally have computer software departments, as do most office supply stores. Even some toy stores, grocery stores, bookstores, and variety stores sell text-processing software for children.

Although children's software can be found on the shelves of many retail stores, the selection is generally limited to a few of the most popular programs targeted to the mass family/home consumer market. In addition, software in retail stores generally is sold in single-user, home versions only. Lab packs, network versions, and site licenses rarely are available through retailers; teacher's guides, lesson plans, and other supplementary teaching materials are also difficult to find in retail stores (see Table 12.2). There are several benefits to shopping for software in retail stores, however, the most obvious being the ability to purchase software and use it immediately without waiting for ordering or shipping. In addition, software prices in retail stores may be lower than prices offered through publishers' catalogues or the Internet. Prices in retail stores vary considerably, however, and educators are wise to shop around before buying, as well as to check whether an educational discount might be available through school sources.

Table 12.2. Software purchasing options

Option	Description
Home version	A version of software designed for use in the home
	Usually includes a single copy of the software
	May include a manual
	Usually costs less than a school version
School version	A version of software designed for use in schools
	Usually includes a single copy of the software plus a back-up copy
	May also include a teacher's guide, blackline masters, lesson plans, and other teaching materials
	May include special teacher options for storing student records
	Usually costs more than a home version
Single-user version	A single copy of software designed for use on one computer
	May be a home version or school version
Lab pack	Multiple copies of same software title packaged together
	May be offered in packages of 5, 10, 15, or other number as defined by publisher
	Usually comes with a single manual
	Designed for use in lab situation with multiple stand-alone computers
	Usually costs less than purchasing multiple single-user versions of same software
Network version	A special version of software that is designed to be installed on a server
	Cost depends on how many computers will be networked to the server
Site license	A single copy of software with permission to install on multiple computers
	Cost depends on number of computers for which permission to install has been granted

Software Publishers

In addition to purchasing software from retail stores, educators can buy software directly from publishers. Most educational software publishers offer consumers a free printed catalogue of their products. Some publishers maintain a mailing list and send out new catalogues automatically as they are updated. Others send updated catalogues only to customers who have purchased software in the past. Educational systems qualify for discounts from some retailers.

There are several ways to request printed publisher catalogues. Most publishers offer a toll-free telephone number for information about their products and maintain a web site through which catalogues may be obtained.

Many publishers offer their products through other software resellers. These resellers usually carry software published by dozens of different publishers. Thus, instead of requesting individual catalogues from many different publishers, educators can request just a few large reseller catalogues. In addition, reseller prices are sometimes lower than direct publisher prices. A disadvantage of using reseller catalogues is that the product information may be incomplete. Whereas publishers' catalogues usually provide detailed information about home versions, school versions, site licenses, networking capabilities, and operating systems with which the software will work, reseller catalogues do not usually provide this same level of detail. We recommend that you call the reseller to get specific product information if it is not contained in the catalogue. Table 12.3 provides contact information for several educational software resellers.

Table 12.3.   Selected software resellers

Creation Engine
http://www.creationengine.com

Educational Resources
http://www.edresources.com

Learning Services
http://www.learnserv.com

Keep in mind that not all publishers market their software through resellers. Some publishers only sell their software directly to consumers. Thus, it is important to get copies of some catalogs directly from primary publishers or to check their web sites.

Internet

Most educational software publishers maintain web sites containing information about their products. We provide links to many of these on our Writing Lab Outreach Project site (http://www.wmich.edu/wlop) and also at www.brookespublishing.com/writinglab. Many publishers offer on-line catalogs of their products and allow customers to make electronic purchases through their web sites. Usually, customers must provide a credit card number and a shipping address. Then, depending on the shipping method selected, the software will be delivered via a postal or courier service.

An advantage of shopping for software on the Internet is that publishers' on-line catalogues generally are more up to date than their printed catalogues. Although software titles may change more frequently, most publishers update their printed catalogues at most every few months. Web sites, on the other hand, can be updated more frequently.

Several web sites provide information to assist consumers in their search for software information. The PEP Registry of Educational Software Publishers (http://www.microweb.com/pepsite/Software/publishers.html), for example, provides an alphabetical list of links to more than 1,000 software publishers. Of course, visitors to this web site must know which publisher they are interested in finding. Some sites, like The School House Software Review (http://www.worldvillage.com/wv/school/html/scholrev.htm), offer on-line software reviews so that potential users can read evaluations of software titles before buying. Table 12.4 contains a list of selected web sites that offer resources and tools to assist educators in their search for educational software.

EVALUATING TEXT-PROCESSING SOFTWARE

After locating potential text-processing software titles, instructors need to examine each for the presence of critical design features. Chapters 7–10 provide a comprehensive taxonomy of text-processing tool features that may be found in children's programs. That is, software tools may include features designed to support students during the planning and organizing stage, the drafting stage, the revising and editing stage, or the publishing stage.

Table 12.4. Selected web sites for educational software information

Children's Software and New Media Revue
http://www.childrenssoftware.com

Choosing Children's Software
http://www.choosingchildrenssoftware.com

The Educational Software Selector
http://www.epie.org/epie_tess.htm

Northwest Educational Technology Consortium
http://www.netc.org

PEP: Parents–Educators–Publishers
http://www.microweb.com/pepsite

The School House Software Review
http://www.worldvillage.com/wv/school/html/scholrev.htm

Smart Kids Software
http://smartkidssoftware.com

SuperKids Educational Software Review
http://www.superkids.com

Technology and Learning Online—Searchable Software Reviews
http://www.techlearning.com/review.html

Several methods can be used to evaluate software for design features without actually purchasing copies of the programs. First, as mentioned earlier, one can access online reviews of software programs. Many web sites publish evaluations of educational software. These reviews may be conducted by individuals who send them in unsolicited, by in-house staff, by professional organizations, or by software evaluation projects. Although reading reviews is not the same as actually using the software, software reviews can provide initial information about critical design features.

In addition to accessing software reviews on-line, educational software reviews appear in some professional journals and educational magazines. For example, the journal *Learning and Leading with Technology*, published by the International Society for Technology in Education, publishes a regular software review column. Although software reviews can be quite helpful for obtaining initial information about programs, it is important to remember that the reviewers may or may not share the values, perspectives, or priorities of the instructional team. Thus, published evaluations may provide information about software features but may rate those features differently than the team would after having tried the software or used it with students.

Several strategies may be used to try out software before buying. First, some retail stores load educational software on their demonstration computers and allow customers to try out selected titles in the store. Some universities, particularly those with teacher education programs, maintain software evaluation laboratories where students can try out software as a learning experience. Educators in the community may be able to access these facilities. Some intermediate or cooperative school systems also maintain instructional materials resource centers that include educational software previewing facilities. Checking with the local school system can lead to the closest facility. Also, some educational software publishers offer a limited preview option to schools. Others allow schools to purchase software, try it out, and return it for a refund if they decide not to use it. Finally, many publishers offer demonstration ("demo") versions of their programs. Some publishers compile a CD-ROM of selected demos and mail it to customers on request. Others allow potential customers to download demo versions of individual software titles from their web sites.

Whether you read software evaluations written by other users or try out software tools yourself, the next step is to document the critical design features of the software. Figure 12.1 provides a form for recording the results of the evaluation process. Documentation is extremely important when reviewing more than one program. As quickly becomes evident, many of the programs have similar titles, and each has a different array of features. Without documentation, it is easy to forget which program has which features.

MATCHING SOFTWARE FEATURES TO STUDENT NEEDS

The final step in selecting text-processing software is to match software features to students' individual writing needs. Several questions arise at this point:

- Who should determine which tools students will use?

- To what extent should student preferences dictate choices?

- Should all students use the same software at the same time?

- Should students use one program or several over the course of a school year or semester?

These are just a few of the pragmatic questions that teachers and clinicians ask when initiating computer-supported writing opportunities. Although there are no universal answers to these questions, we offer several suggestions based on our experiences in a variety of computer-supported writing environments.

Selecting Software to Address Instructional Goals

First, we suggest that it is the responsibility of the instructional team to select appropriate writing software for individuals or groups of students. In some school systems, a software committee chooses educational software, including text-processing tools, for the entire district, school, department, or grade level. This committee might include teachers, administrators, related services staff, parents, and even students. If possible, we encourage members of teams who plan to use the software with their students to become members of these committees. Doing so may be an educator's most effective method of influencing what is purchased for students.

Software selection committees have advantages and disadvantages. On one hand, it is helpful to have the collective input of many people when making large-scale software purchases. With a committee structure, all members can share their perspectives, and there is a good chance that what is selected will meet the needs of a large percentage of students. On the other hand, committees must address the needs of the majority of students they serve; therefore, they may overlook the needs of individual students who struggle with specific aspects of the writing process. For example, a software selection committee might choose a writing program that meets the needs of the majority of students in an elementary school, including clip art, scene creation tools, a

Name of program: _____

Publisher: _____ Version: HOME   SCHOOL

Directions: In the left column, place a checkmark next to all features that are contained in the program. In the right column, provide details to help you remember the program later.

Planning and organizing—Idea generation features

__ Stimulus pictures _____

__ Clip art _____

__ Scene creation tools _____

__ Drawing and painting tools _____

__ Multimedia authoring _____

__ Brainstorming _____

__ Mixed-up phrases _____

__ Idea lists _____

__ Story starters _____

__ On-screen notepad _____

Planning and organizing—Organizational aid features

__ Graphic organizers _____

__ Outliner _____

__ Prompted writing _____

__ Templates _____

Drafting features

__ Picture symbols _____

__ Word prediction or word bank _____

__ Abbreviation expansion and macros _____

__ Collaborative writing _____

__ Speech recognition _____

Revising and editing features

__ Standard editing tools _____

__ Thesaurus tool _____

__ Rhyming word tool _____

__ Spelling checker _____

__ Homonym checker _____

__ Grammar checker _____

__ Speech synthesis _____

__ On-screen manual _____

Publishing—Desktop publishing features

__ Desktop publishing features _____

__ Book formatting _____

__ Alternative publishing formats _____

Publishing—Desktop presentation features

__ Multimedia options _____

__ Electronic book formatting _____

__ Publishing on the web _____

Other Considerations

Platform: __ Macintosh   __ PowerPC   __ PC (Windows)

Format: __ 3.5" disk   __ CD-ROM   __ Mac/Windows CD-ROM

Operating System: __ Mac OS version _____   __ Windows version _____

Memory Required: ____ Mb   ____ Gb

Price: ____ Home ____ School ____ Single ____ Lab Pack ____ Site License ____ Network

The Writing Lab Approach to Language Instruction and Intervention, by Nickola Wolf Nelson, Christine M. Bahr, and Adelia M. Van Meter
Copyright © 2004 Paul H. Brookes Publishing Co., Inc. All rights reserved.

Figure 12.1. Software design features documentation form.

spelling checker, a thesaurus, and an outlining feature. The committee may unwittingly overlook the needs of a few students who have severe spelling difficulties, however, by not considering or selecting programs that have on-screen word banks, word prediction, or speech output features. Thus, it is important for teachers and clinicians who work with students with LLDs to serve on local software committees to ensure that the needs of all students are addressed in the selection process.

Selecting Software to Meet Students' Needs

Our second suggestion is to consider students' written expression goals and objectives when selecting software tools. Some students need help generating writing topics and ideas. Without scaffolding, they tend to write about the same topics over and over, and they have difficulty with text organization. These students might benefit from software that includes stimulus pictures, scene creation tools, idea banks, prompted writing, or other features that support the prewriting stage of the writing process.

Other students have goals and objectives related to increasing their written vocabulary. These students might benefit from software that includes a word bank feature or word prediction. Still others struggle primarily with sentence structure and may have objectives related to writing compound or complex sentences. For these students, hearing aloud what they have written through speech synthesis might be the most important feature. Teachers and clinicians must consider carefully students' individual goals and objectives when making software selections. Reflecting on students' writing goals and objectives, teams can ask:

- In which stage of the writing process does this student require the most scaffolding?

- Which software features can support that stage?

Selecting Software to Provide Variety

Our third suggestion is to make a variety of software tools available to students. Ideally, students should be introduced to several programs over the course of a school year and allowed to select the ones they prefer to use. In our years of working with students in computer-supported writing labs, we have seen many children express specific preferences for one tool over another. What may be appealing to one student is not necessarily appealing to others. Like adults, students have individual preferences, and many of them know what features help them most. When possible, teachers and clinicians should make a variety of tools available to support personal choices and learning needs, as well as different stages of the writing process.

Another aspect of this suggestion is that all students should not have to use the same tools at the same time. At any given time, individual students may be working on different stages of the writing process or on completely different writing assignments. Likewise, they may be using different text-processing programs. One student might be creating a picture with a program that includes scene creation tools, while another is revising his piece with a program that includes a grammar checker. Particularly when software funding is limited, one possibility is to purchase several different tools instead of multiple copies of a single program, thus providing students with a variety of options. Although the keep it simple principle might argue against such an approach, more practiced teams can handle greater variety with less difficulty.

We would caution, however, that an inclusive service delivery model works best when students are working on similar projects. In addition, although the expectations may vary for students with disabilities, all students should be held to high standards and provided the support they need to meet them.

OTHER SOFTWARE SELECTION CONSIDERATIONS

When selecting writing tools, several factors should be considered that extend beyond finding the best fit for curricular goals and for students' individual writing strengths and needs. Those include 1) computer platform and format, 2) operating system, 3) memory, 4) networking capabilities, and 5) cost.

Many educational software programs are offered for both Macintosh and PC (Windows) platforms; however, some are available for just one platform. Programs may also offer both Macintosh and PC versions on a single "hybrid" CD-ROM. This information usually is available in the publisher's catalog or web site, or it may be printed on the software box itself.

Instructors also need to consider the operating system on the computer where the writing software is to be installed. If a Macintosh computer will be used, the operating system will be Mac OS, with a version number. If a PC computer will be used, the operating system probably is some version of Windows (e.g., Windows 98, Windows XP). Again, it is necessary to ensure that the intended software will work with the available operating system. If not, it may be necessary to purchase and install a newer operating system to run the latest software.

In addition to the operating system, the random access memory (RAM) requirements of the software must be considered. Each computer has a specific amount of RAM installed. It may be 16 Mb, 32 Mb, 128 Mb, or more. The intended software will require a certain amount of RAM. If the computer does not have enough RAM, the software will not run. For most computers, it is possible to purchase and install additional memory if necessary.

Before purchasing software, teams should determine whether networking capabilities will be needed. Some software programs can be installed on a server that runs many computers linked together through a network. For others, a special network version of the software must be purchased to install it on a server. Yet others cannot be installed on a network server and instead must be installed on individual hard drives. In this case, it is necessary to purchase multiple single-user copies of a program or purchase a site license that permits duplication of sufficient copies for all computers in the system.

Finally, cost is an unavoidable factor affecting decisions. Most children's word processing tools cost between $30 and $100 per single-user copy. If schools purchase multiple copies (lab packs) or a site license for permission to install the software on multiple computers or a network server, the cost per unit likely will be less. This is because most publishers offer discounts for larger orders or special pricing programs for schools.

SUMMARY

The process of selecting text-processing software for the writing lab starts with a sense of purpose for meeting curricular goals and responding to students' strengths and needs. Retail stores, software publishers, and the Internet all can be sources of information and places of purchase. It is advisable to examine software before purchase and to use the form provided in Figure 12.1 to catalog software features. This chapter describes a number of strategies for conducting the evaluation prior to purchase. Several considerations for individualizing software to students' needs, and for satisfying a need for variety, are introduced. Finally, a set of technological concerns is explained that can influence whether or not software can function properly in a particular environment.

Using Collaborative Teams to Implement Inclusive, Individualized Services

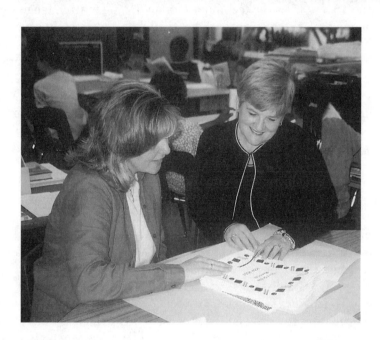

The writing lab approach fosters shared ownership for students' learning among general and special educators and SLPs and the students themselves. Parents also play an important role in helping their children develop as authors and competent communicators. To accomplish shared ownership requires teamwork and collaborative planning. Section III provides information about how to set up collaborative working relationships with the aim of including students with disabilities in achieving general education goals. It also provides detail on the assessment activities that guide instruction, the establishment of individualized objectives, and the use of these objectives to monitor outcomes and document process.

Chapter 13 focuses on supporting inclusion through collaboration. It describes levels of inclusion, using the case study of a student, Spencer, who initially was perceived as a visitor in his general education classroom but became a fully accepted resident. Another feature of Chapter 13 is the inclusion of quotations taken from interviews held by our project evaluator, Dr. Katherine Kinnucan-Welsch, with many of the educators who have worked with us in developing the writing lab approach. Using qualitative research techniques, we reviewed and coded these interview transcripts to provide insights from the viewpoints of others about how the collaborative process and the writing lab works. The voices of students also are heard in Chapter 13, drawing on interviews conducted by Kara McAlister as part of her master's thesis research.

Chapter 14 describes formal and informal assessment processes. It includes a table with formal assessment tools that focus on the assessment of written language development, and it offers a review of commonly used methods for scoring written language samples—holistic, analytic or trait scoring (with rubrics), and quantitative measures. The chapter also describes a variety of informal assessment methods, including the use of portfolio samples of work gathered from curricular projects, as well as how to gather written language probes for the express purpose of assessing needs and marking progress.

Chapter 15 describes the techniques for analyzing written language probes and offers developmental progressions, where available, for assessing needs and knowing which advances to target next. It is built around an assessment process for analyzing writing processes; written products (at discourse-, sentence-, and word-levels, as well as writing conventions); and spoken communication. We provide a case example using our recommended narrative probe to illustrate these procedures, but we also point out that similar methods could be used to analyze other forms of discourse or to analyze portfolio samples gathered during curricular activities. The appendix to Chapter 15 provides a blank worksheet and summary and objectives form for readers to use with their students.

Chapter 16 focuses on the process of establishing individualized goals, objectives, and benchmarks for guiding instruction and marking progress. It describes how to take the information from the assessment process and weave it into a comprehensive plan. This chapter illustrates the process with a series of brief excerpts from case examples, as well as a more comprehensive example. Chapter 16 ends with a procedure and a form for engaging students in evaluating their own written products, documenting their progress, and establishing next stage goals for themselves.

Chapter 17 provides two types of evidence to support the effectiveness of the writing lab approach. It provides qualitative case study evidence from students with special needs to demonstrate the progress that can be made when students with varying degrees and types of disability are engaged in a writing lab approach. It also presents the quantitative evidence from a series of three probes gathered across the school year in a group of third-grade classrooms in an inner-city school. Although these evaluation data do not meet the research standards of a fully controlled clinical trial, they do show evidence of growth for all students. The increments in language skills for students with disabilities are comparable to those for students without disabilities, and all made significant progress.

Although we do not claim that a computer-supported writing process approach should take the place of all other intervention methods and contexts, we do believe that it can contribute to sustainable improvements in the language and learning potential of all students. This approach is good for students and satisfying to educators. We also hope that the written language samples provided in the case studies will convey the message to our readers that the writing lab approach can be quite entertaining (no dull drills here), as the originality and creativity of young authors never ceases to surprise, amaze, and delight!

13

Supporting Inclusion Through Collaboration

A truly inclusive classroom culture gives all students opportunities to participate and to be challenged appropriately to grow linguistically, academically, and socially. The collaborative process needed to create this environment depends on building a foundation of working relationships. It succeeds when general and special educators and SLPs, together with parents and students, collaborate to establish a culture where existing abilities are appreciated, new abilities are targeted, and change is expected. That is, it requires the development of a team. This chapter is about the team process and how it evolves over time to support inclusive, collaborative practices.

As discussed in Chapter 3, an unintended consequence of labeling students as "special" may be that their teachers, peers, and even they themselves begin to believe that learning is impossible for them within the typical classroom environment. To establish an inclusive writing lab based on the balance principle, general education teachers and special service providers must work together to design and implement a program that meets two criteria:

- All students have opportunities to participate and to feel part of a dynamic learning community.

- All students are challenged to grow linguistically, academically, and socially.

Building a collaborative team is a process that involves establishing and maintaining relationships that support student-centered goal setting and shared responsibility for instruction. When implemented successfully, the writing lab approach com-

We appreciate the contributions of Dr. Katherine Kinnucan-Welsch to this chapter; she conducted the interviews and initiated the selection of representative comments.

bines curriculum-based learning activities and student-centered teaching methods to advance the language and cognitive development of all students (see Chapter 17).

This chapter discusses how to establish and build relationships for guiding inclusive practices. Teams are encouraged to adhere to the patience principle as they work through the early awkward stages that often characterize new collaborative relationships. Turning points that can signal systemic change are described in this chapter, and suggestions are provided about how to stimulate such change.

Excerpts from interviews with teachers are included in this chapter to bring to life the stories of transition as teams learn the true meaning of *inclusion* and become more comfortable with collaboration. Direct quotations are taken from the authors' and graduate students' journals and from interviews conducted by Dr. Katherine Kinnucan-Welsch in her role as evaluator for the Writing Lab Outreach Project. Kinnucan-Welsch pointed out that "the voices of the teachers are particularly illuminating in describing the evolution of the collaborative process." These are the voices of development team members who collaborated with us in the Writing Lab Outreach Project. They were general or special education instructors or SLPs who worked directly with us and our graduate students to develop and test the writing lab approach in elementary schools in our partner school district. They described their experiences implementing writing process instruction, using computers to support all stages of the writing process, and including students with special needs while individualizing instruction for all of their students.

The voices of students also are present in the form of interview comments gathered and documented by Kara McAlister, as part of her master's thesis research (McAlister, 1995; McAlister et al., 1999). McAlister interviewed fourth- through eighth-grade students who had been participating in an after-school writing lab about their knowledge of writing processes and attitudes toward writing lab activities. The chapter ends with a tool and a process that teams can use for guiding their reflections on how well they are implementing all components of the writing lab approach.

LEVELS OF INCLUSION: FROM VISITOR TO RESIDENT

In truly inclusive classrooms, students with disabilities are viewed as residents rather than visitors. Although it is a constant goal of the writing lab approach, a number of barriers make this ideal difficult to achieve. As comments in this chapter show, many schools are in the early stages of implementing more inclusive practices. Logistic barriers often prevent special educators and SLPs from having as much time to work with general educators as they would like. Other barriers are attitudinal, which usually decrease as people learn to work together toward common goals. Addressing attitudinal barriers also can lead collaborative teams to tackle logistic barriers or to work around them, even when they cannot be together physically to provide instruction in the same room at the same time. True inclusion extends beyond the classroom and into society as a whole.

General educators, SLPs, and special education teachers share goals for their students to progress in language and cognitive skills and to master curriculum benchmarks. All instructors are critical to the ultimate success of their joint students (Bland & Prelock, 1996; Ebert & Prelock, 1994). Many, however, approach the idea of including students with disabilities during general education instruction with varying degrees of enthusiasm. Differences often stem from differences in prior experiences with and understanding of students with special needs (Praisner, 2003). General education teachers, for example, may voice concern that students with disabilities require teaching methods or materials that are possibly beyond their scope of training or practice. Special education teachers and other specialists may support inclusive education practices but lack understanding of general education routines and curriculum. The first portion of this chapter discusses how the collaborative process can support more comprehensive levels of inclusion for students with special needs in general education classrooms.

Introducing Spencer

To some educators and parents, the concept of inclusion may mean that students with special needs are physically present—but not necessarily intellectually engaged—in the classroom. One example comes from the story of Spencer, a third-grade boy with severe learning disabilities. Because his reading and writing abilities were at a pre-primer level, he was included in his classroom for science and social studies but received pull-out special education services for reading, writing, and math. When Spencer's teacher was first approached about including him in the general education classroom for writing lab, she was not convinced that his needs could be met. Nevertheless, she encouraged the SLP to observe Spencer's performance in her classroom.

On his first day in the writing lab, Spencer showed that he was a master avoider. He rummaged through his desk, played with paper clips, and disturbed students next to him by poking them, throwing paper wads, and making funny faces. In fact, Spencer made little pretense of writing. His desk was clear of paper and pencil for most of the session. Unlike other avoidant writers in his classroom, however, the teacher did not question Spencer's behavior, nor did she redirect it.

At some point during this writing time, Spencer informed his teacher—who was surprised but did not question him—that he was expected back in his special education room, and he left. His special education teacher, equally surprised to see him return prematurely, did not question him, assuming he had been sent back for behavior issues. Spencer was calling the shots. Later when the general education teacher was asked about her classroom expectations for Spencer, she replied, "He's just a visitor in my room. He can't do anything!"

Spencer's story illustrates some of the breakdowns that occur when educators do not act as a team. Although the instructors understood that Spencer would be present in the general education classroom during writing lab, they did not set clear student goals and objectives to be addressed across learning environments. There were no clear roles and responsibilities for the general education teacher, and there was no opportunity to discuss any specialized instructional methods Spencer might need. Spencer, in turn, used the lack of communication between his general and special education teachers to manipulate them and to avoid situations he perceived as difficult.

Identifying Barriers to Collaboration

Why did this situation occur? One easy hypothesis would be that the teachers simply did not care; however, their willingness to collaborate when this breakdown was brought to their attention suggests otherwise. The most likely explanation is misconception about the inclusion process. We have been in many classrooms where teachers—both general and special education teachers—have expressed good intentions toward inclusion but have been frustrated by logistics. Out of these frustrations, however, have come conversations that have brought renewed commitment to viewing all children as residents.

In separate interviews at the conclusion of the school year, Spencer's teachers reflected on their understanding of what inclusion meant. These quotations reveal that teachers understand the basic premise of inclusion but do not have a firm understanding of the team approach necessary for inclusion to be successful. The special education teacher understood inclusion as,

> *We were going to integrate the special needs children in with their regular ed. class, some time in the class for writing and also in the lab for writing and working on language skills. [We are] doing that instead of pulling them out, as they are part of the regular classroom.*

The general education teacher also had a general understanding of inclusion, which she explained as,

> *The special ed. kids would come into the room to [be exposed to] the lessons and perspectives of all the other children. They would be included, and that would be a good thing.*

Beyond the basic understanding of inclusion, confusion arose about the special educator's role. Both teachers also had initial discomfort and insecurity in relating to each other. Significant time constraints complicated the ability of these teachers to collaborate. The general education teacher admitted,

> *I didn't really think the special ed. teacher would do that part of it. I thought the child would [come into my classroom], but not the teacher.*

The special education teacher explained her dilemma as,

> *It was going to be that all the children were going to be in with their classes across all the grades, first through third. . . . That has not been able to materialize because not all the teachers came aboard that were originally planned. I had 11 teachers, and not all wanted to come aboard. Because of that time frame, I have so many of the kids in the morning, it hasn't been possible to come up*

> *with a schedule where I can get into the other classrooms without*
> *sending my kids back to their regular ed. classes.*

Toward the end of the school year, she was working on a plan that would allow her to collaborate directly with the first-grade teacher and the SLP in the first-grade classroom in which several of her students (including one with autism spectrum disorder) were participating in writing lab activities. She expressed concern about the general education teachers' acceptance of those students:

> *[General education teachers] think of [students with disabilities]*
> *as separate instead of as a whole. But this is one of the main things*
> *of what the project was doing was to break that barrier, the bar-*
> *rier of having special ed. kids in regular ed. classrooms.*

Despite her reservations, the special education teacher remained hopeful about inclusion and said,

> *I think that it has been wonderful for the children with special*
> *needs to feel part of their [general education] classroom. To have*
> *ownership in their classroom and to feel proud that they are able to*
> *actually participate in something and that they are doing it well.*

The goal of inclusion is for all children to experience membership and learning opportunities and for teachers to feel ownership for all children in their classrooms. It is a goal toward which the collaboration supported through the writing lab approach has been directed. How to build those collaborative relationships and structures so that more children will experience being residents, instead of visitors, is the next topic of discussion.

BUILDING COLLABORATIVE RELATIONSHIPS

Building collaborative relationships involves establishing communicative pathways among the key players. In this section, we focus on how to stimulate growth in relationships that involve 1) members of the instructional team; 2) instructors and their students; 3) students and their peers; and 4) parents, educators, and students.

Building Relationships Among Members of the Instructional Team

Instructional teams supporting students with special needs are complex entities. General education teachers, special service providers at the school and district level, and building administrators all play key roles in the successful inclusion of children with disabilities. How do the members of these teams approach the crucial process of building collaborative relationships? Just as each child is unique in this process, so are the members of the instructional team.

Some general education teachers enter the collaborative process anxious to talk about their most challenging students as integral members of their classrooms. They provide rich descriptions of students' learning strengths and needs, and they share techniques they have tried to help their students with special needs participate fully in their classrooms. Such teachers express their openness to new ideas and anticipation of working as a team. Other teachers are more hesitant to jump into the inclusive enterprise—either out of inexperience and uncertainty regarding students with special needs, or because they view such students to be the responsibility of others.

Likewise, special service providers, such as special education teachers and SLPs, have varying degrees of understanding of general education classroom expectations. They may feel more comfortable suggesting techniques and strategies for their general education colleagues to use rather than working side-by-side with them in the classroom. As Spencer's special education teacher expressed, some are concerned about the welfare of their students in less protective environments. In addition, some may be reluctant to give up the autonomy of their own therapy or resource rooms to support students more directly in general education classrooms. One SLP talked about the advice she would give to other special service providers embarking on inclusive intervention, noting how the same objectives might be addressed in different ways:

> *Just know right away that you might not see the same type of progress in an inclusion setting or pull out. For instance, [in pull-out therapy] I really want a kid to work on pronouns, and we are just going to drill, you know: he, she, they. And we are going to look at pictures and talk about them and set up props. You don't do that kind of therapy in the classroom. You build it into the curriculum. Don't be afraid that just because you're not drilling, the child won't get it. You can still have small-group time or one-on-one time where they are reading a piece of writing or talking about it, and you can build a little lesson into that. So [pull-out therapy and drilling is] a hard thing for a lot of speech pathologists to not do because we are so used to drilling, and we are so used to working in isolation where we have our lovely language worksheets, and we have our great lessons that are really wonderful, but do they really apply to the curriculum?*

Another SLP described how she was able to work with students with disabilities in general education classrooms. She noted:

> *I would ask the teacher when they were having writing workshop and ask if I could work with the student on my caseload at that time. In a second-grade classroom, the teacher let me come in once a week and let me move freely around the room, working with all of the students. I would work primarily with my particular student, but I would also observe [the student] working independ-*

ently and with others while I worked with other students. The same was true for a first-grade classroom. The teacher would let me come in and wander, working with all the students. I had a student with speech goals and a student with speech and language goals. For the speech student, I was able to observe her articulation skills while she read her story and conversed with peers. I was able to give her reminders and to model (overemphasize) the correct speech sound while I worked with her. I was also able to model for the teacher how to provide [scaffolding] within the classroom and basically let the teacher see what we were addressing in speech therapy. The same was true for the language-impaired students. Interestingly enough, often the other students would hear the questions I was asking the language-impaired student and the models I was providing; then, they in turn would do the same and became excellent little helpers—a definite plus for working in the classroom!

School principals may be unsure of the role they play in the process of facilitating collaborative relationships, but they are essential. Often administrators see themselves as responsible for the administration of programs, but they are less comfortable in the role of instructional leader or contributor to collaborative team efforts. Yet, principals can make a huge difference in facilitating the collaborative process. In acknowledging acceptance of this role, one principal commented,

> *We are pitiful in helping teachers grow. I needed to support what they needed.*

Building a team requires strategies for overcoming logistic and attitudinal barriers. Three elements that can support professionals to build their relationships as a collaborative team are to establish mutual goals, find a time and place to plan, and negotiate a common vocabulary.

Establish Mutual Goals

It is good to start the collaborative process by identifying mutual expectations and needs. Most general education teachers are pleased when they learn that a special education teacher or SLP is willing to work with them in the context of activities that are already central to their teaching mission. Likewise, most special education teachers and SLPs are encouraged when invited into a general education classroom to address student goals in a highly relevant context.

What are some of the goals that teachers and special service providers share that can be addressed through a writing lab approach? When professionals collaborate, more opportunity to provide individual attention to students occurs. In fact, having help is a primary motivator for teachers to collaborate. The "extra pair of hands" theme was one that came up frequently when Kinnucan-Welsch interviewed teachers about factors that would lead them to recommend the writing lab approach to others. One third-grade teacher commented,

> *I have taught writing for quite a long time and have done the writing process. What I wanted was someone else in the room with me, whether I did all the work or they did some of it or I helped or whatever—I didn't care. I wanted more people in my room. I have a lot of [students with attention-deficit/hyperactivity disorder], and I have a lot of [third graders] who don't want to [write]. They need lots and lots of encouragement. So when people come into my room and help, this is very good for me. I think it's great!*

A third-grade teacher noted that more adults can bring in different perspectives, as well as an extra pair of hands:

> *I like having more people involved with the students. The students benefited from having the interaction and having more people and different perspectives with dealing with their writing. That part was very helpful for the project from start to finish. And it really gives you lots of support having so many different adults to work with the children.*

A second-grade teacher made a similar observation when asked what made her want to collaborate in the writing lab approach:

> *Having another perspective. When you're teaching, sometimes you have concepts and you know what you want to teach, but somehow you can't get across what it is I want. Having her [the SLP] come in and then give her feedback was really neat because a lot of times teachers don't get other feedback. It's basically what my understanding of what I'm teaching is, and so I teach it. So kids never get another perspective so when [the SLP] would come in, she'd say, "Well what about this?" or "I've got this neat way to do this." And it gave me a better perspective of what I was teaching. For a lot of kids, that different way, or that slight variation may have meant the difference of them understanding what to do or them looking at me like they [didn't understand]. So it's nice to bounce ideas off people.*

Teachers also were more likely to want to take the trouble to collaborate when they saw the writing lab approach as a means of meeting their regular curricular goals. The last thing teachers need is an add-on to already impossibly busy days. In some cases, the curricular goals are directly aimed at helping children improve their writing. As we noted in Chapter 1, more teachers are seeing writing as a valid part of the language arts curriculum, and they value writing across the curriculum. One of our development team schools had recently become a magnet school writers' academy. Thus, the fit was automatic. A first-grade teacher in that school talked about how addressing common goals meant avoiding the add-on approach she had feared at first:

> *I was kind of skeptical of doing this in the beginning because I thought, "Oh boy, here we go again. Here is another add on. I don't know how much more of this I can take." And I was very pleased with them coming in . . . . I just look forward to doing it next year, starting at the beginning of the year.*

The second-grade teacher also described how her collaborative relationship worked regarding fitting the writing lab approach into the regular curriculum:

> *One thing I am really impressed with is how well they come in and work with my existing curriculum and embellish the things I am already doing. [The SLP] will come in and say, "What are you doing? What can we do? How can we tie this into the computers? How can we go about either changing or adding to it so the kids get a well-rounded view of the concept you are teaching or the story you are teaching, or whatever it is you are teaching?" And that really helped a lot.*

This teacher then provided an example of the way writing of a persuasive piece was integrated into the second-grade language arts curriculum. Although persuasive discourse writing is often viewed as partially difficult and saved for later grades (Scott, 1999), the team collaborated to design a project appropriate for second graders:

> *One particular project we were talking about, the story was about building a robot, so they built these robots in the art room, and then the task in the computer room was to write and print out a for-sale sign. They had to describe their robot, what it did, how much it costs, and then they had to do a little paragraph at the bottom selling their robot—why they think it would be beneficial for you to buy their particular robot. And that was really neat because they got into changing fonts and size and making it look presentable and flashy and those sorts of things, so that was fun.*

A third-grade teacher at a different school also saw the value of working on writing within the curriculum. She was influenced to collaborate when another third-grade teacher shared some of the products her students had produced within her team's writing lab activities. The new school was fully inclusive in that no students were pulled out for special education services [although they were pulled out for speech-language services]. Not much writing had been occurring in the third grade, however, until this teacher and the other third-grade teachers became part of a writing lab development team. The teacher described her initial positive impressions and motivation to participate:

> *I looked at it as an opportunity for kids to get in and do more writing within the curriculum, not as an "add-on," not as something extra that we had to do but to get them to think more thoroughly and be more observant about things we were learning in the classroom.*

One way the teachers we have worked with accomplished curriculum integration was to look at the district writing curriculum to see what specific objectives in the curriculum were appropriate for students with special needs. Special education teachers, SLPs, and classroom teachers engaged in this process together. It was interesting to watch the dynamic back-and-forth exchange of the conversations, as the curriculum became a context within which IEP objectives could be addressed. One third-grade teacher said that it has been beneficial for her to collaborate with the special education teacher on ways to achieve the goals of the curriculum and that the collaboration resulted in "working together to make everything we did authentic."

An SLP working in one development team school described how her interest in collaborating grew as she experienced success working on her students' IEP goals in the inclusive contexts of the writing lab approach. When asked to give examples, she said,

> *One in particular was the author's chair experience that usually happened when we would do free writing or when we were at the end of a unit we were sharing. And a couple of my children . . . with speech and language needs and other labels, wouldn't have had that same opportunity to speak in front of their class at that same time if they were pulled out in their special ed. room. So it seems like it was nice to help them use strategies like making eye contact, practicing a couple of times before they went up there, talking about ways to deliver themselves in front of people. And that was really important for me to see, and I felt like I actually put some strategies into play that worked. So that was encouraging for me, and I think the students. I've got five students [with disabilities] in the classroom, and they seem to raise their hands and want to be part of [author chair].*

Find a Time and Place to Plan

A second point to consider in fostering collaborative relationships among professionals is that doing so requires time and space for the people involved. As part of the patience principle, we remind ourselves that collaboration is a relationship, and relationships do not develop immediately. The members of instructional teams begin to see themselves as teams when time and attention are committed to that process. These are challenging aspects of collaboration, particularly for special education teachers who may have children included in several different classrooms.

One special education teacher, who (like Spencer's special education teacher) could not schedule time in the general education classrooms of her students, remarked that she often unintentionally took her students in a different direction than what had been started in the classroom because she had not had time to talk or plan with the general education teachers. One of the third-grade teachers who shared students with this special educator recognized her colleague's dilemma:

> *She did as well as she could because she has some other children in there and different needs. We couldn't get that worked out so that she could be around for some preplanning and be in contact with us about something that the kids could work on with her.*

The special education teacher described how the team had addressed this problem:

> *Toward the end, we were doing a much better job. We were sending things back and forth. We had a writing folder that went back and forth between us. And that helped a lot.*

Other logistics that can ease the barriers to planning and collaborating involve clustering several students with disabilities in one or a few general education classrooms. As an SLP commented,

> *A biggie for special education teachers and SLPs is to almost have the students clumped together if possible, and if you could get that done before the start of the school year, then you could try to have a bulk of your students in one classroom . . . without having to be in two separate rooms for one or two. That really helped me, and that just kind of happened because [the third-grade teachers] were team teaching, and they just happened to have a lot of my kids in their room.*

Opportunity to meet, however, still is critical, and that is one arena in which school principals can play a key role, assisting with scheduling and finding space for teams to meet. Creative scheduling through common blocks of time is one avenue leading to successful collaborative relationships. Often, collaborative teams find ingenious ways to address the issue of time to collaborate. After school, over lunch, early in the morning—each of these has possibilities when professionals work together. A second-grade teacher said:

> *[The SLP] particularly would come in and ask what I was doing, what she could do. Sometimes we would make up a template of a concept I was trying to teach and then how to tie it in to the computer writing. She would say, "Well, let me make up a template for*

you; let me put this on there for you so we can give the kids some
added guided practice on how to do what it is you want them to
do on the computer with less time than having to write it out.
They can just punch it right in."

When asked about the times when this kind of planning would occur, the teacher said,

There were times she came in after school, right after the kids left,
and then there were times when she came in before school.

Principals who see collaboration as a powerful context for professional development will make the structures available to support collaborative instructional teams. Some principals, for example, support more intensive planning and special activities, such as joint evaluation of writing probes and goal setting, by hiring substitute teachers at key points to give instructors several hours to work together as a team.

As important as time is for building collaborative teams, it is not a panacea. Not everyone is willing to collaborate. In fact, the early stages of team building are rough for most teams. The exception may be teams who are able to build on existing positive personal relationships. Readers should be aware, however, that some educators voice strong preferences for maintaining independent practices and do not choose to be members of collaborative teams. Others commit to participating at lesser levels of consultation. In such cases, principals can play a role in making administrative decisions to place students in classrooms with teachers who are interested in collaborating and working with students with disabilities in their classrooms.

Negotiate a Common Vocabulary

A third aspect of developing interprofessional relationships for collaborating across discipline boundaries hinges on the negotiation of a common vocabulary. A common vocabulary is necessary both for adults communicating with students and for adults communicating with each other.

To facilitate communication with children, special service providers should study the vocabulary of the general curriculum, observe teachers carefully, and adopt the classroom vocabulary when working with students with disabilities. The team also can work together to assess students' vocabulary understandings and to find alternative ways to help students gain understandings of the words their teachers and classmates use.

In addition, educators from different backgrounds should be aware of the need to clarify vocabulary specific to their disciplines and to make sure they are using shared terms to mean the same thing. They also need models to see how unfamiliar concepts or activities look in practice. One third-grade teacher commented,

I'm really a visual person, and so I need to see . . . what the author
chair looks like. I need to see what a minilesson looks like, what
kind of things you do. I'm very visual, and I know that there are a
thousand kids out there that are the exact same way.

Educators and special service providers on collaborative teams represent diverse areas of expertise and differing philosophical orientations. Differences in perspectives and interactive styles can be both challenging and rewarding. This process of becoming a team takes patience, as well as dynamic flexibility. The SLP on one team recommended,

> ***Be patient because it takes a lot to collaborate among many professionals with many diverse personalities, which you are always going to find in a group. Know that it's okay to do some alternative things . . . I think it's okay to do [activities in] both [environments]—do some pull-out and some in the classroom, which I do with children, especially if I'm just starting them out. And most of all, just be open to teaching each other about what you do because people don't know what you do in your little room until you tell them and show them . . . So don't be afraid to give suggestions to the teachers [and to tell them] that you might need some help but you are willing to work in the classroom.***

When differences of opinion occur, it is important to respect others' perspectives. Teams can keep conflicts from becoming personal by labeling theoretical positions—not people. One area of common ground most professionals share is a passion for help-

---

Box 13.1.   Negotiating Differences in Perspective and Philosophy

Chelsea, a 7-year-old first grader with autism, spent most of her day in the special education classroom with a personal aide. Her classroom language activities focused on following simple directions and naming a large set of pictures. Although Chelsea could name several pictures, she produced almost no spontaneous speech. Chelsea screamed frequently to refuse activities imposed on her and to convey that her needs were not being met. When this occurred, her teacher or paraprofessional teaching assistant reprimanded her firmly and put her in time-out.

The SLP introduced the idea of teaching vocabulary to Chelsea in contextualized and interactional activities with a social interactionist approach. This differed from the previous approach in which vocabulary was taught with a discrete-skills picture naming approach. Instead, the SLP suggested that Chelsea participate in play with toys using words represented on her picture cards. In addition, she suggested that, rather than quickly moving Chelsea to time-out when screaming occurred, screaming could be viewed as an opportunity to teach words that could be substituted for screaming. The special education teacher was skeptical and worried that, if not punished immediately, the screaming would intensify. The mutual trust that had been built between the two educators made it safe for them to share and label their different philosophical approaches as behaviorist and social interactionist. They agreed to integrate elements of both approaches in what the educators referred to as "The Grand Experiment." As Chelsea began to use more words and scream less, it was easier for the special education teacher to accept the social-interactionist methods.

ing students learn. Keeping this communal goal at the forefront of thinking and talking about differences openly eases the collaborative process. The team can then discuss a strategy for using the research principle to investigate systematically which paths to try, and how to gather data that will help them decide whether one path works better than another. Box 13.1 provides an example of how this experimental process worked to resolve a disagreement between whether to teach vocabulary using a discrete trials behaviorist approach or a more contextualized social-interactionist approach.

It helps if early discussions focus on shared values, philosophies, ideas, and strategies, along with logistics. In fact, such discussions can take place in the specific context of planning lessons or working to implement them. Gradually, through discussion and side-by-side classroom work, instructors come to recognize individual competencies in each other and to develop shared competencies. This time is when the team model can be considered transdisciplinary rather than merely multidisciplinary, or even interdisciplinary (see Chapter 4).

Although collaboration is not easy and there is no way that all professionals can be on exactly the same page at the beginning of the process, our findings indicate that inclusive, relevant practices and the resulting effects for students make the effort worthwhile. As teams evolve, the benefits of collaboration become more visible. In Chapter 17, we present evidence of the benefits of the writing lab approach for all students. At the point when these benefits become evident, many educators reconsider their commitment to the team process, and they begin to participate at higher levels, thus contributing to intersystemic growth. Although collaboration cannot be forced, willingness to collaborate can grow over time if initial experiences are positive and if mutual goals for students, as well as professionals' goals for their own personal productivity, are being met.

Building Relationships Between Instructors and Students

General education teachers play important roles in welcoming students into classrooms and integrating them into the classroom culture. Special education teachers and SLPs can support general education teachers in playing this key role by helping them build relationships with students with disabilities. Three suggestions for assisting general education teachers to view students with disabilities as residents, rather than visitors, are to 1) expect all students to follow classroom routines, 2) expect all students to progress in language and literacy development, and 3) take advantage of the computer as a neutral change agent.

Expect All Students to Follow Classroom Routines

Students who are pulled out for special education or speech-language services may miss opportunities to learn classroom routines and procedures. They also are more likely to need classroom routines and procedures to be communicated explicitly and repeated frequently. Most students with special needs can learn classroom routines, however, and should be expected to follow them.

Beyond routines, students need to understand clearly the academic and social expectations that come with being a part of the classroom. Special service providers can work with students with disabilities, if necessary, to prepare them to confer with their general education teachers to develop personal goals. For example, students may set goals to work independently for longer periods of time, read their own stories in the author chair, use a planning web, or participate more fully in some other way. Teachers and students also can confer about how students can monitor change in their own skills. In this way, students can gain increased ownership for progress. Fully developed relationships mean that students with special needs are treated as full members of the class, even though they may require more intensive attention in some ways. Spencer's third-grade teacher described her understanding of what he needed from her:

> *You have to make sure that there's a background of whatever you're going to be writing about. He needs to clearly understand what you're talking about. When he does understand, you have to keep him focused. He needs one-on-one. There's no saying, "Spencer sit there and write for 3–4 minutes by yourself, and then we'll come back." Someone must sit right next to him and help him the whole entire way. If you leave him, then he's done. With some other students you can leave them, but with Spencer, he's gone.*

Partial evidence for students becoming residents, rather than visitors, is that they are held accountable for participation and for complying with the same rules as the other students in the class. Spencer's special education teacher described how this looked when his general education teacher started demonstrating increased ownership for him and confidence in her role with him:

> *Now she is disciplining him more and asking him questions during the writing time. She has asked him to share more, so there's been more ownership. I think that it has broken the barrier.*

Expect All Students to Progress

Another way special service providers can support relationship building for general education teachers and students with disabilities is to help teachers set higher expectations for their students to progress within the general education curriculum—and to achieve them. There are two ways to influence this process. First, teams might confer in team meetings about raising expectations, and if necessary, use the research principle to risk higher expectations and to gather data about the success of the approach. Second, team members might model scaffolding techniques that any of them can use to help students attempt tasks and progress in ways previously viewed as impossible.

Chapters 5 and 6 present suggestions for providing scaffolding and other supports that foster language learning (spoken and written) and greater independence. One example for students with limited reading and writing skills is to take dictation initially to allow them to get their own words on paper (rather than to perform copying tasks while their classmates wrote, as many of our students with special needs were doing originally). Another example is to allow peers to support students with limited literacy skills to read their own stories, standing by to whisper words in the students' ears during early author chair experiences and gradually providing less support as the children's skill and confidence develop. A third is to help slightly more advanced students brainstorm lists of words they will need for a particular piece to create personal word lists (on paper or with the computer) the students can use while writing. Providing support to show the general education teacher how to scaffold such events can be especially conducive to relationship building.

An SLP described how the process of revised expectations took place for one third-grade teacher. She told how, when she started to work with the students with special needs, the teacher said, "You can't work with those kids. Those kids are special. They don't do writing in here." The special education teacher had to go into to the teacher's classroom to say, "No, actually they're supposed to do writing in here," to help this teacher accept that the students with disabilities were to be held to the same standards as his other students.

The SLP then described this teacher's relationships with his students with disabilities toward the end of the school year as an example:

> *[The teacher had] gone over and embraced his special ed. kids' needs. In [this teacher's] class, where he said, "I'm having trouble with this student. I need to work with him a little bit more." The next day I came in, and he was sitting on the floor working with that student.*

The teacher himself described changes in his perceptions after being a member of a writing lab development team for the school year:

> *I guess I'm a greater believer in the children and their learning. They can do a lot when you build their expectations just a little higher. . . . It's widened and broadened my perspective with what I can do with a group of children.*

A special education teacher whose children were included in a third-grade teacher's classroom talked about the difference in student–teacher relationships for students who participated in the inclusive writing lab approach, compared with those who did not:

> *It did a nice job of having [the teachers] know what [the students] can and cannot do. My other kids pulled that "I can't do that" [routine]—when they can—and then [they still] get away with it.*

We have found that the process of helping teachers realistically target IEP goals within classroom curriculum has been a powerful means of changing such perceptions. In this way, the writing lab approach differs from many uses of the term *realistic*, which is often a euphemism for lowered expectations. That is, it may be necessary for the language and communication specialists on the team to help other members see that they can realistically raise their expectations for higher levels of language and literacy learning, rather than to be "realistic" by lowering them.

The prior special education teacher also commented on how her students reached their IEP goals and then exceeded her own expectations:

> *Just to give you some insights on the students—social skills were not there. Sentence structures in just speaking—I mean if we had a complete sentence come out of someone's mouth, it was amazing. Their thoughts were so scattered. So, our objective—well, my objectives—for the year were, in the beginning, very low. I had expectations where I just wanted them to think clear thoughts and be able to communicate them verbally, and when they're talking, to make eye contact with each other and wait until it's their turn; to be able to sit still when other people are sharing, to sit in front of a peer—and they went way beyond that!*

The multi-grade language arts consultant at one school summarized the effects of holding high expectations for students with disabilities within inclusive settings:

> *I saw support for what I've always read in mainstreaming literature—that when kids are able to interact with their peers, everyone succeeds. The bar really got held up for the special needs kids. I mean they really had to work, and they rose admirably to meet the challenge.*

Take Advantage of the Computer as a Neutral Change Agent

The computer as a component of the writing lab approach is a tool with the potential to modify relationships between instructors and students. Instructors can take advantage, for example, of speech synthesis features for revising and editing. In this case, the computer feedback can change the perception from making corrections in punctuation, syntax, or spelling in order to please the teacher to making changes so that the computer will read the text the way the student intended.

The computer lab teacher at one of the development team schools described the effect of using computer features on her relationship with the students this way:

> *They don't mind being corrected. I feel that I'm teaching them. I ask them specific things about their sentences, such as "What do you need here? Okay, a capital. Let's go change that." I let them do that. It doesn't seem to bother them at all that it's a grammar correction. It's not like putting a red circle around it on a piece of paper and handing it back. You don't get a lot of red marks on the computer, you just go back and fix them. I don't think there's that negative response with the computer, as opposed to a piece of paper that the teacher might mark up with a bunch of red lines. On the computer, you just erase or fix it and nobody ever knew.*

Building Relationships Among Students

In computer-supported inclusive settings, students with special needs experience increased opportunities to interact with typically developing peers. Their identification as special, however, may lead peers to create a different set of academic, behavioral, and social expectations. As a result, the students with disabilities may feel distanced. When children are included as residents, however, the classroom becomes a place where children with special needs can demonstrate their language competence and be recognized as full-fledged members of the class by their peers. As one third-grade teacher observed,

> *[Students with disabilities] all had a chance to experience becoming writers, emerging writers, and having their work recognized and appreciated and celebrated.*

Techniques for building better peer-to-peer relationships involve a multipronged approach to 1) model and scaffold acceptance of students with special needs among general education peers, 2) scaffold students with disabilities to improve their social acceptability by building their pragmatic communication skills, 3) scaffold all students to see each other as an important audience (and source) for ideas, and 4) use the power of computer expertise to level the playing field.

Model and Scaffold Acceptance of Students with Special Needs

All educators on the team play active roles in building understanding for individual similarities and differences. Writing lab activities, such as author group and peer conferencing, provide opportunities for targeting objectives addressing social communication. Educators also scaffold peer-to-peer interactions, withdrawing support when it is no longer required. The results can be remarkable in terms of greater peer acceptance. One computer lab teacher commented,

> *I saw [one child with cognitive-linguistic disabilities], in particular, in [a third-grade teacher's] room really stretching to meet and do what the other kids did, and I saw his peers supporting him in all his efforts. And in terms of kids that did come with their classrooms [to the computer lab]—and I have other classrooms that did not bring their special needs students—there is a marked difference in terms of how much special needs students have achieved this year. And I'm going to advocate that all classrooms follow that pattern next year.*

Supportive relationships among diverse students are wonderful to observe, but they cannot be taken for granted. They require intentional scaffolding and specific modeling. General education students may need encouragement at first to become peer-editing partners with students who are clearly different from them. One technique for encouraging acceptance is to model respect for each student's individual efforts.

Box 13.2.   Scaffolding Social Skills in an Inclusive Setting

Discord arose during drafting time in the third-grade classroom. Tom pushed and ridiculed Spencer, who was attempting to look at Tom's paper. The SLP scaffolded the following conversation to assist both boys to construct new knowledge about the pragmatics of social distance (proxemics) and to use positive words rather than negative actions to communicate about a problem. Then, she helped the boys practice using the knowledge to generate a new set of skills for solving social problems.

SLP: What's going on?

Tom: He's messing with me.

Spencer: I just want to see his story.

SLP: Tom, you said Spencer is messing with you. What is making you uncomfortable?

Tom: He didn't ask. He's on my back, and he's touching me.

SLP: You want him to ask.

Tom: Yes.

SLP: And you don't like him touching you?

Tom: No.

SLP: You think he is too close?

Tom: Yes.

SLP: How can you let Spencer know he is too close.

Tom: I'll push him out of my face.

SLP: That's one way, but what might happen?

Tom: I'll get in trouble, but I don't care, if he's messing with me.

SLP: What could you say to Spencer so he knows what you want him to do?

Tom: "Back off."

SLP: Yes, you could say, "You're too close. Step back." Spencer, look at Tom. What does it look like when he's uncomfortable?

Spencer: Mad.

SLP: Yes, he's making a mad face. What can you do when you see that?

Spencer: Stop.

SLP: Yes, you can stop. You can take a step back. You can ask, "Why are you mad?" Let's talk to Tom and see if we can learn how close is comfortable and what feels too close?

After some trial and error experimenting, the two boys agreed that an arm's length felt comfortable, and they practiced measuring this distance several times.

SLP: Okay, Spencer and Tom. Let's practice. Spencer, how can you get Tom's attention without silly faces?

Spencer: Tom?

Tom: Yeah.

Spencer: Can I see your paper?

Tom: Maybe later.

Spencer was able to accept this outcome for the moment.

Another is to scaffold interactions in such writing lab activities as peer conferencing or author groups. If necessary, a capable student might be pulled aside and told that the teachers would like him or her to take on this role because of the student's knack for being an interested listener. The message is one of confidence in this student's ability to help other students make good planning choices and come up with original ideas.

Scaffold Appropriate Social Skills for Students with Special Needs

In some cases, students with special needs want desperately to be accepted by their peers, but they do not know how to make that happen. This was the case for Spencer. Helping Spencer to learn the social routines for relating in the general education classroom involved scaffolding both him and his peers to use of a broader range of interpersonal communication strategies.

The process started with a large group minilesson to encourage students to reflect on individual similarities and differences between them. This lesson was designed to build understanding of diverse strengths and needs. Small-group minilessons followed to make more explicit some of the rules that govern social communication. Topics addressed how close to stand next to someone, when and how to touch people, how to read body language, and how to get someone's attention.

Many opportunities were found to scaffold use of the strategies discussed in the minilessons during peer-to-peer interactions. The example in Box 13.2 illustrates scaffolding that occurred following an argument between Spencer and Tom, a peer who had little tolerance for Spencer's unusual communication style. The SLP engaged both students in reflecting on language and communication. Spencer needed to be directed to attend to nonverbal as well as verbal aspects of communication. Tom needed to be scaffolded to use feedback more specific than pushing and ridiculing.

Scaffold Peers to Appreciate One Another as Audience and Idea Sources

The learning contexts of the writing lab, particularly peer conferencing, author groups, author chair, and computer-use experiences, are designed to facilitate students' appreciation of each other as important members of the audience and sources for ideas. It may require some scaffolding to help general education students accept their special education peers in this way and vice versa, but the relationship has to go both ways for students with disabilities to become true residents of their classrooms, rather than visitors.

McAlister's interviews with fourth- through eighth-grade students yielded insights into how older students viewed their interactions with peers in writing lab contexts (McAlister et al., 1999). When discussing author groups, for example,

> David reported that author groups are "people who work with you to do stories." Another student, Alison, stated that author groups are "where you can discuss your stories with other people in your group."
>
> In response to a question about why we have author groups, Alison stated, "So we can try to help other people out." Susan [a girl with Down syndrome] reported that the reason we have author groups is "because people might have ideas for other people's stories." Steve provided a similar response but added the point, "to make sure your story makes sense and it makes the other kids have an idea for another story." (McAlister et al., 1999, p. 164)

These comments show that the students not only understood the purpose of author groups; they also had emerging concepts of peers as audience. Later, when asked about revising and editing—rarely students' favorite activity—more students displayed a sense of audience awareness:

> [Students said editing and revising was] "so people can read your story better" and "we do it because, if we didn't revise and edit, the people that were reading it wouldn't know what we were talking about." Other students appeared to see the surface level meaning only, suggesting the reason as "so that when the stories come out, they won't be wrong, won't on the printer be wrong." (McAlister et al., 1999, p. 169)

The language arts/computer lab teacher in one elementary school described the essence of peer interaction for her. She related it to a photograph of two students, one with cognitive limitations and another with learning risks:

> *I have this great picture from the poetry center . . . with [this student] reading his poetry at the poetry slam, and [another student] is up there with him, and she has her little arm around him, and they are reading together. I mean, to me, that is sort of a core image of this year.*

Use the Power of Computer Expertise to Level the Field

Computer use can support improved peer-to-peer relations as well as improved instructor-to-student relations. At one point, Spencer experienced the special power of being able to demonstrate a computer software feature he had been taught before in the special education classroom for his less knowledgeable peers. The computer lab teacher described how Spencer used this special knowledge:

> *In the computer lab, they're all equal . . . [Spencer] was slow, but when he came in, he was showing us the audio portion of the software. He was showing us how to click around and get different sounds and voices. I didn't realize where he was at [in the special education room] and what his disabilities were until that happened. Then, it was explained to me that he had used the microphone in his special ed. room to record his story. He had learned this in his special ed. room, and then he could share this with everyone else. I had no idea that he was unable to write the words.*

The computer lab teacher also described this leveling power of the computer lab experience more generally:

> *I think because computers are something everyone enjoys no matter what their intelligence level, everyone comes into the computer lab feeling very good. Everyone is excited about coming in. There's not one person that has said, "Oh, I hate this!" That speaks wonders for teachers to hear. No matter what their intelligence level is, [students] can come in and work on the computer. They can look similar as far as the overall appearance of the product that gets printed out. If you look at details, you might see differences in the*

vocabulary usage or the spelling, with something like that. I real-
ized I did not know who the special ed. students were in the class-
rooms that came in. I had no idea who they were. No one told me
ahead of time. So I just looked at it when working with them that
some were slower than others. I still am not sure. Until we started
naming some of them at meetings, I didn't know who the special
ed. kids were. So maybe that's a position I'm in of advantage. I just
work with all students who come in there, and go with whatever
place they're at.

Building Relationships Between Parents, Educators, and Students

Parents are important members of educational teams. They can provide special insights into their child's strengths, needs, and sources of motivation and pride. Parents can be expected to advocate for programs and instructional methods they feel are best matched to their child's learning needs. Some regularly attend school gatherings and monitor curriculum content and progress closely. Other parents have limited interaction with school teams and need to be brought into the process. It is important to communicate with parents the writing lab language and literacy learning opportunities. Parents of students receiving pull-out special education services need information about how IEP objectives will be addressed in the inclusive writing lab context.

Parents also are key participants in celebrating successes. Publishing parties that showcase students' work are important community events that bring together young writers and their appreciative audiences. As described next, Spencer's mother was present when he willingly read his own story from the author's chair—a proud moment, and a turning point, for both of them.

ACHIEVING RESIDENT STATUS: TURNING POINTS

In spite of their mutual concerns about Spencer's developing language and literacy skills, when the school year began, neither his general education teacher nor his special education teacher had initiated the collaborative process to coordinate their efforts. Instead, each did her best in her own classroom to meet Spencer's needs, relatively blind to the goals, intervention strategies, and desired outcomes of the other teacher. In this particular case, the SLP consulted in both rooms, and she stimulated the collaborative process by sharing information back and forth between teachers. Both teachers then found that they appreciated the broader picture of Spencer's needs and abilities reported by the SLP.

Building a Team While Planning for Spencer

Together with the SLP, the two teachers met and began the process of collaborating to support Spencer's language and literacy learning. The special education teacher commented on the importance of this intermediary, or bridging, role:

> *Unfortunately, when special needs kids come in and out of the classroom, and they come in during a lesson, and maybe they don't know what's going on, they don't always feel good about themselves because they are questioning what's going on. [The writing lab experience] has been helpful because there has been help, and they definitely need that in writing.*

Spencer participated with his general education peers in the baseline writing probe activities discussed in Chapter 15. With heavy scaffolding, he generated four possible story ideas, all involving physical fights but with different players. Because he was reluctant to write connected text and his spelling skills were limited to sounding out a few initial letters, he dictated his first story. In this way, he took the first step toward becoming an author.

When it was time to present this story in author chair, however, Spencer refused. He also would not participate in author chair opportunities to comment or ask questions about work shared by his peers. Spencer's dictated baseline probe, which was analyzed using the methods described in Chapter 15, showed how Spencer struggled to generate story ideas. He linked his story ideas causally to relate a story about a fight with another child. He communicated the main ideas, but he did not identify the other child by name, only *he*. His language was simple but adequate. His special education teacher contributed that he had incomplete learning of sound–symbol relationships for reading and spelling and that this was a primary focus area in his special education curriculum.

Spencer's general education teacher observed that although he was eager to interact with his typically developing peers, he was not well accepted by them. His primary antagonist, Tom, actively rejected him. Tom acted-out whenever Spencer was seated next to him, and taunted, "He can't even read."

To understand the peer rejection, Spencer's SLP observed him interact with his peers in his general education classroom. She noticed that Spencer initiated interaction by making silly faces and sound effects. In addition, he showed a tendency to violate comfortable proximity distances when talking, by standing too close and touching his peers. The SLP also observed the culture of the special education classroom, which included more physical contact in the form of hugging among peers and with the teacher than was acceptable in the general education classroom. As described in Box 13.2, Spencer needed some explicit scaffolding to bridge the two classroom cultures.

Based on baseline observations, the team generated the following objectives for Spencer. To improve reading and writing skills, Spencer would

1. Generate multiple topic ideas during the planning stage

2. Use sound–symbol relationships in decoding and encoding

3. Read and write new sight vocabulary and word parts related to each writing project

4. Draft text with minimal to moderate support using word lists generated during dictation, personal dictionary, word walls, and invented spelling

5. Revise written work for logical organization and adequate information

6. Summarize reading to check for comprehension and sense making

To improve social and spoken language skills Spencer would

1. Maintain appropriate proximity during peer conversation independently

2. Use social language routines for initiating a conversation

3. Participate in classroom discussions

4. Present work in author chair with minimal support

After reaching consensus on these goals for Spencer, the team discussed intervention strategies and teacher roles. They decided that Spencer needed additional direct teaching and practice with sound–symbol associations to improve his word generation skills. He also needed to learn high-frequency words and word chunks. The plan was for his special education teacher to provide direct instruction aimed at these specific difficulties in the resource room. The SLP would take initial responsibility for scaffolding Spencer's written and spoken language during writing lab activities. As his teacher felt more comfortable in this role and confident that she could manage individual scaffolding in the context of the larger group, she would increasingly assume this role. A section in Spencer's author notebook would be dedicated to spelling information and would list sounds, words, and word parts that were familiar to him. It was decided that the notebook would travel back and forth with Spencer so that he could use it as a support in both rooms. Indirectly, the author notebook provided a means for each teacher to see what activities occurred in the other's room.

The general education teacher and the SLP decided to share responsibility for classroom minilessons. Although Spencer's special education teacher was unable to be in the classroom during writing lab time due to other scheduling demands, she planned to support his ongoing writing process work in her classroom. This support included preteaching some language concepts and software features (e.g., descriptive language and how to use the recording feature) and revisiting concepts introduced in the general education room (e.g., the stages of the writing process, generating a list of topic ideas). To enhance continuity and promote learning across settings, all agreed to use the same instructional language when possible and to meet on a regular basis to compare notes and fine-tune Spencer's program.

Table 13.1. Turning points from visitor to resident status for included students

Students	Teachers
Participate socially and are accepted by peers	Share responsibility for
Show self-awareness of class membership • Say "I'm in . . ." rather than "I go to . . ." • Are willing to take new risks	• Student objectives • Classroom lesson plans • Instructional strategies • Scaffolding individual students • Anticipating needs during scheduling and planning
Participate in the larger group of learners • Make contributions to group activities • Share ideas, reflections, and learning strategies	Share materials
Challenge themselves to new levels of independence	Acknowledge students; hold them accountable for • Classroom procedure • Academic work
Take pride in seeing their own success	Celebrate student success together

Turning Points and Stories of Change

Table 13.1 summarizes the signals of turning points for students and teachers. These are signs groups can look for as they become a team. In the case of Spencer, the process was gradual—he began to participate in shared writing, then to write more independently. He worked for longer periods of time independently and showed preference for asking peers for spelling supports rather than asking adults. After a group mini-lesson on descriptive language, Spencer described a watermelon as looking like a beach ball (see Figure 13.1).

His teacher responded enthusiastically to his colorful description and used his simile as an example of the kinds of descriptive language she valued. Later in the year, Spencer wrote a story about being teased. Spencer's use of descriptive, figurative language blossomed in this "Angry Mad" story (see Figure 13.2), in which he wrote about how his "temperature rised." Although Spencer received scaffolding to support spelling during computer editing, the ideas and words were his own. Upon completion, he told his teacher with a broad smile, "You are going to love this," reveling in his sense of audience and growth as a writer.

A turning point in peer acceptance for Spencer came in the computer lab when he was able to demonstrate for peers sitting next to him how to change color and font. This was a skill Spencer's special education teacher had taught in her classroom, but it had not yet been introduced formally in the general education classroom. Peers flocked to Spencer's computer to learn how to make their work more visually interesting. He became a bit of a celebrity that day.

A few days later when Spencer's turn came during author chair presentations, however, he again refused to read his story in front of the group. After much encouragement, Spencer's teachers and peers persuaded him to approach the author chair. As he did so, he turned suddenly and bolted from the room, saying he needed to use the bathroom. When the class broke into laughter, Tom came to Spencer's defense and explained to the class that he had been scared to read in front of the group at first, too. Picking up on this comment, the general education teacher led the group in a discussion about how it feels emotionally and physically to be afraid. When Spencer returned, the room quieted, and another peer walked to the front of the room to assist him to read his story. Spencer read his story to an appreciative and respectful audience. At that point, and later in the day, he glowed when reliving the moment and retelling it to his special education teacher (a moment signaling major growth of his spoken communication skills as well).

Turning points also occurred for Spencer's teachers. As his general education teacher began to recognize him as a true resident in her classroom, she took more responsibility for scaffolding his communication attempts. In addition, she taught some of Spencer's classroom peers how to scaffold his written language without encroaching on his independence. When describing Spencer to the interviewer, at first, she started to say, "He doesn't really write," in the old, absolutist mode typical of when she had viewed Spencer as a visitor. Then, she immediately revised her comment:

> *He has very limited writing skills and reading skills, but he does think, and [the SLP and graduate assistant] do write down the*

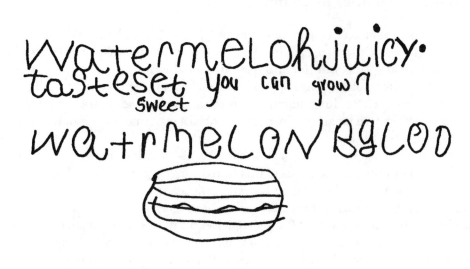

Figure 13.1.   Spencer's watermelon story.

words that he says. The first time that they wrote his story down for him, he wasn't willing to share it. Then, one of the students said she would help him. They practiced a bit, and [the peer] stood there. When he hesitated on the beginning of words, [the other student] whispered them to him. He was pretty proud of himself, that

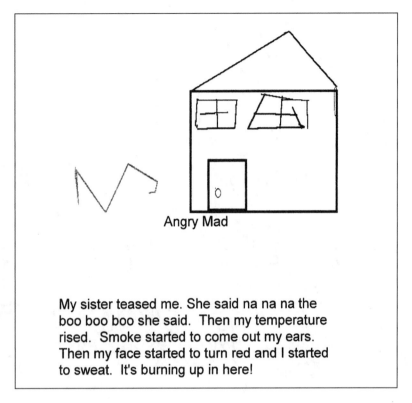

Angry Mad

My sister teased me. She said na na na the
boo boo boo she said. Then my temperature
rised. Smoke started to come out my ears.
Then my face started to turn red and I started
to sweat. It's burning up in here!

Figure 13.2. Spencer's "Angry Mad" story.

*he could do that. Now, when it comes time for sharing stories, he
really likes it. He practices what has been written.*

The special education teacher, seeing Spencer's motivation to work with classroom
peers, made efforts to provide services to him in his general education classroom for brief
periods each week. As the general education teacher and the special education teacher
communicated more, they were able to adjust Spencer's schedule so that he could participate during classroom lessons that would later be topics for student writing.

The special education teacher described how the general education teachers had
begun to reconceptualize their roles with the students with disabilities in her classroom:

*I think some of the teachers are looking at special needs kids in a
different light. I know one in particular has actually seen one of
the students that are in her classroom being able to actually participate in the writing and enjoy being in there.*

What began as a collaboration to support inclusion in writing activities gradually
expanded to include more classroom learning opportunities. Spencer expressed a desire
to participate in a math activity that involved learning math tables and culminated in
a classroom ice cream party with his general education classmates. His teachers found

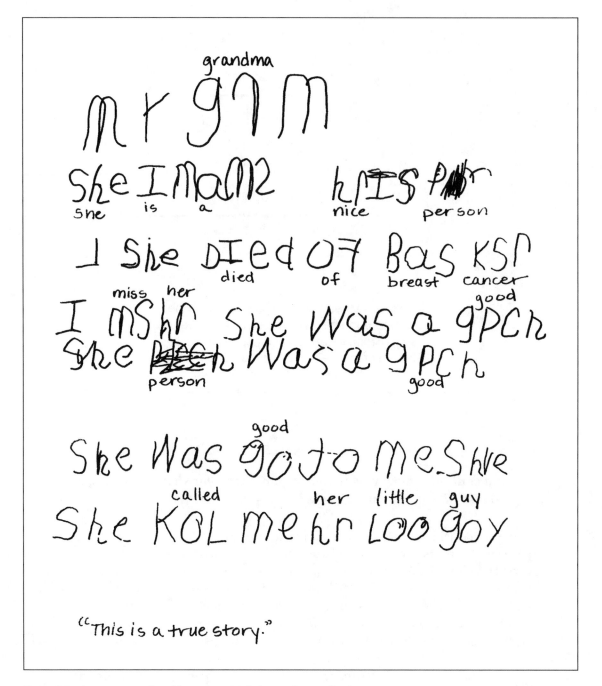

grandma
mr g1m

She I MaM2   h I S PMr
she   is   a   nice   person

1 She DIed O7 Bas KSr
     died   of   breast cancer

       miss   her   good
I mShr She Was a gPCh
She ~~PMCh~~ Was a gPCh
       person   good

She Was goJo me Shre
         good

       called   her little guy
She KOL me hr LOO goy

"This is a true story."

Figure 13.3. Spencer's story about his grandma. Original was written on lined paper.

that with minimal support in class, he could participate fully in this activity with his peers, who shared his joy at reaching a new goal.

At the end of the school year, Spencer wrote a poignant story about his grandmother, who had died of breast cancer (see Figure 13.3). He generated his topic independently and explained to his teacher that he was writing a true story. He used invented spelling to write independently. During a publishing party with his proud mother present, he willingly read his own story to the group. After finishing, Spencer exclaimed, "I'm so happy today!" His transition from visitor to resident was complete.

It would be misleading to suggest that the collaboration of the team in Spencer's school (or any of the other development teams) progressed easily to each turning point. It did not. This collaboration began as part of a professional development research-to-practice grant from the U.S. Department of Education to teach and support the writing lab approach. The teachers involved did not fully embrace inclusive practices at first, and none of our teams started with a working relationship among general educators and special service providers. All of the educators cared, however, about the literacy success of their students. As reported previously, many were encouraged to participate when offered the in-class support of one of the authors and a graduate student. Along the way there were difficulties scheduling meetings, disagreements in educational philosophies, and occasional misunderstandings. Despite the challenges of this new working situation, all team members gained new insights on the collaborative process and its potential for supporting all students.

SELF-EVALUATION TOOL FOR TEAMS

We developed the self-assessment tool (see Figure 13.4) to support teams in implementing the writing lab approach and evaluating their success in doing so. This tool takes the components of the writing lab approach (presented in Figure I.1) and places them in the form of a checklist.

Although we have used this tool in our research on the writing lab approach, we designed it originally to fill a need to step back as a development team and analyze how well we were doing in implementing the approach. The checklist can be used after several months of implementation when a team takes a moment to engage in self-reflection. This evaluation occurs best at a meeting set aside from the pressures of deciding what the next project and minilessons will be (see Chapter 4). Each of the team members first completes the form individually, then the group holds a round-robin discussion to talk about how each rated the implementation of components and to develop a group summary of successes, barriers, and needs.

Another strategy that we have used successfully is for each member of the team to take a moment to jot down a personal "wish list" of things they would like the team and students to accomplish in the next few weeks. Then, the team goes around the circle to consider everyone's primary wish first, then second wish, and so on. Discussions that result from this process are richer than would have been possible without the systematic reflection on the process. Table 13.2 provides examples of reflections two different teams produced as they completed this process.

SUMMARY

This chapter has focused on team building and inclusive, collaborative practices. We have described the process as one of relationship building among professionals, between teachers and students, among peers, and among the broader team that includes

Name: _____ Date: _____

Underlying values			
Have we built the components on a BACKDROP of principles, including:			
Balance, in acceptance/challenge; wholes/parts; teacher-directed/student-centered?	Y	P	N
Authentic audience, so that students recognize writing as a form of communication?	Y	P	N
Constructive learning, so that students are led to make discoveries "on their own" ?	Y	P	N
Keep it simple, so that we don't overload students or ourselves with too many new demands at once?	Y	P	N
Dynamic, with flexibility to respond to teachable moments and current needs?	Y	P	N
Research and reflective practice, so that it is guided by a questioning attitude about what works?	Y	P	N
Ownership, so that students assume increasing control of their own writing processes and learning?	Y	P	N
Patience, by allowing student ownership, focusing on process as much as product, and being patient with each other as we build new collaborative relationships?	Y	P	N

Successes	Barriers

Writing process instruction			
Authentic writing projects. Have we			
• Provided opportunities for students to choose topics and generate their own text?	Y	P	N
• Provided a range of audiences for written and oral presentations?	Y	P	N
• Helped students to focus on using language to share meaning?	Y	P	N
• Accepted students where they are while challenging them to reach higher levels?	Y	P	N
Recursive process. Have we			
• Focused on process as much as product?	Y	P	N
• Structured writing time to allow students to move recursively writing process stages?	Y	P	N
Language levels. Have we given attention to			
• Discourse level?	Y	P	N
• Sentence level?	Y	P	N
• Word level?	Y	P	N
• Conventions	Y	P	N
• Oral communication?	Y	P	N
Learning components. Have we maximized use of			
• Individual scaffolding?	Y	P	N
• Scaffolding worksheets?	Y	P	N
• Minilessons on writing process, writing skills and strategies, computer supports?	Y	P	N
• Teacher/peer conferencing?	Y	P	N
• Author's chair?	Y	P	N

Successes	Barriers

The Writing Lab Approach to Language Instruction and Intervention, by Nickola Wolf Nelson, Christine M. Bahr, and Adelia M. Van Meter
Copyright © 2004 Paul H. Brookes Publishing Co., Inc. All rights reserved.

Figure 13.4. Writing lab team evaluation checklist.

Computer support			
Software features. Have we used specific software features to support students in different stages of the writing process?	Y	P	N
Keyboarding. Have we provided adequate opportunity for students to practice keyboarding skills?	Y	P	N
Specialized access. Have we considered computer and software modifications to assist students with disabilities?	Y	P	N
Physical environment. Have we made classroom and lab modifications to improve student participation and learning?	Y	P	N

Successes	Barriers

Inclusive instructional practices			
Educational outcomes. Have we			
• Included all students in the language learning activities of the writing process?	Y	P	N
• Modified objectives, strategies, supports to meet individual needs?	Y	P	N
• Monitored student outcomes?	Y	P	N
Collaborative team development. Have we			
• Collaborated regarding instructional planning for projects?	Y	P	N
• Developed action research questions, methods, and outcomes?	Y	P	N
• Shared learning to promote systemic change?	Y	P	N

Successes	Barriers

What I would most like to see in the next project(s) we attempt:

The Writing Lab Approach to Language Instruction and Intervention, by Nickola Wolf Nelson, Christine M. Bahr, and Adelia M. Van Meter
Copyright © 2004 Paul H. Brookes Publishing Co., Inc. All rights reserved.

Table 13.2. Examples of collaborative planning resulting from team self-evaluation

	Team One	Team Two
Areas of need	Writing processes and language targets Focus on language: • Interesting words • Word chunks • Varied sentences • Paragraph organization • Parts of a particular genre Computer supports: • Use of computers for drafting • Use of computers for revising and editing Inclusion: • Inclusion of all students in process • Greater collaboration between general and special education	Writing processes: • More peer conferencing with a minilesson to teach how-to • Connect proofreading skills to editing their own work • Greater independence in using the stages of the writing process • Make sure we mark/celebrate the end of projects Language targets: • Make story grammar explicit • Teach spelling strategies • Construct sentences from notes in expository projects • Develop individual supports for student reference (e.g., word lists, brainstorm lists, how-to notes for punctuation) Computer supports: • Need keyboarding practice • Teach editing features
Ideas/goals for future projects	Consider: • What elements do successful projects share? • What are the best ways to teach conventions? • How do we scaffold student writing at computers?	Consider: • Science writing • Poetry • Stories
Wish list (What do we want to accomplish before the end of the school year?)	We want to: • Give students an opportunity to complete a project of their own choice • Give more experience in peer conferencing • Use computers for all stages of the writing process • Evaluate success in reaching students' individual objectives • Complete a final probe	We want to: • Have more amplification for author chair, and an amplification system for the computer lab • Provide clips on computers for holding notes and drafts • Give the students personal dictionary pages with third-grade spelling words for their author notebooks

parents, teachers, and students. Elements have been described that can facilitate the building of these relationships, many of which draw on other components of the writing lab approach.

The voices of professionals who have worked with us on development teams are heard in this chapter, describing their own perceptions and changed expectations as they participated on writing lab teams. Students' voices also are heard. Scaffolding techniques and turning points are described for each. The chapter uses the stories of students, one in particular—Spencer—to illustrate the mutually facilitative processes of team building and inclusive practices. Spencer entered his general education classroom as a visitor at the beginning of the school year and ended it as a resident.

14

Identifying Needs Through Formal and Informal Assessment

Students with special needs often participate in extensive assessment activities. The goals of assessment include

- To determine eligibility for special services

- To construct reading, writing, and spoken language profiles

- To establish intervention objectives

- To guide instruction

- To measure change over time

- To document outcomes

Just as the purposes for assessing writing and other language forms are varied, so, too, are the types of assessment tools and strategies available. The best method of assessment for a given student depends on the questions professionals seek to answer. This chapter addresses the assessment process by introducing varied approaches to written language assessment. The process begins with the formulation of questions that serve as a framework for matching assessment needs to appropriate tools and strategies.

ASSESSMENT CONCERNS

Assessment involves the process of gathering information and analyzing it for multiple purposes. Students in some school districts are routinely tested to meet public goals. These might include measuring how one group performs compared with another or how a group progresses over time. Results frequently are used to determine policy or to implement policy (e.g., failing school districts lose their privileges of self-determination and administration). Students also may be tested to compare individual performance on one or several variables to a group of age- or grade-matched peers. Although many of the assessment tools and strategies discussed in this chapter and in Chapter 15 can be administered and scored for a large group, the focus in this chapter is on assessments that are used to meet the specific diagnostic and instructional needs of individual students.

Questions Guide the Process

Assessment questions guide choices of appropriate tools. For example, key questions at various stages of the process might include

1. Norm-referenced questions:

   How does this student's written language compare with age- and grade-matched peers?

   Is this student eligible for special educational services?

2. Baseline questions:

   What is this student's pattern of strengths and needs in spoken and written language?

   What knowledge and use of writing strategies does the student bring to the writing process?

   What current levels of functioning can be documented against which progress can be measured?

3. Planning related questions:

   What language intervention goals and objectives should be targeted?

   What instructional strategies will be most successful with this student?

   What is the next step or challenge for this student?

A comprehensive evaluation might involve answering all of these questions. At other times, educators might choose to be more focused in their assessment procedures, looking only at a few features that relate to individual need, or that correspond to a particular classroom's curricular goals. As Calkins noted,

> It's all too easy to have only the trappings of a student-centered curriculum: the small-group discussions, the optional activities, the hands-on and interactive work. In the end, a classroom is student-centered if and only if our teaching happens in response to individual students. Assessment allows us to be student-centered in our teaching. (1994, p. 314)

For students with special language and learning needs, assessment of written language may grow out of a referral for a comprehensive assessment of general factors affecting educational achievement, or written language may be the primary area of concern. The examples in Box 14.1 illustrate three students, each with a unique profile of language-learning strengths and needs. In each case, the process is entered at a different stage. Sometimes, information is needed for a student failing broadly in multiple areas of language-based activities. At other times, specific information is needed re-

---

Box 14.1. How Assessment Questions Differ for Individual Students

Sarah's parents referred her to our after-school writing lab project when she was 10 years old. Although Sarah had been diagnosed with neurological problems, she had progressed well in most speech and language areas during her early years. When we met Sarah, her primary difficulties were in the areas of fine motor coordination and attention. Sarah's parents reported that she did not experience early language difficulties, but lately she had been having increasing difficulties. When she tried to relate stories verbally, her stories lacked key information, were disorganized, and strayed off topic. Her conversations were similar. Sarah's parents observed, too, that as the language demands of school increased, Sarah showed more difficulty understanding spoken discourse, reading for comprehension, and writing cohesive stories. They wanted to know "What was the relationship between Sarah's spoken and written language abilities?" and "How could Sarah's language-learning needs be best addressed?"

Sudhir was in the seventh grade when he was referred by his special education teacher for extra help in writing. His teacher noticed that he could express his ideas in a simple manner, but his written narration skills, use of grammar, and spelling were less mature than any of his peers. His teacher asked, "What strategies would help Sudhir to progress to the next step in writing maturity?"

Jonah's vivid imagination kept him well fueled with entertaining stories, but spelling difficulties interfered with his attempts to put ideas on paper. At 9 years old, Jonah's writing contained a proportion of spelling errors that distracted readers and at times interfered with their understanding of his text. Jonah also continued to have mild articulation difficulties in his spoken speech. Jonah's parents and special education teacher wanted to know "What was the nature of Jonah's spelling difficulties?" and "How could Jonah best be assisted to improve his spelling skills?"

---

garding the parameters of concern when a student exhibits poor performance in one of several areas specific to writing.

Interviews and Other Conversations

Specific questions for guiding assessment grow out of interactions among the participants: teachers, parents, students, and professionals who will conduct assessment activities. Spending the time to understand the perspectives of the multiple players permits focus on the educational needs presented. In this context, interviews and/or group discussions begin the assessment process, pulling together the insights of those involved in a student's educational planning and teaching. From this process come the questions that will serve as a framework for collecting and analyzing additional information.

Depending on the stage of development of a team and the assessment roles of the professionals participating, an interview format or a discussion format may be used to gather and summarize background information. Prior to the development of a team, an interview format may be necessary. In interviews, professionals from one discipline (e.g., speech-language pathology, school psychology, learning disability) gather information from others, including teachers, parents, and students. They also share information from their own professional perspectives. In situations in which teams have begun to work collaboratively, conversations among the members are more like discussions than interviews. That is, information is shared in multiple directions, and topics are negotiated equally among members of the team. In either case, the primary purpose is to develop a picture of the student as a whole. Other goals at this stage are to

1. Establish the multiple and shared perspectives of students, parents, and teachers.

2. Identify "zones of significance" (i.e., areas multiple participants view as a primary) (Nelson, 1998), based on discussions of the student's strengths and needs.

3. Elicit information on the student's language processing skills, including the relationship between reading, writing, and spoken communication.

4. Identify emotional variables (e.g., anxiety, low self-esteem, perfectionism) and learning constraints (e.g., distractibility, long-term and working memory difficulties, perspective taking) (Singer & Bashir, 1999b).

5. Explore instructional strategies that have been tried to date, along with their corresponding outcomes.

6. Build partnerships and a sense of working together as a team to assist this student and others to improve their language and literacy skills.

With the student, the interview establishes a learning partnership based on trust and caring for the student's insights and learning processes. For parents, it acknowledges the student's insights and contributions, short- and long-term concerns, and hopes and goals for the future. For teachers, the interview process sets the stage for a collaborative relationship that stresses joint problem solving and aims at keeping students in the general curriculum. In this way, special educators and SLPs can steer participants away from the pitfall of multiple curricula.

The framework for the interview or discussion process begins with general questions and gradually becomes more specific and focused. The need for assistance in the area of language and writing already may have been identified as part of the referral for special services or in a previous IEP. Interviews and discussions extend the examiners' understanding of how a student's written language abilities and needs relate to his or her overall language processing skills, the curricular demands of the classroom, and the student's perception of self.

Interviews should be structured and conducted in ways that encourage parents, students, and others to express their own words and concepts, while addressing the goals of the assessment team to cover certain topics (Nelson, 1998; Westby, 1990). Conversations with the referring educator can be conducted in a variety of contexts. In extended conversations, examiners may probe responses for examples and more detail. Although face-to-face and extended conversations have advantages, even a brief telephone conversation or the completion of a written questionnaire can be informative. In cases of an established team, a group that includes parents, the student, and other educators meets face to face and responds to each other's questions and observations about various aspects of the student's language and communication development.

What are your primary concerns about the student's development?

What are the student's strengths?

What are your observations about:
- What is most likely to help the student improve?

- What have you tried that didn't work as well as you would like?

- What have you tried that seems to hold promise for helping the student improve?

If you could change just one thing for this student, what would that be?

Figure 14.1. Parent–teacher questionnaire about general concerns.

The written interview or questionnaire serves as another tool for gathering information. Although generally less desirable than face-to-face conversations, such written responses have the advantage of describing problems and strengths in the original words of the participants and remain available over time. Written interviews also may overcome some of the time-constraint problems of collaborating across disciplines in that teachers may fill out forms even when they do not have time to meet. In addition, students may respond more frankly on written self-evaluation forms that include questions such as

1. What do you like most about writing?

2. What do you not like about writing?

3. What have you learned so far about writing?

4. What do you want to learn next?

Interview forms may be personalized to meet the needs of a particular assessment (Graves, 1983; Singer & Bashir, 1999b). Figures 14.1 and 14.2 offer written interview formats for gathering information regarding general or specific language concerns. Figure 14.3 is a self-assessment tool for students in the early stages of their writing lab experience.

Matching Assessment Purposes and Tools

Just as the purposes for assessing writing are varied, so too are the available assessment tools and strategies. Each method of testing brings specific benefits and limitations. For instance, an assessment tool that works well for determining eligibility may not be the

1. Describe your child's/the student's strengths and needs in reading and writing for the areas below:

   a. Reports and stories

      • How well does your child/the student understand longer texts?

      • How well does your child/the student organize and write stories and reports?

   b. Sentences

      • How well can your child/the student understand complex sentences?

      • How well can your child/the student construct written sentences?

   c. Words

      • How well can your child/the student read words?

      • How well does your child/the student spell words?

      • How well does your child/the student understand words in the general education curriculum?

      • How well does your child/the student use words in writing stories and reports?

2. Describe your child's/the student's strengths and needs in the area of social interaction:

3. What are your observations about:

      • What is most likely to help your child/the student improve?

      • What have you tried that didn't work as well as you would like?

      • What have you tried that seems to hold promise for helping your child/the student improve?

4. What does your child/the student value in writing?

5. If you could change just one thing for your child/the student in the area of reading and writing development, what would it be?

The Writing Lab Approach to Language Instruction and Intervention, by Nickola Wolf Nelson, Christine M. Bahr, and Adelia M. Van Meter
Copyright © 2004 Paul H. Brookes Publishing Co., Inc. All rights reserved.

Figure 14.2. Parent–teacher questionnaire about literacy concerns.

	A lot 😊	Sometimes 😐	Never ☹
I like writing stories.			
I like writing reports.			
I like talking to friends about my writing in author group.			
I like reading my work in author's chair.			
I like planning my writing.			
I like to revise my story and report after I write the first draft.			
I like people helping me while I am writing.			
I like using the computer to write.			
I like drawing with the computer or using it to illustrate my work.			

Figure 14.3. Student questionnaire.

best measure for evaluating change over time. Therefore, educators must determine which method of measurement will best meet the specific goals of assessment. In the following section, we discuss types of tests across three dimensions:

1. Test content—aspects of written language that are measured with various tools and approaches

2. Sampling methods—tasks that are used to sample written and spoken language skills

3. Scoring methods—techniques that are used to evaluate written language samples

As with all discussions of testing, the psychometric issues of validity and reliability of measurements require consideration. Validity refers to whether an assessment tool measures what it purports to measure. This relative concept is based on the question "Valid for what purpose?" One must ask, therefore, "Is this test valid for the purpose I am addressing?" Reliability refers to whether the results of an assessment would be consistent if administered and/or scored by the same person at different times (intrajudge reliability), by two different examiners (interjudge reliability), or at two points relatively close in time (test–retest reliability).

Table 14.1. Formal tests that measure written language development

Test	Publisher	Normative range	Scoring method	Primary areas assessed	Writing sample
Boder Test of Reading-Spelling Patterns (Boder & Jarrico, 1982)	The Psychological Corporation	Kindergarten through Grade 12	Reading grade level and quotient based on single word reading. Percentages are reported for known words spelled correctly and unknown words spelled as good phonetic equivalents (g.f.e.).	Reading single words Spelling single words	Single word spelling lists constructed from reading sample
Oral Written Language Scales (OWLS) (Carrow-Woolfolk, 1996)	American Guidance Service	5–21 years	Some items are multiple choice. Others are scored using item-specific rubrics. Standard scores may be compared with related scores on scales for Oral Expression and Listening Comprehension.	Conventions: letter formation, spelling, capitalization, punctuation Linguistics: modifiers, phrases, question forms, verb forms, complex sentences Content: details, coherence, supporting ideas, word choice	Single items requiring written responses Writing sentences to dictation Story retelling Brief samples written to questions and other prompts
Test of Adolescent & Adult Language–3rd ed. (TOAL–3) (Hammill, Brown, Larsen, & Wiederholt, 1994)	PRO-ED	12 years through 24 years, 11 months	Examples of correct and incorrect responses are given for each item. Raw scores are converted to scaled scores, composite quotients, and percentiles.	Writing/vocabulary Writing/grammar Other subtests measure listening, speaking, and reading.	Ability to use given vocabulary words in sentences Ability to combine two given sentences into one
Test of Early Written Language–2nd ed. (TEWL–2) (Hresko, Herron, & Peak, 1996)	PRO-ED	3 years to 10 years, 11 months	Basic writing subtest criteria are provided for scoring mechanical aspects of writing. Contextual writing samples are scored according to 14 criteria. The two subtests are combined to yield a Global Writing Quotient.	Mechanical aspects: drawing, writing vocabulary, spelling, punctuation, sentence combining, sentence logic Contextual aspects: theme, plot sequence, descriptive details, characters, dialogue, elaboration beyond the picture, spelling, and sentence structure	Basic writing uses individual items. Contextual writing is done to picture prompts (one for younger; one for older).

Test	Publisher	Ages/Grades	Scoring	Areas Assessed	Format
Test of Phonological Awareness (TOPA) (Torgesen & Bryant, 1994)	PRO-ED	Kindergarten version for last half of kindergarten year; Early elementary version for first- through second grades	Not a writing test per se, but a test to measure phonological awareness skills underlying reading and spelling; Items are scored as correct or incorrect; Test takes approximately 10 minutes; Raw scores are converted to percentiles and other standard scores	Phonological awareness	Students mark a picture-based answer in response to items presented orally by examiner.
Test of Written Expression (TOWE) (McGhee, Bryant, Larsen, & Rivera, 1995)	PRO-ED	Ages 6 years, 6 months through 14 years, 11 months	Two parts: Individual items are scored as correct or incorrect; Writing sample is scored on the inclusion of targeted items.	Writing conventions: alphabet-letter writing skill, capitalization, and punctuation. Language elements: ideation, semantics, and syntax. Spelling. Discourse elements: length, presence of paragraphs, plot sequence, descriptive details, spelling, grammatical accuracy	Essay written in response to a story starter (administered to students age 8 years and older).
Test of Written Language—3rd ed. (TOWL–3) (Hammill & Larsen, 1996)	PRO-ED	7 years to 17 years, 11 months	Quantitative measures of features	Vocabulary; Style; Syntax; Thematic maturity	Contrived subtests; Writing sample generated to picture prompt
Writing Process Test (WPT) (Worden & Hutchenson, 1992)	Riverside	Grades 2–12	Analytic scales	Development: purpose, audience, vocabulary, style/tone, support/development, organization/cohesion. Fluency: sentence, variety, grammar/usage, capitalization, punctuation, spelling	Writing sample generated to story starter prompt

FORMAL ASSESSMENT

For purposes of this discussion, we define formal tests as published assessment tools that are more or less structured and that provide normative or criterion-referenced data for comparison purposes. This information may be represented as a single score or as a series of subscores related to specific writing components or skills. Formal tests provide a means for comparing a student's performance with a larger group of students or a predetermined criterion. This type of measurement often provides a basis for decisions of eligibility for services. Caution, however, should be applied in interpreting results when evaluating students from diverse populations, whose peers may not be appropriately represented in normative populations or whose experiences do not match those sampled by the test. Problems also occur in that there is a "fine line between 'normal' and 'disordered' in writing," with the result that "writing difficulties are a matter of degree rather than outright difference" (Scott, 1999, p. 225).

Formal tests, by their nature, contain fixed content and are administered using prescribed methods. Some can be administered to large groups of students simultaneously, whereas others are designed for individual use only. Writing may be one area sampled in subtests of a more comprehensive language evaluation, or it may stand on its own as the focus of a test that looks at multiple components of writing. The tests summarized in Table 14.1 all are commercially available. In the current climate of national focus on writing proficiency, however, many local school districts and state departments of education have developed their own curriculum-based tests and other writing assessments to meet the purposes desired by their respective constituents.

Formal Assessment Purposes and Tools

A significant investment of time and energy is required for the administration, scoring, and interpretation of formal tests. A significant investment of student time also is involved in taking a formal test. Comprehensive formal tests seem best suited to determining how well a student is performing in structured writing tasks as compared with peers. Two questions that may be best answered with formal tests are 1) Does the student have difficulty writing in relation to same-age peers in a normative sample? and 2) Is the student eligible for special education services?

Pros and Cons of Formal Content and Sampling Methods

Formal assessments of written language vary in their choice of skills to assess. "No single test assesses comprehensively all aspects of written language achievement" (Bailet, 2001, p. 221). In a standardized assessment, however, content is fixed. To review a particular test, educators need to ask if the content evaluated is relevant to the purpose of the test and to the team's purpose in evaluating the student. Some tests are comprehensive and provide a means of measuring multiple skills or components that contribute to overall success in writing. Skills traditionally represented in such formal tests include grammar and usage, spelling, vocabulary, and mechanics. When efforts are made to view writing on a discourse level as well, components include theme, focus, organization, and style. Tests that examine component skills provide a way to identify general patterns of skill strengths and needs. Areas of need then may be probed more deeply using measures that focus on a specific area, such as understanding and using story grammar or spelling.

Although standardized testing results have the advantage that they can be compared with normative data, they also have disadvantages due to the limitations of contrived writing tasks. For example, some contrived tasks ask students to make multiple-choice judgments about spelling, word usage, or mechanics. Another contrived testing strategy requires students to demonstrate knowledge of component skills by writing corrected or modified versions of given texts. One of the problems of such approaches is that making decisions about correctness by choosing a best response or rewriting a word or sentence may be better described as testing editing skills rather than as assessing individual writing skills. Validity, therefore, might be called into question when the writing samples being assessed are derived from decontextualized language content and situations.

On the positive side, even though decontextualized tasks lack an authentic writing purpose, some have the positive benefit of challenging students to use skills they might not try in a more spontaneous sample. The results of such tasks also might make it possible to compare a student's knowledge and use of a particular skill to normative data. On the negative side, the contrived nature of these tests does not contribute to an understanding of a student's ability to use component skills in an integrated manner. To observe integrated skills, the sampling method must involve having the student generate his or her own story or report, which is, after all, the end goal of the writing process.

Some formal tests do include a self-generated writing sample. Generally, the writing samples are written in response to a picture or story prompt. These tests respond to a desire among educators to measure written language skill in a more spontaneous but still controlled, writing context. Some of these tests (e.g., the Writing Process Test; Worden & Hutchison, 1992) provide opportunities to evaluate writing processes (including planning, drafting, revising, and editing) as well as written products. On these tests, the quality of formal test writing samples may be compared with samples produced by same age- or grade-level peers. A task that appears on the surface to be the same for all children, however, may actually differ considerably for individual children relative to their personal experiences and preferences. When interpreting the results of such tests, therefore, it is helpful to keep in mind that students may have differential responses to writing prompts depending on cultural differences and other factors.

Pros and Cons of Varied Scoring Methods

Information about a written product can be derived from several scoring methods. Formal assessments that evaluate students' self-generated stories typically are scored using one or a combination of the following scoring methods: 1) holistic, 2) trait or analytic scale scoring using rubrics, and 3) quantitative measures of specific writing features.

Holistic Scoring

Holistic scoring refers to global assessment of written products. The term *holistic* has evolved to encompass a variety of rating strategies. In its simplest form, holistic scoring refers to a guided procedure for ranking stories written on the same topic in relationship to other stories in a pool or group. Scores typically are assigned based on an initial impression a story makes as a whole (Cooper & Odell, 1977). In some cases, the samples are scored on a fixed scale with a predetermined range of points. In other cases, trained reviewers develop a scoring system by ranking example papers to define a customized set of standards. In forming holistic judgments, readers may use a list of features as a general guide, but they are not required to count or tally occurrences of features.

Holistic scoring offers a quick method for assessing a large group of papers. It is limited in that it provides only a single scale value comparing one student's performance with a target group (e.g., to all other same grade-level students in a school district or state). No specific information for development of individual goals and objectives can be gleaned from this method of assessment. Holistic scoring methods serve primarily for evaluating the effectiveness of an educational system or curriculum and whether individual students are meeting curricular expectations as a whole. They also may serve as a screening device for identifying students who need more comprehensive assessments.

Analytic or Trait Scoring Using Rubrics

Analytic or trait scoring modifies the single holistic scoring scheme by focusing on a set of dimensions or features that are rated on a series of scales with a set of "rubrics" defining skills at each ranking. "Rubrics are sets of rules or benchmarks describing different levels of performance" (Westby & Clauser, 1999, p. 265). Rubrics might correspond to components of the curriculum (e.g., paragraph use, subject–verb agreement, punctuation). In such cases, they identify profiles of student strengths and needs as a means of evaluating individual and group change. The results may or may not contribute readily to the development of specific individual objectives. Whether they do depends on the number of features measured and the depth of evaluation at each level assessed by the measurement tool. Alternatively, rubrics might be organized as developmentally sequenced hierarchies. Westby and Clauser (1999) provided developmentally organized rubrics for rating qualities of several discourse genres, including narratives, expository, and persuasive discourse.

Quantitative Measures of Specific Writing Features

Measures that quantify specific writing components (e.g., counts of punctuation elements used correctly, numbers of words spelled correctly) provide the basis for scoring some formal tests. Writing samples taken from the same story prompt might be evaluated based on quantitative measures of specific features of writing. These measures might be normed according to age or grade level and used as indices of a student's writing skill for specific writing elements, such as vocabulary, grammar, and mechanics or as a total combined score. Such assessment tools can provide information related to a student's performance level compared with peers and can lead to the construction of a profile of strengths and needs, possibly contributing also to planning individual goals. Chapter 15 suggests methods for combining quantitative and analytic trait scoring techniques to evaluate writing samples gathered with informal assessment procedures.

Summary of Scoring Methods

In summary, formal assessment can lead educators to appropriate goal areas for students, but they often lack sufficient detail about spontaneous written language capabilities to establish individual performance baselines and specific intervention objectives. More in-depth assessment of one or more specific components using informal measures may be needed to assess patterns of use sufficient for meeting such purposes.

INFORMAL ASSESSMENT

Students reveal something of themselves as people and as developing authors in the stories and articles they write. In both their written work and their reflections on their work, students share their insights, personal experiences, creativity, organizational schemas, and linguistic sophistication. A wealth of information about a student's language and writing skills can be garnered from analysis of an original written language sample. Informal assessment offers an opportunity to look at student performance as both process and product within the context of authentic writing experiences. Goals and objectives derived from such assessments connect to the real writing expectations of classrooms. In addition, change can be tracked by using the same task and procedures at intervals over time. Observations may be comprehensive in nature or focused more selectively on a few specific features.

For some assessment purposes, informal assessment can replace or extend the information gathered through formal testing. On-line observation of a student in the process of writing a story or report, followed by analysis of the completed product, can provide in-depth information about the student's writing processes as well as his or her language skills. A profile of individual strengths and needs can be derived from information related to language skill at different levels of processing (e.g., phoneme level, word level, sentence level, discourse level). In addition, analysis of a student's work provides solid quantitative and qualitative baseline data that serve as a foundation for writing individualized objectives, determining effective instructional strategies, and measuring change over time.

Informal assessment has the added benefit that it is not dependent on a specific story starter or picture stimulus. Assessment procedures can be adapted to any genre. In this way, assessment truly focuses on an authentic writing experience that the student controls from the start by generating an original topic. Informal tasks do not provide scores that can be compared with normative data as formal tests do. They are, therefore, better suited to planning purposes or for documenting progress than for establishing eligibility for services.

Samples of a student's written language do not have to be gathered in specialized contexts in order to provide informal assessment information for goals and objectives. In natural school contexts, students produce written pieces that can be evaluated for multiple purposes. Educators, however, need to plan ahead when using curriculum-based samples for multiple purposes so they observe systematically the students' use of writing processes in addition to analyzing written products.

Portfolio Samples

Portfolio assessment has gained popularity in many schools as a way to demonstrate growth in writing over time. Typically, students reflect on their written products with assistance from teachers and choose their best samples to make a portfolio collection (e.g., Graves, 1991). Examiners can analyze these samples for signs of development in comparison with a local normative group, avoiding issues of cultural-linguistic bias and other constraints often associated with formal testing.

Although preexisting pieces provide one source of material that can be analyzed for written language skills, conditions for writing the story or article may vary according to instructions and stimuli provided. Therefore, it is important to know the context under which samples were produced. This information can be used to plan repeated measures under similar conditions to facilitate assessment of change over time. The advantage of the portfolio strategy is that it reduces the need to create special writing events solely for the purpose of assessment. The disadvantage is that opportunity for observing writing *processes* may be sacrificed if not documented at the time of writing.

When collecting portfolio pieces, it is useful to save finished published pieces with their drafts (dated) in order to preserve a history of the student's planning, drafting, revising, and editing. The inclusion of any worksheets helps to document the quality of the student's independent work and the nature of peer and educator scaffolding. Such evidence provides a concrete means for students and educators to reflect on development in the use of writing processes and language.

Writing Sample Probes

An assessment strategy we often use is to collect brief but complete handwritten samples or probes at various intervals of time. We collect these using similar instructions for each probe but encourage students to generate original topics for each sample. The probe samples are used to determine a student's baseline skill and longitudinal change in independent, unscaffolded writing opportunities. General instructions for gathering a sample are

- You can print or use cursive.

- You have about an hour to plan and organize, draft, revise, and edit. Use the plain sheet of paper to do your planning and the lined paper to draft. It is a good idea to skip every other line.

- We're giving you a pen to use because we want to see the changes you make. Making revisions and edits is part of being an author.

- Spell the best that you can.

- At the end, you will read your story to an adult, and we can write in any words that are too hard to spell.

The time needed for gathering a sample will vary. It has been our experience that 45–60 minutes is satisfactory for most students to complete their baseline stories. Younger students may require less time; older students, more. As students across grade levels build endurance for writing and become more comfortable with the processes and more language proficient, they ask for more time to develop their ideas. Consequently, teachers generally find that students early in the school year utilize less time for this activity than later in the year. Individual students in a class also vary in the length of time needed to complete a sample. For students who finish early, evaluators can plan quiet activities related to the writing process, such as illustrating or starting a second written piece. These activities help maintain a distraction-free environment, as well as encourage students to use the time available. This prevents a tendency for students to adopt the "get it over with quick" strategy in order to participate in a more appealing activity, as permitted by complete free choice.

Directions for collecting the writing sample should include cues that *encourage* students to use all stages of the writing process without *requiring* them to do so. The objective is to see whether children have enough knowledge and control to use such processes as planning, organizing, drafting, revising, and editing without direct scaffolding. Writing processes such as revisions can be observed more easily if students use pens rather than pencils. If computers are available, however, the task could be adapted to word processing with close observation of the processes a student uses to plan, compose, and revise. It is often necessary to clarify that printing is acceptable when gathering handwritten samples as students frequently interpret a request to "write" as a request to use cursive writing.

Some students have strong emotions tied to the use of conventional spelling or clean copies. We encourage such students by conveying that these samples are first drafts only and that we expect that they will contain imperfect spelling and revisions. Some students feel more in control of the process if they can communicate to teachers and others that they know when a word is not spelled correctly, despite not knowing the conventional spelling. For this purpose, teachers may want to remind students that on their drafts they can use editing marks, such as circling a word and marking it with the code "sp."

For some students, encouragement is not enough. Emotions are part of what the student brings to the writing process and should be considered important baseline information. An individual objective for a student who resists using words that he or she cannot spell might be for the student to take more risks in word choice during the drafting stage. Because the goal of informal assessment is to understand what the student does as a writer at a particular point in time, we advocate flexibility in implementing the general instructions. When students are distraught over misspellings, they can be reminded that teachers will write in any spellings that are needed when the students read their completed stories to adults at the end of the session. When this reassurance is not enough and the student cannot proceed without support, we give the needed support and document this baseline need. When students avoid the use of pens because of their need for clean drafts, we allow pencil and erasures and try to note revisions. Such modifications represent the balance and dynamic principles in practice. That is, based on values for establishing a climate of respect and trust, we apply dynamic decision-making to balance the desire to get a sample of independent writing with respect for this student's need for greater scaffolding supports to produce a sample at all.

Some students' original handwritten work may be difficult to read due to poor spelling and penmanship. When several adults are available, we follow a procedure in which students read their finished drafts to an adult prior to turning them in for analysis. At this point, instructors may jot down notes to clarify students' spelling, penmanship, and communicative intent. Often, students will identify missing or extra words during this activity. When this occurs, the student's skill of noticing opportunities for revising and editing while reading work aloud can be noted on the draft.

Prompts for Narrative Probes

Researchers and educators have proposed many methods for eliciting written narrative samples, including 1) story retelling, 2) verbal story starters, 3) picture prompts, 4) a combination story starters and picture prompts, and 5) students generating their own topics. Consistent with the ownership principle—and because generating topics is a significant part of what authors do—we recommend allowing students to formulate their own story ideas as part of the process. It is possible, however, to issue directions for the probe in a manner that is more likely to elicit true narrative discourse than isolated descriptions or sequence stories. For example, the following prompt serves as a means of encouraging students to produce a story with narrative structure without influencing the content too specifically. The wording of this prompt was not arrived at casually:

- We are interested in the stories students write.
- Your story should tell about a problem and what happens.
- Your characters and your story can be real or imaginary.

This prompt has been honed over several years of experience gathering probes across grade levels from first through eighth grade. In particular, asking students to tell a story about characters who have a problem and what happened is most likely to draw forth a goal-oriented narrative with full story grammar structure if the student is capable of producing one.

Prompts for Other Genres

Instructions for gathering samples of expository text must be constructed to guide students to think about the key features of the requested genre and subgenre. Expository discourse provides information. In writing a report, therefore, a student might be asked to consider what is interesting about a topic and relate the main idea and supporting details. A prompt we have used for gathering such a sample is

- Think about a topic that's interesting to you.
- Plan a report on your topic, and write about it.

In a compare/contrast article, students might be asked to plan and organize ideas that relate to ways related topics are the same and different, then draft their paper. Educators might prompt a specific whole text organization (e.g., "Write a report with a beginning, middle, and end") or paragraph organization (e.g., "Include a topic sentence and three supporting details") that parallel classroom teaching and grade expectations.

SUMMARY

This chapter has focused on the multiple purposes for assessment. We have reviewed formal and informal assessment strategies, discussing the pros and cons of each, and have provided directions that we generally use for our own work when gathering writing sample probes. The samples might be gathered for a whole class, but only samples for certain target students might be subjected to complete analysis. Chapter 15 extends this discussion by presenting the analysis framework and methods of measurement that can be applied to portfolio samples or to probes elicited for the purpose of assessing abilities and skills and establishing instructional objectives at repeated points over time. Chapter 16 describes methods for preparing goals, objectives, and benchmarks based on the assessments and observation data. Chapter 17 provides evidence of change for one group of third-grade students who completed such writing probes at three points across a school year.

Written Language Sample Analysis

15

As noted in Chapter 14, written language samples produced in classroom contexts provide one of the best ways for measuring students' knowledge and skills. The literature on writing contains numerous suggestions for analyzing such samples (Isaacson, 1991; Mather & Roberts, 1995; Westby & Clauser, 1999). This chapter describes procedures we recommend to yield a comprehensive profile of a student's strengths and needs in the areas of writing processes, written products, and spoken language abilities. Alternatively, a more focused analysis can be conducted using selected procedures to fit individual needs that have been identified through interviews and related to classroom instruction. In other words, the assessment procedure is designed to be a flexible framework that professionals can modify for their own purposes.

To build an understanding of how to use these procedures and to illustrate their application, we introduce Arreyona. Arreyona was a third-grade student in a classroom that was part of a collaborative inclusive computer-supported writing lab that met 3 days per week. Arreyona's general education teacher expressed concern that although some of Arreyona's written work reflected grade-level expectations, she was difficult to motivate to write, had difficulty completing written tasks, and was easily distracted.

The sample of Arreyona's writing found in Figure 15.1 was gathered mid-year for documenting mid-term outcomes and individualizing language goals. The story prompt and procedures described in Chapter 14 were used to gather the sample. At several points in this chapter, we return to Arreyona's written sample story to demonstrate how the assessment methods presented in this chapter are used to analyze and to interpret written language skills.

My Cosin Briceson still had
his baby ~~teet~~ teeth
when he was six years old.
~~they~~ He always acks
~~to~~ his mother was his
~~teeth~~ toeth ~~lose~~ loes.
His sister ~~Asia~~ allways
~~laft~~ at ~~him~~ him.
One day his toeth came
out anther One came
out and antherOne
came out three of
    them came out he was
so happy.

Figure 15.1.   Arreyona's story.

My sister laft ~~at I~~
at ~~the~~ him ~~too~~ too
I did not laf at
him becase if his teeth
did not come out
~~I~~ evry body would
call him ~~I~~ a baby
and he is ~~I~~ seven
he know how to count
by 25 and tiye is shoes
we are best cosins
I love my ~~cos~~ cosin

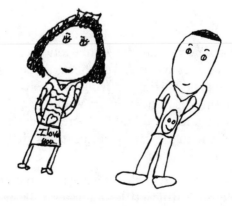

ANALYSIS FRAMEWORK

We devised the Writing Process and Product Worksheet to serve as an assessment tool for summarizing data regarding a student's written and spoken language skills as demonstrated through a writing sample. A blank, photocopiable worksheet appears in the appendix to the chapter along with its companion, the Writing Assessment Summary and Objectives Worksheet. Both writing and reading assessment tools are discussed in Nelson and Van Meter (2002), and downloadable versions of both forms are available on http://www.wmich.edu/wlop and http://www.brookespublishing.com/WLA. The Writing Assessment Summary and Objectives Worksheet is organized to guide examiners to gather information in three primary areas: 1) writing processes (planning and organizing, drafting, and revising and editing); 2) language levels related to written products (discourse, sentence, word, and conventions); and 3) spoken language skills (as observed in formal presentations and within the interpersonal spoken activities of the writing lab). Within each section of the worksheet, process and product features can be described using both quantitative measures and qualitative descriptions. A rubric at the bottom of the worksheet provides a simple means for documenting a student's overall level of independence with a particular skill: a plus sign (+) indicates a feature that is clearly evident and independent; a tilde (~) indicates a feature that is partially evident and still needs scaffolding; and a minus sign (–) indicates a feature that has not yet emerged. A blank indicates that a feature was not specifically observed. Figure 15.2 provides an example of this worksheet completed for Arreyona's writing sample.

The Writing Assessment Summary and Objectives Worksheet provides an organizing framework to integrate results of assessment to describing a student's writing profile and determining objectives that will guide instruction. In parallel to the worksheet, the summary sheet allows examiners to summarize information and establish objectives in the three areas: 1) writing processes, 2) language levels, and 3) spoken language skills. Figure 15.3 provides an example of this worksheet completed for Arreyona's writing sample.

ASSESSING WRITING PROCESSES

On-line observation of the student's use of writing process strategies (or lack thereof) can identify strengths and needs that may not be reflected in written end products. Observations of writing processes are guided by the organizing question: Does the student use the stages of planning, organizing, drafting, and revising and editing in a recursive manner while constructing his or her written work?

Responses to this question will build a better understanding of how the student approaches the task of writing. Additional questions that emerge from this focused observation might include

- What type of planning does this student use (e.g., mapping ideas, making an outline, drawing a picture, writing a title and notes, talking aloud, reflecting for a few minutes)?

- What type of support does the student need to successfully complete the drafting process (e.g., spelling, idea generation, grammatical formulation, audience feedback)?

Writing Process and Product Worksheet

Student name _Arreyona_   Teacher _Mrs. W_   School _WE_   Grade _3rd_   Birth date _October 5_   Age _8:3_

Date of sample _January 4_   Sampling activity _Midyear narrative probe 2_   Observer _AVM_

Assessing writing processes

Planning and organizing
~ Approaches writing tasks willingly
~ Arrives at topic independently
+ Picture—after drafting
— Graphic organizer Type
— Notes
— Dictates

Drafting
— Refers to planning
+ Proceeds quickly from start to finish
+ Pauses periodically
+ Revises along the way—changes spelling and word choice
— Dependent on others for spelling

+ Rereads work
+ Adds information*
— Rewords ideas
— Clarifies references
— Reorganizes content
*extended story with more intro.

Revising and editing
— Corrects grammar
~ Corrects spelling
— Corrects punctuation
— # edits

Assessing written products

Discourse Level

Fluency
<u>102</u> Total # words
— # words/T-unit

Structural Organization
+ True to genre: _narrative_
Maturity level:
Abbreviated episode

Cohesion
+ Clarity within sentences
~ Clarity across text—_repeats idea_
+ Pronoun reference cohesion
~ Verb tense cohesion

Sense of Audience
— Title ~ End
+ Creative and original
+ Relevant information
~ Adequate information
— Dialogue/ Other literary devices

Sentence Level

T-units
<u>14</u> Total # T-units
<u>7.3</u> # words/T-unit
— Range of T-unit length

Types of Sentences
— # Simple incorrect
— # Simple correct
— # Complex incorrect
<u>3</u> # Complex correct
— # run-on clauses (after 2 coord.)

Variability
~ Varied sentence types
+ Overreliance on a particular construction
Attempting complex forms
Some difficulty with verb tense
Some dialectal forms

Word Level

Word Choice
— Mature and interesting choices
— Overreliance on particular words
— Usage errors
simple appropriate choices
Spelling Accuracy
— % incorrect

Spelling developmental stage
— Prephonetic
— Semiphonetic
— Phonetic
x Transitional
— Conventional

Examples:
allways/always
acks/asks
laft/laughed
becase/because
evrybody/everybody
tiye/tie
toeth/tooth
loes/loose

Conventions

Capitalization
+ Initial letter of sentence
— Titles — Proper nouns

End punctuation
~ Periods — Question marks
1st portion, challenges marked, then less consistent

Commas
— Divide series — Divide clauses

Apostrophes
— Contractions — Possessives

Quotation marks
— Direct quotes

Formatting
— Paragraphs
— Poetry/other

Assessing spoken language in writing process contexts

Listening and comprehension
+ Makes eye contact with speaker
~ Listens without interrupting
~ Seeks clarification when needed
+ Follows directions

Manner
+ Articulates clearly
+ Speaks fluently
+ Uses natural prosody
+ Appropriate eye gaze
+ Appropriate loudness

Topic maintenance
+ Situationally appropriate
+ Provides adequate information
+ Asks relevant questions
+ Shares opinions
~ Reflects on own work and others'
+ Engages in conversational turn-taking

Linguistic skill
~ Organizes ideas adequately
+ Completes utterances
+ Uses specific vocabulary

Figure 15.2. Writing Process and Product Worksheet completed for Arreyona's story. Copyright © 2001, N.W. Nelson, A.M. Van Meter, and C.M. Bahr.

Writing Assessment Summary and Objectives Worksheet

Student _Arreyona_ Grade _3_ Teacher _Ms. W._

Assessment sample _Midyear probe_ Genre _Narrative_ Date _January 4_

Observations and impressions	Goals and objectives
Writing processes	
Planning and organizing No overt planning. Initially had difficulty generating an idea.	Brainstorm list of story ideas. Use graphic organizer to plan and organize story prior to writing.
Drafting	
Revising and editing Corrected spelling and word choice while drafting. Extended story at end. * Drew illustration at end.	Reread work when done with drafting to revise for amount and ordering of information. Use editing symbols to add, move, and delete information.
Written products	
Discourse level Wrote abbreviated episode. Ordering problems.	Write full episode by adding character planning and attempts to solve problem. Order ideas logically with minial scaffolding.
Sentence level Complex sentences present. Inconsistent verb agreement (some dialect).	Increase the number of complex sentence constructions with subject–verb agreement across sentences.
Word level Simple appropriate vocabulary present. No use of descriptors or colorful words. Phonetic to transitional stage of spelling.	Include three descriptive words in story. Use -ed morpheme consistently. Learn and apply rule for double letters. Independently use a spelling dictionary to support spelling.
Conventions Inconsistent use of end punctuation and initial letter capitalization. No paragraph formatting.	Identify and mark sentence boundaries independently.
Oral language	
Writing process oral contexts Inconsistent atention to speakers in author chair and peer conferencing.	Ask one question or make one relevent comment pertaining to peer work in author chair or peer conferencing activities.
Genre specific	

Figure 15.3. Writing Assessment Summary and Objectives Worksheet completed for Arreyona. Copyright © 2001, N.W. Nelson, A.M. Van Meter, and C.M. Bahr.

- Does the student reread his or her work, looking for opportunities to revise content as well as to edit for spelling and punctuation?

The writing process portion of the assessment worksheet provides a framework for documenting the results of direct observations and provides a small space for qualitative descriptions of the student's approach to the tasks of planning and organizing, drafting, and revising and editing. If asked, either during the process or at its completion, students often contribute insights about a strategy they used. For example, a sampling of some observations solicited from different students in one planning session included

- "I'm not writing anything down for planning because I have it organized in my head."

- "I don't like story maps because they are confusing. I like to just write notes."

- "I just told my story to the teacher so I don't need to write anything down."

- "My teacher makes us do story maps, so I guess that's okay."

Eliciting reflections such as these contribute to a better overall understanding of the student as a writer and learner and suggest areas to target in intervention.

In the area of planning and organizing, we observe the independent use of executive strategies that students show as they initiate the writing process. There is space to document the use of planning supports such as graphic organizers, dictation to a peer or teacher, or notes. When a student uses a graphic organizer, the observer includes information on the type, complexity, and organizing strategies present, such as numbering and using arrows to indicate sequence.

In the area of drafting, observers report whether students refer to their planning during drafting and how they proceed from start to finish. Students more dependent on others for spelling may request spelling support and pause to wait for it. A desirable behavior is for students to pause periodically to reflect while drafting and to reread and rework their stories along the way.

In the worksheet box for recording evidence of revising and editing processes, the left column is a checklist for revising, and the right column is a checklist for editing. To capture revising efforts, observers should note when students reread and rework their stories to add, clarify, or reorganize information. To capture editing, observers should record when students attempt to correct grammar, spelling, punctuation, and formatting. Although on-line observing is best for gaining a clear picture, evidence of revising and editing processes also can be gleaned from finished products. This is why we give students pens to write with and directions to cross out edits with a single line, rather than erasing or scribbling out revisions darkly. We also give students the option of circling any words they think they may have spelled incorrectly.

The Assessing Writing Processes section of Figure 15.2 reports that Arreyona needed scaffolding to approach written tasks. She initially used negative self-talk (e.g., "I don't want to write today. I can't think of anything to write about"). Then, she put her head down on the table and hid under her arms. After several minutes of not participating, she was approached by an instructor and persuaded to interact. She was encouraged to review a list of previously brainstormed story topics kept in her author's notebook. After warming up to the possibilities, Arreyona independently generated a story topic. She refused any formal planning but illustrated her story after she completed her writing. While drafting her story, Arreyona paused periodically and reread her work. She was eager to share her work with peers and adults in the room and extended her story by adding more information in response to listener enthusiasm and questions. She made twelve edits that included seven spelling changes, four word-choice changes, and a grammatical agreement change. She circled the word *lafts* and marked it "sp" to indicate her uncertainty about its spelling.

ASSESSING WRITTEN PRODUCTS

Educators and researchers have used several strategies for creating meaningful writing component categories (e.g., Isaacson, 1991; Mather & Roberts, 1995, Westby & Clauser, 1999). Consistent with our own goal of using writing as a context for building language skills, we propose a framework that encourages systematic evaluation of language skills at multiple levels. In Chapter 2, we describe a five-target framework for analyzing language at the discourse level, sentence level, word level, writing conventions level, and a level that targets spoken language interactions. In this chapter, we present tools and "how to" suggestions for assessing strengths and needs at each of these levels. Chapter 5 provides suggestions for related scaffolding techniques.

The assessment worksheet parallels this framework. Educators first observe and analyze a written sample at the whole discourse level, then gradually move to smaller language units. This approach balances looking at specific skills while maintaining a sense of the whole. Although each level of language processing can be viewed independently, it is important to look at ways the levels are interrelated. For instance, in order to write a story that relates ideas causally, a student needs to write complex sentences that contain words that link information causally (e.g., *because, if . . . then*). Therefore, assessment must move recursively between individual language levels or writing components and the story or article as a whole. The idea is to gain a balanced picture of significant details against the backdrop of the essence and effectiveness of the entire story.

Developmental Guidelines

Where available, developmental guidelines for interpreting data in relationship to peers for each of these five target areas appear in tables. Such developmental guidelines should be used with caution, however. Samples that have provided the data have been gathered under diverse conditions and not necessarily with recognition of diversity in culture, language, and dialect. In our own work, we have found that the same student can provide samples that vary widely from one day to the next depending on such factors as interest in a particular topic or situational motivation to do his or her best work. It is best to think of comparing a student's work with his or her own prior work, rather than against set developmental standards, but with the recognition that even this approach is flawed because of the day-to-day variability within students, particularly those with LLDs.

Gathering and Preparing Samples for Analysis

Samples of student work may be taken from a variety of classroom writing activities, which may be aimed at producing narratives, expository texts, or other genres. The goal is to observe a student's highest level of independent work in the intended genre. The assessment genre chosen by the collaborative team typically is based on general curricular objectives. If teachers have no clear preference, the narrative sampling procedure described in Chapter 14 works well. It also addresses the purpose of collecting a sample of independent written language skills for a class of students for whom comparisons can be made over time, and it does so without taking time out for "testing." Aspects and techniques of the probe may be modified to look at other genres and sub-genres of writing.

When students produce little or no text after the first 15–20 minutes, we implement dynamic assessment techniques (discussed in Chapter 5) to evaluate a student's language abilities with scaffolding support. This evaluation can yield information about whether the student's difficulty stems from problems generating topics to write about (as in Arreyona's case), or from a sentence- or word-level problem in generating written language. If the student has a sentence- or word-level problem, the examiner can scaffold him or her to generate the story orally, using dictation or the shared pen strategy to get the student started, but encouraging the student to write as much and as independently as possible. With students at higher levels of independence, dynamic assessment techniques can assist examiners to identify and confirm areas of strength to support change and to observe responsiveness to scaffolding in potential target areas. Information about the amount and type of scaffolding provided is documented on the transcript.

Although the probe activity is designed primarily as a curriculum-based assessment tool, we generally tell students that they will have an opportunity to share their work in author chair on a subsequent day. Students tend to be more motivated to do their best work with the promise of an audience that goes beyond the teacher.

Samples can be coded in several ways: 1) directly on a child's handwritten or computer printout sample for ease of time, 2) on photocopies in order to preserve originals (Figure 15.4), and 3) using computer analysis programs such as the *Systematic Analysis of Language Transcripts* (SALT; Miller & Chapman, 2000) (Figure 15.5). A computer analysis system takes more time initially because the story must be transcribed, but the trade-off may be worth the extra preparation time for some students because of the depth of information that can be coded, counted, and printed out. Using the conventions of SALT, each T-unit (a term defined and discussed later in this chapter) is given its own line, and bound morphemes are noted with a slash mark. Words are typed using correct spellings, with student spellings in brackets immediately following. This allows the software to count the number of different words accurately. The student's use of writing conventions is preserved in the transcription, although end punctuation must be added to each line to make SALT perform correctly. Missing morphemes are coded with a slash and an asterisk to indicate where they should have been. Additional analysis codes are placed in brackets and counted by the software program.

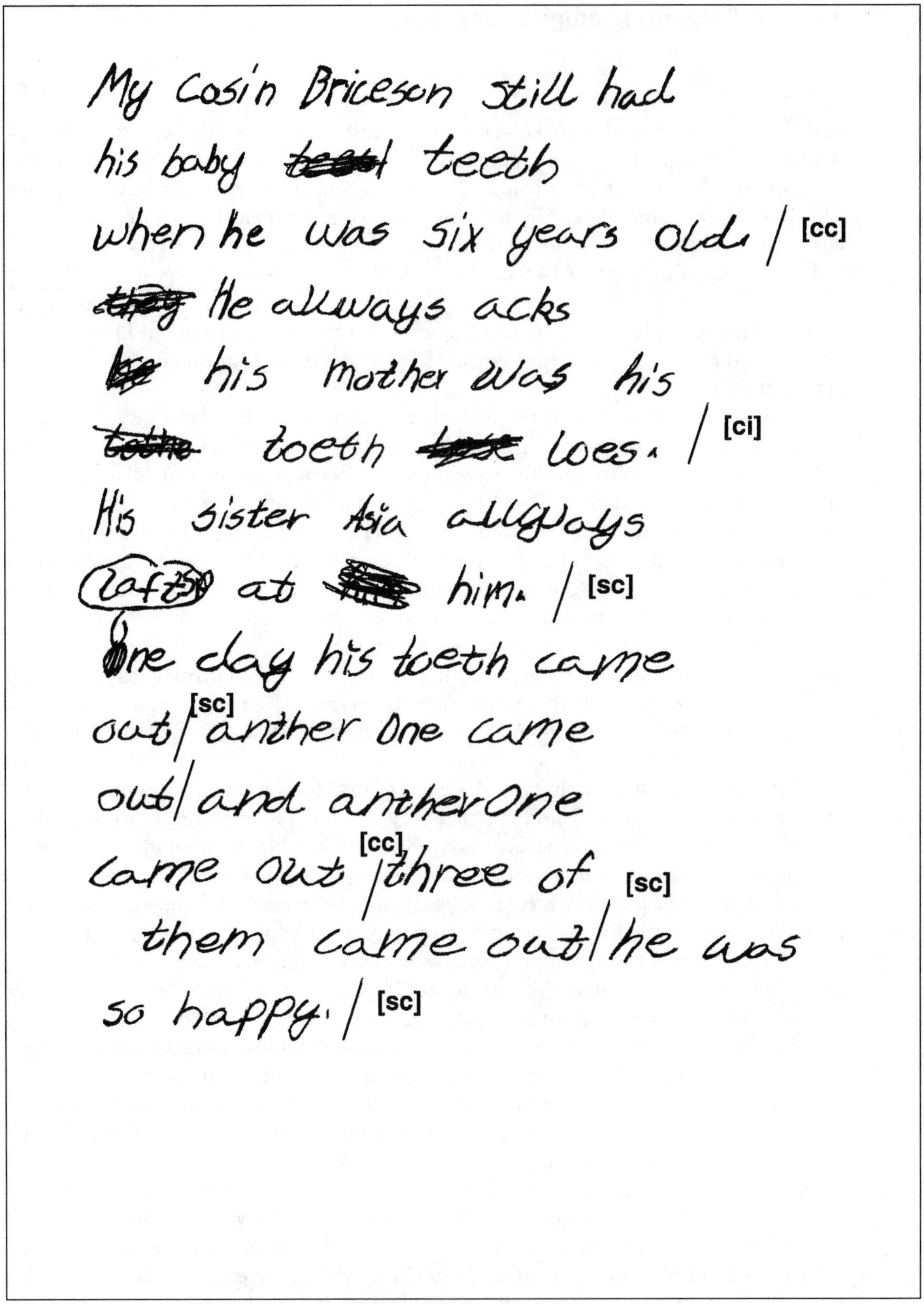

My Cosin Briceson still had
his baby ~~teeth~~ teeth
when he was six years old. / [cc]
~~they~~ He allways acks
~~his~~ his mother was his's
~~teeth~~ toeth ~~loes~~ loes. / [ci]
His sister Asia allways
(loft) at ~~this~~ him. / [sc]
One day his toeth came
out /[sc] anther One came
out / and anther One
came out /[cc] three of [sc]
them came out / he was
so happy. / [sc]

Figure 15.4. Arreyona's story coded for T-units and sentence codes (explained in Table 15.7).

My sister laft ~~at~~
at ~~he~~ him ~~too~~ too / [sc]
I did not laf at
him becase if his teeth
did not come out
~~I~~ evry body would
call him ~~a~~ a baby /
and he is ~~t~~ seven / [cc]
he know [d] how to count
by 25 and tiye is shoes / [ci]
we are best cosins / [sc]
I love my ~~cos~~ cosin / [sc]

Discourse-Level Analysis

Discourse-level analysis considers the global organization of the work and how the story or topic elements are combined to create a clear, logical, and interesting piece. Discourse-level assessment begins with observing how well a piece conveys meaning to the reader. Questions that guide the team's judgment of success at the discourse level might include

- Does this piece make sense?

- Is it interesting?

- Does it meet the writer's intended goals?

- Does it conform to the discourse genre solicited by the directions for the probe?

Subcomponents of assessment at the discourse level include several methods for analyzing discourse level skill related to the sample's 1) productivity and fluency,

```
$ Arreyona
+ Name: Arreyona
+ Gender: F
+ DOB:
+ DOE:
+ CA: 8;3
+ Context: narrative writing sample - 2nd probe
+ Examiner:
+ Transcriber: Anna Putnam
+ Grade: 3rd
+ edits: 17
+ word count: 102
- 0:00

A [pic].
A My cousin[sp]{cosin} Briceson still had his baby teeth when he was six year/s old [cc].
A He always[sp]{allways} ask/ed[sp]{acks} his mother was[d]{if} his tooth[sp]{toeth} {was}
   loose[sp]{loes} [ci].
A His sister Asia always[sp]{allways} laugh/ed[sp]{laft} at him [sc].
A One day his tooth[sp]{toeth} came out[p] [sc].
A another[sp]{anther} one came out.
A and another[sp]{anther} one came out[p] [cc].
A three of them came out[p] [sc].
A he was so happy [sc].
A My sister laugh/ed[sp]{laft} at him too[p] [sc].
A I did not laugh[sp]{laf} at him because[sp]{becuse} if his teeth did not come out every-
   body[sp]{evrybody} would[v] call him a baby[p].
A he is seven[p] [cc].
A he know/*3s [d] how to count by twos and tie[sp]{tiye} his[sp]{is} shoe/s[p] [ci].
A We are best cousin/s[sp]{cosins}[p] [sc].
A I love my cousin[sp]{cosin}[p] [sc].
```

Figure 15.5.   Coded SALT transcript.

2) discourse structure and maturity, 3) cohesion, and 4) sense of audience and voice. Some or all of the features may be analyzed depending on the focus of the assessment and how much time the examiner can devote to the analysis. Each area is represented on the assessment worksheet.

Productivity and Fluency

Many students initially have difficulty generating text. Such students may struggle to generate words and to compose simple sentences. Although longer does not necessarily translate into better, tracking individual productivity measures can capture a student's ease of generating text over time.

Productivity is a simple measure of text length that can be calculated in a couple of ways. One way is to tally the total number of words in a sample. A second way is to tally the total number of sentences or T-units (as described subsequently) in a sample. Productivity related to a unit of time, as in our 60-minute narrative probes, is considered a fluency measure (Scott & Windsor, 2000).

Fluency measures provide an easy way for quantifying growth, particularly in the early stages of writing development. Such measures can be compared with classroom, district, or state averages, and group data can be used to develop local norms for appropriate developmental levels in a particular community or school (see Chapter 17 for group data showing evidence of change for one group of third-grade students in an inner-city school). Scott and Windsor (2000) found that school-age students with LLDs produced written narrative summaries of a film they had watched that were 62% as long as their same-age peers and expository summaries that were only 49% as long. A review of the fluency elements of Arreyona's sample shows that she wrote a total of 102 words during the hour probe. Her words were presented in a total of 14 T-units.

Narrative Organization and Maturity Measures

As discussed in Chapter 2, text structure and organization within paragraphs and across paragraphs varies with the genre and subgenre of a work. Given the structural differences represented in the large variety of genres and subgenres, no single tool or even small set of tools can be used to measure overall development of any given genre. In this section, we discuss the structural and organization maturity measures for evaluating stories or narratives. This is consistent with our preference to use a narrative probe (as described in Chapter 14) to gather informal written language samples. Later in this section, we address other genres represented in writing curricula and offer suggestions for creating structural and organizational assessment tools that parallel classroom teaching and expected outcomes.

Developmental models are designed to describe the progression of developmental maturity in a particular genre. Frequently, referenced developmental models for narratives can be found in the works of Applebee (1978), who described centering and chaining; McCabe and her colleagues (McCabe & Peterson, 1991; McCabe & Rollins, 1994; Peterson & McCabe, 1983), who described high-point analysis based on Labov (1972); and Stein and Glenn (1979), who described story grammar analysis. Others who have interpreted these approaches and provided clinical tools for using them include Hedberg and Westby (1993) and Hughes, McGillivray, and Schmidek (1997).

In addition, as mentioned in Chapter 2, Bruner (1986) suggested that narratives differ in the degree to which they include a *landscape of consciousness*, or subjectivity, such that characters respond emotionally and reflect on the events of a story, as well as a *landscape of action*, essentially the plot, or the unevaluated events of the story. These elements appear in varying degrees in the analysis methods mentioned in the previous paragraph, but they deserve some consideration of their own. Beyond their use as language indicators, they may connect to the degree to which children and adolescents reflect on and bear responsibility for their own actions and decisions.

Kemper and Edwards wrote, "It is not until age 6 that children's narratives are causally coherent in that they consist of a causally connected sequence of actions, physical states, and mental states that explain the antecedents and consequences of characters' actions" (1986, p. 18). According to Sutton-Smith, by age 7 years, children generally tell stories with a plot, "that is, their stories have some beginning, some characters who have to deal with villainy or deprivation, who then seek to right the wrongs they suffer, and in due course resolve the issues at hand" (1986, p. 7). By the time most children reach 9 years, they are able to represent multiple characters' perceptions and feelings in the majority of their stories (Westby, 1994). In our own research (Nelson, Bahr, & Van Meter, 2002; Nelson, Van Meter, & Bahr, 2002), we have found that children as young as at the end of first grade can produce complete narratives, and some fifth graders who have not been taught story grammar elements may write isolated descriptions about themselves and their friends. Based on typical performance, however, it is reasonable to expect first- and second graders to produce at least temporal sequences, third graders to produce at least causal sequences, and fourth- and fifth graders to produce at least abbreviated episodes.

Each narrative analysis procedure has advantages for focusing the team on a particular aspect of development. The procedures also overlap considerably when one looks at them closely. We include a developmental progression table for each approach and recommend that teams select the approach (or modification/combination of approaches) that works best for their students. Our preference has been to apply the story grammar analysis approach adapted by Hedberg and Westby (1993) from Stein and Glenn (1979), but we often refer to one of the other approaches to capture the essence of a story. The chapter appendix includes examples that readers can use to check their impressions against ours. Although numerical scores can be assigned to any of these scales, their primary value is descriptive. By capturing elements of a student's organizational strengths and then asking, "What characteristic is missing that would take this student to the next higher level of maturity?" teams have information for establishing objectives and knowing where to begin to scaffold each student to a higher level of discourse maturity.

Centering and Chaining Analysis

Applebee (1978) characterized spoken story development from the ages of 2 to 6 years as six increasingly advanced narrative forms produced by combining the organizational strategies of centering and chaining. *Centering* refers to relating story elements around a central core feature, which could be a character or noncharacter element, such as an action or scene. *Chaining* refers to linking ideas in a temporal or logical way that connects ideas from one step to the next (see Figure 15.6). This model captures children's abilities to attribute their characters with more consistent features and motivations as they evolve into mature storytellers (Sutton-Smith, 1986). It also represents progress from organizing ideas around a central focus, to chaining ideas temporally, then causally. True narratives maintain a conceptual center in the form of a theme or moral that evolves across the story's sequence of events. This type of narrative maturity scale may be particularly helpful in describing early stages of narrative development, especially for children with more dramatic special needs.

High-Point Analysis

McCabe and her colleagues (McCabe & Peterson, 1991; McCabe & Rollins, 1994; Peterson & McCabe, 1983) used a slightly different approach to capture the developmental sequence for narratives. They described how *high-point narratives* differ from *chronological narratives*. In chronological narratives, which do not qualify as true narratives, children and adults of all ages simply string together an unevaluated sequence of actions, with no event selected for particular focus or detailed description. This differs from the classic high-point, or true, narrative which includes an event that is full of drama and accompanied by a concentrated set of evaluative comments. Table 15.1 provides examples of stories scored according to this model.

Considering how the various analysis models fit together is useful. For example, relative to story grammar analysis, the chronological narrative would be analyzed as an *action sequence*. A high point in a narrative can generally be traced to the presence of a problem, which leads the audience to be interested in the outcome—hence, our em-

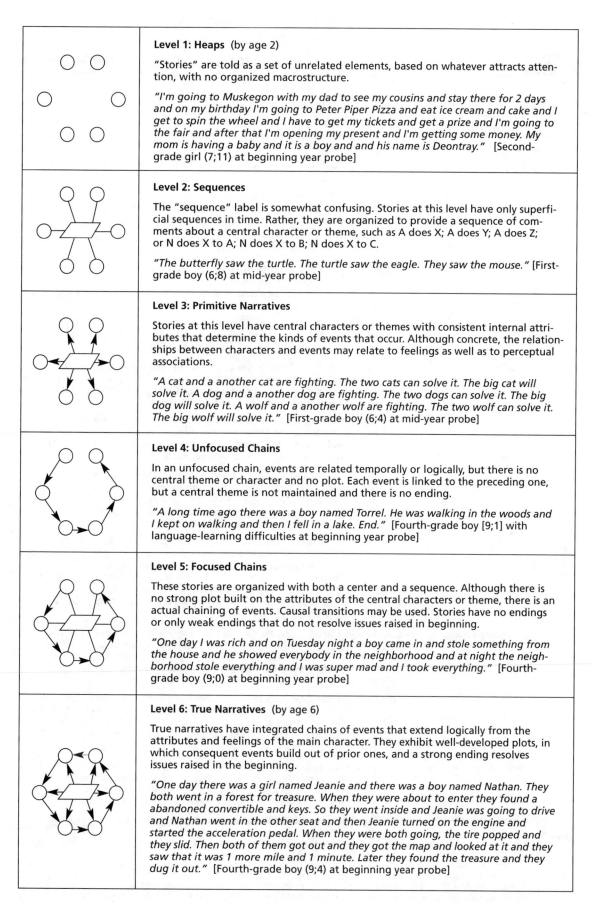

Level 1: Heaps (by age 2)

"Stories" are told as a set of unrelated elements, based on whatever attracts attention, with no organized macrostructure.

"I'm going to Muskegon with my dad to see my cousins and stay there for 2 days and on my birthday I'm going to Peter Piper Pizza and eat ice cream and cake and I get to spin the wheel and I have to get my tickets and get a prize and I'm going to the fair and after that I'm opening my present and I'm getting some money. My mom is having a baby and it is a boy and and his name is Deontray." [Second-grade girl (7;11) at beginning year probe]

Level 2: Sequences

The "sequence" label is somewhat confusing. Stories at this level have only superficial sequences in time. Rather, they are organized to provide a sequence of comments about a central character or theme, such as A does X; A does Y; A does Z; or N does X to A; N does X to B; N does X to C.

"The butterfly saw the turtle. The turtle saw the eagle. They saw the mouse." [First-grade boy (6;8) at mid-year probe]

Level 3: Primitive Narratives

Stories at this level have central characters or themes with consistent internal attributes that determine the kinds of events that occur. Although concrete, the relationships between characters and events may relate to feelings as well as to perceptual associations.

"A cat and a another cat are fighting. The two cats can solve it. The big cat will solve it. A dog and a another dog are fighting. The two dogs can solve it. The big dog will solve it. A wolf and a another wolf are fighting. The two wolf can solve it. The big wolf will solve it." [First-grade boy (6;4) at mid-year probe]

Level 4: Unfocused Chains

In an unfocused chain, events are related temporally or logically, but there is no central theme or character and no plot. Each event is linked to the preceding one, but a central theme is not maintained and there is no ending.

"A long time ago there was a boy named Torrel. He was walking in the woods and I kept on walking and then I fell in a lake. End." [Fourth-grade boy [9;1] with language-learning difficulties at beginning year probe]

Level 5: Focused Chains

These stories are organized with both a center and a sequence. Although there is no strong plot built on the attributes of the central characters or theme, there is an actual chaining of events. Causal transitions may be used. Stories have no endings or only weak endings that do not resolve issues raised in beginning.

"One day I was rich and on Tuesday night a boy came in and stole something from the house and he showed everybody in the neighborhood and at night the neighborhood stole everything and I was super mad and I took everything." [Fourth-grade boy (9;0) at beginning year probe]

Level 6: True Narratives (by age 6)

True narratives have integrated chains of events that extend logically from the attributes and feelings of the main character. They exhibit well-developed plots, in which consequent events build out of prior ones, and a strong ending resolves issues raised in the beginning.

"One day there was a girl named Jeanie and there was a boy named Nathan. They both went in a forest for treasure. When they were about to enter they found a abandoned convertible and keys. So they went inside and Jeanie was going to drive and Nathan went in the other seat and then Jeanie turned on the engine and started the acceleration pedal. When they were both going, the tire popped and they slid. Then both of them got out and they got the map and looked at it and they saw that it was 1 more mile and 1 minute. Later they found the treasure and they dug it out." [Fourth-grade boy (9;4) at beginning year probe]

Figure 15.6. Center and chaining model. (Adapted from Nelson and Friedman [1988]. ©1988 by N.W. Nelson. Shared by permission of the author. Based on descriptions by Applebee [1978], Botvin and Sutton-Smith [1977], and Westby [1984]. Spelling and punctuation of student writing samples have been corrected.)

Table 15.1.   High-point model of narrative development

One-event narrative	At about 22 months, children begin to refer to past events, with much adult scaffolding. By age 2, their narratives often concern negative past events, such as injuries.
	"Three bears went back home and ate food." [First-grade girl (6;2) at mid-year probe]
Two-event narrative	By age 3½, children's longest narratives consist of two events, and more than half of their conversational narratives concern real personal experiences.
	"I had to give away my cat to a pet shop. I had to give away my cat to my sister." [First-grade girl (6;10) at year-end probe]
Miscellaneous narrative	McCabe and Rollins (1994) inserted this category as a structure between 2-event and leap-frog narratives. They characterized it as one in which there are more than two past-tense events, but there is not yet a logical or causal sequence.
	"I was afraid to ride a dirt bike and dad teased. Me and my dad popped a wheelie and then I rode it." [Third-grade boy (7;9) at beginning year probe]
Leap-frog narrative	By age 4, children's narratives tend to consist of more than two events that occurred on one occasion. There is a logical or causal sequence to the events, but events may be narrated out of sequence, and events necessary for the narrative to make sense often are omitted.
	"I got hit by a car. I was two years old but I went to a hospital and my mom was sad and the girl went to jail and I was outside. I rode my bike and I was in a coma for 3 weeks and the girl work at my mom job. The end." [Third-grade boy (8;9) at mid-year probe]
Chronological narrative	McCabe and Rollins (1994) pointed out that a chronological narrative can occur at any age, but they placed it developmentally between leap-frog and end-at-high-point narratives in their progression. In such narratives, the order of events mirrors the sequence in which they logically must have occurred, but there is no high point.
	"Once I went camping in the woods with my auntie Robin and my friends. I stayed there for 5 days. The first day I went we had to get wood for the food or we couldn't get food. When we got done eating we played a game. Then when it was dark time we ate snacks and stayed up for a long time. When me and my friends got in a tent we played games. We played cards and all other stuff. When I went home I told my family about what I did." [Third-grade girl (8;7) at mid-year probe]
End-at-high-point narrative	By age 5, children rarely have difficulty sequencing the events of their oral narratives, and they can provide evaluative remarks about a high point. They tend to end their narratives prematurely at the high point, however, dwelling on a dramatic event and failing to provide a conclusion.
	"When I was little I got stuck in the elevator and it was locked and I was scared and I was screaming help, help, someone help me get out of here. In the elevator it was a phone and I picked it up and I pressed a button and someone said something and I said I'm stuck in here get me out." [Third-grade girl (8;3) at mid-year probe]
Classic narrative	By age 6, children can tell a well-formed story and orient the listener to who, what, and where something happened; narrate a sequence of events that leads to some sort of climax or high point; and then provide a resolution by telling how things turned out after the crisis point.
	"At my aunt Kathy's house there are bunnies and I got to hold them. One of them got out and ran away into the woods. I told my aunt Kathy and we ran into the woods and we got the bunny. The end." [First-grade girl (7;0) at year-end probe]

Sources: Descriptions and age of emergence data are from McCabe and Peterson (1991), McCabe and Rollins (1994), and Peterson and McCabe (1983). Student writing samples are from our research, but spelling and punctuation have been corrected. *Note:* It is *not* accurate to say that a third-grade student writing a leap-frog narrative, for example, is functioning at a 4-year-old level.

phasis on gathering written narratives by asking students to tell a story about a problem and what happened. The *evaluative comments* of high-point analysis might be called the "landscape of consciousness," following Bruner (1986), or the "internal response to the problem" and "clear goal-oriented planning" by those who advocate a story grammar approach (Glenn & Stein, 1980; Stein & Glenn, 1979). In other words, the fact that examiners notice features of subjectivity and encourage their development matters more than the name examiners give to these features.

Story Grammar Analysis

Story grammar elements are combined to produce mature narrative structures that are familiar and predictable. In Western European cultures, the dominant story type has characters that participate in goal-directed behavior (Stein & Glenn, 1979). Several variations have been proposed to describe the elements that make up a classic episode within the narrative genre (Mandler & Johnson, 1977; Stein & Glenn, 1979; Thorndyke, 1977). A summary appears in Table 15.2. Merely counting the number of these elements that appear in a particular story can be a means of judging the story's com-

Table 15.2. Story grammar elements included in a complete episode

Story grammar element	Description	Example
Setting	Time Place Characters	Once upon a time there was a girl named Jasmine. One night on October 30th (Devils Night) we went out to tee-pee houses, soap windows, and egg houses.
Problem (initiating event)	A problem or conflict that sets events of story into motion	One day I said, "Mama, I want a horse." She said, "No." The worst part of being a princess was that you had to marry a prince by your 10th birthday. He grabbed me and took me to the spaceship.
Internal response	Character feelings in response to problem	I got mad. They were suspicious of one person, Dan. Allison was so humiliated by her friends.
Internal plan	Statement of ideas or plans to address problem	I'm just going to ignore him. Some people wanted to leave it alone, but most of the counsel wanted to change their ways. The girls decided to make an even bigger team.
Attempt/action	Action taken to solve problem	I called my grandma, and she said, "Don't worry." She hit the fence with it and left it there. Tamara went to find them.
Resolution/ outcome	What happens as a result of actions	I only made the first free throw. They won by one basket. Fireball hit G.W. Script off the John Hancock building. He died. So she married him.
Ending/conclusion	Story closing and ending	They learned a lot from the game. Ralf joined the family. Ralf and Rover lived happily ever after.

Sources: Glenn and Stein (1980); Hedberg and Westby (1993); Mandler and Johnson (1977); Stein and Glenn (1979); Thorndyke (1977).

Table 15.3. Narrative maturity rating using story grammar levels

Level 1. Isolated description

Ask: "Is this story limited to an isolated description of people, places, and events?"
- May have setting
- No sequence of events
- A less mature isolated description might just involve heaps of unrelated information.
- A more mature isolated description might provide considerable information around a central topic.

Example
I like birds. My favorite kind of bird is a parrot. They are a problem because they copy a lot of people. But I like their pretty feathers. They have red, blue, orange, purple, green, brown, and black.

Level 2. Temporal sequence

Ask: "Is this story limited to a temporally related sequence of events or actions?"
- Series of actions that are temporally linked in a "what next" strategy
- Ideas often linked by *and, so,* and *then*

Example
I went to a football game and I had a good time. I saw someone get hurt. I ate good. And then we won the game two times.

Level 3. Causal sequence

Ask: "Is this story limited to a causally related sequence of events?"
- Series of actions that are causally linked but without planning
- Causal relationships can be implied, but must characterize most of story.

Example
Me and Anna and Kasey got in an argument. We got so mad at each other that we weren't friends any more. The next day we were not upset anymore, so we were friends again.

Level 4. Abbreviated episode

Ask: "Does this story imply goal direction?"
- Problem is stated
- Characters' aims or intentions are implied or stated in word choices such as *decided* and *wanted to.*

Example
One day I went to Full Blast. I was only five. I was going on a slide. And they said you need a parent. So I wanted to go find my parent. And I looked and I went to the wrong place. I went up. And they said you can go. I was drowning. I got saved by a lifeguard.

Level 5. Complete episode

Ask: "Does planning achieve a clear goal?"
- Includes characters' stated plan to reach a goal
- Ending brings clear closure.

Example
One day I was walking through the woods and I had my bow and arrow because my name is Robin Hood. And I have a side kick named John. And suddenly some men was riding on a horse and started chasing us. We had something they wanted. We had gold. The started shooting their bow and arrows at us. Me and John knew we had to put the gold up somewhere so we put it in our hideout. So the next day, I woke up early so I could think. I thought that we should split the gold. I told John that. I said then they won't be chasing us. That would be a good idea. So the next day we went to the camp where they live and knocked on the door and we said we can split the money. And you know what they said? That would be a good idea. So we will both be rich and we went home and had a happy ending.

Level 6. Complex/multiple episodes

Ask: "Is there an obstacle in the goal path? Is there at least one complete episode, accompanied by additional abbreviated or complete episodes?"
- Complete episode elaborated with multiple plans, attempts, or consequences
- Obstacle in path of reaching goal
- Series of complete plus abbreviated episodes, or embedded episodes

Example
On a summer day about 3 years ago a top secret submarine was stolen from Navy headquarters. The police looked for clues but did not have any, so the Sheriff said "Sorry we can't help you with no clues it's just up to you." After that the leader of a Navy seal gang got the gang to go out looking for the submarine. Bill one of the seals found a piece of the submarine exterior. That wasn't any help to the seals so they kept swimming and saw the submarine on the surface of the water. Bill tried to get into the submarine but it was locked shut and only the thief had the key. Bill and Mike tried to open the submarine by kicking the latch and throwing stuff at the lock. Finally Bill said "Skip it" and pulled out his 45 magnum and shot open the lock and climbed in. When the gang got back to headquarters they all got medals and certificates. After that brake in the navy decided to keep their top secret stuff in a top secret place. The end.

Level 7. Interactive episodes
Ask: "Are there two major characters with separate goals, whose actions each influence the actions of the other?"
- Complete episode
- Clear planning and perspective taking of at least two characters who are working at cross purposes.

Example

Chapter 1   The Witch
Once upon a time there was a mean old witch. She was so mean she would capture little children and tell them she was going to cook them in the pot in the fireplace for supper. She could do all kinds of magic on humans, but they were scare/ed of the witch. They all stayed in their houses.

Chapter 2   The Witch's Home
The witch's home was so nasty. It was filled with cobwebs. She had lots of cats especially Black cats. She loved her house and her cats and everything that she did, but the people in the town did not. They hated it. So one night they all went to her house in the woods.

Chapter 3   The Townspeople
The townspeople got there and knocked on the door. The witch answered it. They all had guns, and they tried to shoot her. She dodged every bullet. All the cats jumped on the townspeople and were biting them. The witch used her powers to throw them from the woods to their own home.

Chapter 4   The Witch's Curse
They all came back the next day. They read a passage that said: Beware whoever steps beyond this line will be placed under a deep, deep curse forever. None of them believed it. So they all stepped past the line, and boom, they were all in a new country, and they didn't know how to get back.

Chapter 5   The Witch's Death
Finally they all were back. They went to the police and told them they want/ed the witch dead. So the cop/s came back with the townspeople, and they went to the witch's house and threw bombs. The witch blew up, but there was one more curse. Whoever killed the witch would become a witch, but there was one more curse. Whoever lit the black flamed candle would bring the witch back to life.

Sources: Glenn and Stein (1980); Hedberg and Stoel-Gammon (1986); Hedberg and Westby (1993); Hughes, McGillivray, and Schmidek (1997).

By school age, it is possible to see narratives at any level. Although early elementary students produce stories at the lower end of the maturity scale, even second graders can produce a level 6 story with complex or multiple episodes. Example narratives with notes regarding scoring are in the chapter appendix.

plexity. The developmental progression is more than just additive, however. Rather, it represents a deeper shift in the nature of narration as storytellers learn to perceive the world in increasingly complex ways.

The rating method we propose is based on story grammar analysis using a developmental progression proposed by Glenn and Stein (1980) and adapted by others (Hedberg & Stoel-Gammon, 1986; Hedberg & Westby, 1993; Hughes et al., 1997). To assign developmental levels, this approach uses a binary choice strategy for answering the series of analysis questions in Table 15.3. The questions are designed to lead examiners to make a series of decisions about whether a story contains certain story grammar elements associated with progressing maturity. The highest level to which "yes" can be answered is judged to be the developmental level of the story. In Chapter 6, we suggest techniques for scaffolding students from their current level of narrative maturity to the next higher level based on framing and focusing missed cues in this sequence.

The story grammar developmental progression (Glenn & Stein, 1980) starts with an isolated description, which could be subdivided, following Applebee (1978), into isolated descriptions that are heaps of unrelated information, as compared with slightly more mature descriptions that are clearly centered on a common theme. The next step in the developmental progression is to tell a story with a temporal sequence (which Glenn and Stein [1980] called *action sequence*). A temporal sequence often involves less mature *and then* transitions to link the events of the story. Applebee (1978) might call such an attempt an *unfocused chain*. McCabe and Rollins (1994) might classify it as a *chronological narrative*.

When storytellers add causal elements to their stories, they have reached the next higher level of causal sequence (which Glenn and Stein [1980] called *reactive sequence*). When narrators state the problem explicitly and imply that there is some goal setting going on by talking about what their characters "wanted to" or "decided to" do, they have produced an abbreviated episode. When they make it clear that their characters are planning to reach the goal and provide a clear resolution to the problem that provides the crux (or "high point") of the story, they have reached the level of complete episode. Of note, a landscape of consciousness begins to appear in abbreviated episodes but becomes more explicit and is stated directly in complete episodes. The sixth level is one in which narratives have complex or multiple episodes. A clear obstacle in the path, or multiple attempts complicates the problem solving in these. Glenn and Stein (1980) also described a seventh level of interactive episodes, in which the story reflects the perspectives and planning of two characters at cross purposes, with the actions of one influencing the actions and perceptions of another.

When using a similar variation, based on the original description of episodic structure by Stein and Glenn (1979), Roth and Spekman (1986) analyzed spontaneously generated narratives told by students with and without learning disabilities (from ages 8 years to 13 years, 11 months). They found older students to use significantly more complete and embedded episodes. They also found the students with learning disabilities to produce fewer propositions and fewer complete episodes, as well as fewer response, attempt, and plan statements.

Difficult-to-Rate Stories

Establishing reliability for judging developmental levels takes practice on the part of educators. We routinely obtain reliability percentages of 80%–90% agreement for narrative maturity ratings, and disagreements are never more than one level apart. Collaborative partners who take time to calibrate ratings with each other can establish shared understanding and use of tools. When students produce stories that clearly fit the categories according to the given guidelines, calibrating ratings is an easy task. Not all stories, however, fit neatly into categories on developmental scales. Frequently, a student's work shows evidence of emerging, though not fully developed, higher-level skills.

McCabe and Rollins (1994) recommended rating a story as a "leap-frog" narrative when it has included multiple related events but violated temporal or logical order. We have seen many stories with such glimmers of higher-level narration combined with clearly less mature forms. In some cases, the limitations appear to be related to running out of time to complete an idea, but not always.

Students with limited fluency skills may not produce enough text for a true pattern to be recognized. When this occurs, we take dictation at some point during the assessment period to learn more about the student's discourse organization skills apart from the limitations in fluency. As noted, students with LLDs also are prone to producing a series of reactive sequences or abbreviated episodes without ever producing a complete episode (Hedberg & Westby, 1993; Roth & Spekman, 1986). Some students begin a story appropriately, then shift focus. In some cases, stories are so confusing that a pattern is difficult to decipher. In any of these cases, single hierarchy scores do not capture the essence of the written work, and an educator's brief description may better reflect the quality of the work produced. Although such stories generally are credited formally with the level of skill mastery at the lower level (i.e., highest level judged complete), emerging skills are noted and used as a bridge to scaffold higher-level abilities. The appendix to the chapter presents several examples of this nature.

To apply the narrative rating scale to Arreyona's story, we read her story with a primary focus on the story elements. Like many early developing writers, Arreyona did not fully integrate information across her story. In the first part of her text, she related a simple endearing story about her cousin's struggle with being teased. In the second half of her text, Arryona elaborated on the problem stated earlier in the story and described some of her cousin's strengths. Arreyona's story was evaluated as an abbreviated episode. It demonstrated story elements beyond an isolated description of people, places, and events. In addition, Arreyona connected a series of events temporally, and she both implied and directly stated causal relationships in her story. Consistent with an abbreviated episode, Arreyona stated a clear problem in her story in that her cousin was teased because he still had his baby teeth. She also showed some goal direction on the part of the main character when he asked his mother if his tooth was loose. Arreyona's story cannot be rated as a complete episode, however, because there is no clear planning or reflection on the part of the characters to achieve the goal.

Structural Organization and Maturity for Other Genres

Our narrative assessment probe allows teams to evaluate written language development over time by repeating the same writing task and measures at periodic intervals. Students, however, participate in writing activities that require knowledge of genres other than narratives. These include opinion pieces, report writing, persuasive writing, and poetry. Educators who desire to measure structural maturity development for other genres can adapt assessment measures specific to the required genre. The genre planning worksheet found in Figure 15.7 provides writing lab teams with questions that can act as guides for developing curriculum- and grade-relevant assessment tools to illuminate strengths and lead to individualized objectives.

A good way to begin to answer these questions and to design an assessment tool is to attempt to write in the genre yourself and to reflect on what you do as you think about a specific genre. Educators also can use available curriculum resources to craft structural maturity measures. For example, many schools have in place expected benchmarks and outcomes for writing development for particular genres at each grade level. Students with LLDs also will have expected outcomes documented on their IEPs.

In one collaboration, the third-grade benchmarks for writing required students to produce a persuasive article that included an introduction with a thesis statement, three supporting arguments, and a conclusion. Consistent with this benchmark, the collaborative team modified the structural maturity scale to capture these structural and organizational features. In later meetings, the team reflected on the persuasive writing pieces produced by its students. They observed the range of development represented in their students' writing and characterized the structural features of less and more mature papers to create a developmental progression. For example, in less-mature pieces, writers listed simple arguments. The arguments in these pieces tended to be from the student's perspective and lacked elaboration. More mature pieces typically included a higher number of arguments with greater variation, demonstrating the ability to take

Genre _____

What structural elements and global organization are associated with this genre?
What paragraph-level organization is expected?
What developmental progression characterizes growth in this genre?

Figure 15.7. Genre planning worksheet.

multiple perspectives. In addition, the arguments were supported with more details and examples. In this case, the team began with an assessment of persuasive genre structure and organization taken from grade-level outcomes. These outcomes dictated the classroom objectives. Over time, the team elaborated the developmental continuum to allow more in-depth understanding and next-step objectives for individual students.

In addition to grade-level outcomes, many school districts and states have developed rubrics to evaluate student writing for specific genres. Other resources are available through educational literature and language arts series. As discussed in Chapter 14, rubrics may describe characteristics of written language at different levels of ability in a global or holistic manner by assigning a single score to represent a written work. Although such global measures are not ideal for identifying specific educational needs of students, certain features at each developmental level can be teased apart to create a hierarchy of skills specific to a particular target area. Rubrics that use analytic or trait scoring provide a means to analyze selected elements or features. In one writing lab for upper elementary students, for example, we focused on advancing written-language skills for presenting factual information. To do so, we adapted parts of a rubric designed by Westby and Clauser (1999) to measure the structural and organizational developmental maturity of informational report writing. This hierarchy combined developmental information detailed in the Organization and Content/Theme sections of the rubric (see Table 15.4).

Table 15.4. Expository discourse maturity rating

Level 1	Brief with little development. May have narrative developments although exposition was intended. All content may not relate directly to topic.
Level 2	Brief, but paragraph includes attempts to center or chain ideas related to a topic. Ideas lack elaboration, cohesive connections, and transitions.
Level 3	Structure shows clear evidence of centering or chaining. Some support and elaboration of ideas is evident. Introductions and conclusions may lack clarity.
Level 4	Structure contains coordinated centering, chaining, and paragraphing, although there may be uneven development of ideas and shallow depth of content within paragraphs.
Level 5	Structure is clear, with appropriate introduction, transitions between paragraphs, and conclusion. Paragraphs have topic sentences and supporting details.

Source: Westby and Clauser, 1999.

Cohesion Measures

Cohesive ties enhance how a student relates elements in a story within a sentence and across sentences. As discussed in Chapter 2, cohesive ties connect ideas in a logical way by providing immediate links between two items, by relating several items in immediate sequence, or by connecting ideas that are more remote or out of sequence, such as those separated by one or more sentences or paragraphs. For a text to be coherent, related information must weave together in a nonambiguous way to create cohesive harmony. More sophisticated linking of ideas demonstrates growing competence in the area of cohesion.

Breakdowns in cohesion result in reader confusion stemming from illogical referencing, inadequate connections, or the need for more information. Frequent problems observed in maintaining cohesion include

- Pronoun referencing errors (e.g., using a pronoun before identifying its referent, using an inappropriate pronoun)

- Article errors (e.g., confusing occasions to use the definite *the* and indefinite *a*)

- Word-choice errors (e.g., being nonspecific, using inappropriate relational words)

- Deictic choice errors for maintaining appropriate perspective regarding person (e.g., switching from first- to third-person point of view), time (e.g., switching verb tense between present and past), or place (e.g., switching directional point of view, *here* and *there*)

- Problems of logic (e.g., using connectors incorrectly: *if . . . then, however, therefore, although*).

One strategy for assessing cohesion is to count the instances of breakdown. We do this by marking where breakdowns occur within a sample with a cohesion code (e.g., [coh]). We then look for patterns of breakdown to better understand and address instructional needs. Teams also might identify overlooked opportunities for using a cohesive tie. Although not an error, missed opportunities may signal a readiness for language instruction to move to the next level of competence in using cohesive ties.

Arreyona's story shows shifting verb tense, as well as difficulty with ordering of information. That is, after she related the conclusion to the simple story about her cousin's teeth falling out, Arreyona elaborated on the story's problem and gave descriptive information about her cousin. This may reflect a more topic-associative style frequently observed in African American narratives (Hester, 1996; Michaels, 1981). Some evidence of Arreyona's use of African American Vernacular English also was observed. Goals for Arreyona included having her reread her work to show standard verb agreement, to integrate descriptive information, and to ask herself whether the information is presented in the best order during the revising process. These were not treated as signs of disorder but as goals of the general education curriculum.

Sense of Audience and Voice

As students learn to consider audiences beyond themselves and the teacher, their purposes for writing broaden. Likewise, students' strategies for engaging this wider audience increase. There are qualities and features of written works that distinguish them as entertaining, informative, interesting, or moving. Such qualities cannot be captured with a focus strictly on linguistic features. Written pieces demand to be read for the ideas and style they convey, not just the linguistic features that act to shape and bind them. The content of a story can be analyzed in an informal descriptive manner. Questions that direct attention to the salient features of content and style in an individual sample might include

- Does this work have a theme, moral, or thesis?

- Is the work creative and original?

- Does the student stay true to the intended genre?

- Is the information relevant and adequate?

- Is there an attempt at humor, dialogue, or other literary devices?

Descriptive information related to a student's strengths and weaknesses in this more general approach can be used to develop individual objectives, and examples from the student's written works can be used to document progress. The self-questioning approach also can be used to develop student self-evaluation strategies and goals to reach their own higher benchmarks.

Arreyona wrote an original narrative about a personal experience. She chose a topic that engaged her peers. She also attempted some character description. Although Arreyona provided relevant information, she could have provided additional information by elaborating on ideas. Individual objectives for Arreyona in the summary sheet (see Figure 15.3) addressed adding description, including a title, and attempting dialogue.

Sentence-Level Analysis

As students' language skills develop, a gradual increase in sentence length and complexity takes place. As discussed in Chapter 2, students move from a dependence on simple sentences, to linking ideas by coordination (i.e., clauses joined with *and*) to the more sophisticated strategies of subordinating and embedding information. How well students formulate a variety of sentences influences their ability to relate ideas within and across sentences.

To produce coherent sentences, students know the rules for combining words to show relationships between elements. To produce texts that are interesting as well as clear, students must have skill in manipulating words and phrases. Questions that guide better understanding of sentence-level skill include

- What range of syntactic maturity is demonstrated?

- How skilled is the student at relating syntactic units within a sentence (e.g., grammatical agreement, embedding, dependent clauses)?

- Can the student code switch between formal standard English and nonstandard English forms (if relevant)? Is there an overreliance on spoken colloquial forms?

In some assessment protocols, evaluation of syntax at the sentence level and conventions for punctuation and capitalization are combined. Our view is that, although the student's use of end punctuation and initial letter capitalization can provide insight into students' awareness of sentence boundaries, the measure is not totally reliable. Students can produce structurally sound sentences despite immature use of punctuation. In this discussion of sentence-level skill, therefore, sentences are judged based on their syntactic qualities, essentially ignoring the student's choice of punctuation. Punctuation is evaluated at the conventions level. A combined problem in syntax and use of writing conventions may render a sample difficult to read and interpret. In such cases, areas of overlap and interdependence can be noted on the worksheet in the area most appropriate.

The worksheet's Written Products section provides opportunities to categorize, quantify, and describe sentence-level skills, including number of words per T-unit, types of sentences, percentage of correct to incorrect sentences, and grammatical pattern diversity.

Sentences, T-units, and Communication Units

To determine the maturity of grammar used in a sample, examiners need a meaningful method for dividing syntactic units. Counting the number of words per sentence as punctuated by the student is one option. This measure, however, does not accurately capture a student's syntactic skill. Students prone to run-on sentences would receive credit for one or a few very long sentences. Students who insert end punctuation mid-sentence would be penalized.

A better way to divide syntactic units is the T-unit, which was introduced in Chapter 2. This method is described with examples in Table 15.5. T-units or "minimal terminal units" are defined by Hunt (1970) as "one main clause plus the subordinate clauses attached to or embedded within it" (p. 49). A main clause, also called an independent clause, includes a noun and verb in a subject–predicate relationship. As sentences become more complex with embedding and complex verb forms, the mean (or average) length of utterance per T-unit (MLTU) increases (Hunt, 1965; Scott, 1988b). Because each independent clause in a run-on sentence is treated as a separate T-unit, T-unit measures reward syntactic maturity without overcrediting run-on sentences. While marking off separate T-units with slash marks (/), examiners also attend to sentence constructions that have remarkable complexity or particular limitations.

Table 15.5. Methods for analyzing T-units

T-unit definition
One main clause and any other clauses embedded in it or subordinated to it is a "minimal terminal unit" (Hunt, 1965, p. 141). Each independent clause (subject + verb phrase, conjoined with *and, but, or, so*) is a separate T-unit.

Dividing T-units
1. For dividing T-units, ignore students' punctuation (or lack thereof) and pay attention to the grammatical structure. Writing conventions, including punctuation, are analyzed separately.
2. Place a slash at the end of each independent clause and any related dependent clauses.
   My name is Ami/ [1 T-unit]
   I like God because he helps me/ [1 T-unit]
   Art is fun because we paint/ but when we come back to our classroom we do our work/ [2 T-units]
   I am 8 years old/ and I am in the third grade/ [2-T-units]
   The boy who is my friend started working after I was done/ [1 T-unit]

Computing Mean Length of T-Unit (MLTU)
1. Count the total number of words in the discourse.
2. Count the number of T-units marked off by slashes.
3. Divide total words/total T-units to yield MLTU.

Potential sources of bias
1. Although examiners could count bound morphemes separately, most researchers use word counts during the school-age years to compute MLTU. Word counts, therefore, are more easily compared with available normative data. They also are easier to compute and are less subject to dialectal bias.
2. It may be advisable to leave intentional grammatical fragments out of MLTU counts so as not to bias the sample, but to include agrammatic fragments attributable to grammatical formulation deficits.
3. Adjustments may be made for other unusual situations that might inflate the MLTU, such as the production of lists (e.g., *I got up, made my bed, took a shower, and brushed my teeth*).

Arreyona used a total of 14 T-units. As Figure 15.2 reflects, several of the T-units were not punctuated as complete syntactic units (e.g., "One day his toeth came out/ another one came out/and another one came out."). The MLTU in Arreyona's sample is 7.3. She constructed several short T-units (five 4-word T-units), as well as a few longer units, including one 20 words in length (i.e., "I did not laf at him becuse if his teeth did not come out evry body would call him a baby.").

A *communication unit* (C-unit) is comparable to a T-unit, but it is designed for dividing complete spoken utterances, some of which would be judged incomplete according to formal written communication standards. Similar to a T-unit, a C-unit is defined as "each independent clause with its modifiers" (Loban, 1976, p. 9). Clauses that are predicated on previous utterances, such as elliptical answers to questions, are considered C-units, despite the lack of a full noun–verb phrase within the utterance. For example, the response to the question, "What are you doing?" might be "Waiting for you." This response is a C-unit.

Authors sometimes produce grammatical fragments that are independent and can stand alone even though they are not complete. These may be grammatically appropriate, as in the case of titles, exclamations, asides, and elliptical single-word or short-phrase responses to questions or comments in dialogue. When such fragments are used as a mature author would, the examiner may decide to note them but not to incorporate them in T-unit computations so as not to lower the MLTU artificially. Titles and "the end" phrases, in particular, are treated this way. When incomplete T-units or fragments represent a breakdown in grammatical formulation, however, they are included in the T-unit count and are analyzed to provide an accurate picture of sentence-level development for a student. Developmental data for MLTU in spoken and written communication appear in Table 15.6, which shows a gradual building of MLTU, albeit with some overlap across age levels, for both spoken and written discourse.

Table 15.6. Mean word per T-unit levels from previous studies

Grade	Type	Score	Comments
1	Written	6.49	(SD=1.90); Source: J
2	Written	6.57	(SD = 1.92); Source: J
3	Spoken	7.62	Source: A
		8.73	Source: B
		9.5	(narrative); Source: I
		10.5	(expository); Source: I
3	Written	7.60	Source: A
		7.67	Source: B
		7.45	Source: G
		9.3	(narrative); Source: I
		9.9	(expository); Source: I
		7.6	(SD = 2.08); Source: J
4	Spoken	9.00	Source: A
		8.52	Source: D
4	Written	8.02	Source: A
		8.60	Source: E
		5.21	Source: F
		8.18	(SD = 1.79); Source: J
5	Spoken	8.82	Source: A
		8.90	Source: B
5	Written	8.76	Source: A
		9.34	Source: B
		8.81	Source: G
		10.7	(male); Source: H
		11.4	(female); Source: H
		8.37	(SD = 1.70); Source: J
6	Spoken	9.82	Source: A
		9.03	Source: C
		8.10	Source: D
		9.1	(narrative, students with LLDs); Source: I
		9.7	(expository, students with LLDs); Source: I
		10.03	(narrative, students without LLDs); Source: I
		11.04	(expository, students without LLDs); Source: I
6	Written	9.04	Source: A
		7.32	Source: F
		8.53	Source: G
		8.9	(narrative, students with LLDs); Source: I
		8.9	(expository, students with LLDs); Source: I
		10.4	(narrative, students without LLDs); Source: I
		12.1	(expository, students without LLDs); Source: I
7	Spoken	9.72	Source: A
		9.80	Source: B
7	Written	8.98	Source: A
		9.99	Source: B
8	Spoken	10.71	Source: A
8	Written	10.37	Source: A
		11.50	Source: E
		10.34	Source: F
		11.68	Source: G
9	Spoken	10.96	Source: A
9	Written	10.05	Source: A

continued

Table 15.6   *(continued)*

Grade	Type	Score	Comments
10	Spoken	10.68	Source: A
		10.15	Source: C
10	Written	11.79	Source: A
		10.46	Source: F
11	Spoken	11.17	Source: A
11	Written	10.67	Source: A
12	Spoken	11.70	Source: A
12	Written	13.27	Source: A
		14.40	Source: E
		11.45	Source: F

From Scott, C.M. (1988b). Spoken and written syntax. In M.A. Nippold (Ed.), *Later language development: Ages nine through nineteen* (2nd ed., p. 56). Austin, TX: PRO-ED; adapted by permission.

Note: The scores listed above represent the mean scores for mean length of T-unit measures for spoken and written discourse from a variety of studies with differing sampling conditions. The studies labeled D, F, G, and I reported data for age only. The data from these studies were entered in the table using the formula: grade = age (rounded) – 6 years.

A. Loban (1976). *N* = 35 at each grade. Data were also provided for high and low ability groups. Spoken scores involved adult–child informal interviews. Written scores involved school compositions.

B. O'Donnell, et al. (1967). *N* = 30 at each grade. Study involved spoken and written retelling/rewriting of a silent fable (narrative).

C. Klecan-Acker and Hedrick (1985). *N* = 24 at each grade. Study involved retelling of a favorite film (narrative).

D. Scott (1984). *N* = 25 10-year-olds, *N* = 29 12-year-olds. Study involved retelling of a favorite book, television episode, or film (narrative).

E. Hunt (1965). *N* = 18 at each grade. Study involved school compositions.

F. Hunt (1970). *N* = 50 at each grade. Study involved a sentence combining exercise.

G. Morris and Crump (1982). *N* = 18 at each age (9.6, 11.25, 12.54, 14.08 years). Study involved rewriting of a silent film (narrative).

H. Richardson et al. (1976). *N* = 257 11-year-old boys; *N*=264 11-year-old girls. Study involved school compositions.

I. Scott and Windsor (2000). *N* = 20 students in each of three matched groups; 20 students with LLDs (mean age 11;5), 20 chronological age–matched peers (mean age 11;6 years), and 20 language ability–matched peers (mean age 8;11).

J. Nelson and Van Meter (2003). *N* = 333 (59 first graders; 69 second graders; 113 third graders; 51 fourth graders; 41 fifth graders); spontaneous narrative probe samples gathered mid year (except first-grade probes at end of the school year) from racially mixed group (50.7% African American; 43% White/non-Hispanic; 5.6% Hispanic; 0.5% Asian/Pacific Island; 0.2 Native American), gathered and analyzed using the methods described in Chapters 14–15. Data for young students (first graders) and students with special needs (all grades) were included only when students became independent enough to write their own words (i.e., dictated samples are not included in the data).

Sentence Types

Although average length of T-unit provides a general index of a student's sentence-level maturity, a closer observation of sentence level-skills can be accomplished by coding and counting different sentences types. As described in Chapter 2, we code the number of simple and complex sentences that are produced both correctly and incorrectly. Sentence codes are added after we divide a student's written language sample into separate T-units. At that point, we make a second pass at the sample to code sentences as [sc] for simple correct, [si] for simple incorrect, [cc] for complex correct, or [ci] for complex incorrect. We code samples by marking codes directly on photocopies of students' original samples or on SALT (Miller & Chapman, 2000) transcripts (review Figures 15.4 and 15.5).

Consistent with the general education literacy curriculum, a sentence is coded as correct or incorrect based on the rules of standard edited English. We attempt to capture dialect differences, however, and code these with a [d]. We then directly address dialect differences and when and how to code-switch from dialect to standard edited English in individual objectives and instruction. This educational decision supports the aim of academic success for all students (Delpit, 1995), and it is consistent with special service providers working in inclusive settings with general educators. It differs from assessment decisions made while diagnosing disability, when it is essential to treat dialectical variants as completely acceptable to avoid confusing language difference with language disorder.

Definitions and examples of sentence codes are presented in Table 15.7. A single T-unit (independent clause) is rated as simple if it has only one verb, but complex if it includes more than one. The second verb might appear as a finite verb (main verb) in a compound verb phrase (e.g., *She hid it and forgot about it*) or subordinated clause (e.g., *After she hid it, she forgot where*), or it might appear as a nonfinite verb (secondary verb) as an embedded infinitive (to + verb, e.g., *She decided to look for it*), gerund (verb used as noun, e.g., *Looking for it proved difficult*), or participle (verb used as adjective, e.g., *Looking for it, she forgot about the time*).

We have established a rule for coding in which we give children credit for a complex (or compound) sentence that uses a coordinating conjunction (*and, but, or, so*) to

Table 15.7. Sentence-coding levels

Simple incorrect [si]

A grammatically incorrect simple sentence. Dialectal speakers may be scored two ways: according to standard edited English expectations and allowing for dialectal variation.
- Then there 10 seconds left in the game. [si]
- The boy knowed it. [si] [d]
- He got kick out of the store. [si] [d]

Simple correct [sc]

A grammatically correct sentence with one independent clause (subject + verb phrase construction), possibly including adjectives, adverbs, prepositional phrases, and compound subjects or objects
- Tiger and Coco were best buddies. [sc]
- The next day we played a trick on the X-men. [sc]
- There were fireballs and laser blasts. [sc]
- Have you seen it? [sc]

Complex incorrect [ci]

A grammatically incorrect complex sentence. In the case of run-on sentences (sentences with more than two independent clauses joined together), only two clauses at a time are considered part of the same compound sentence. If this sentence has a grammatical error anywhere, it is coded [ci].
- She like to sneeked out of the house when the door is open. [ci][d]
- Once upon a time ago there was a girl name Jack Nicholas. [ci][d]
- One day the mother said to her baby chickens that you have to live by yourself now. [ci]

Complex correct [cc]

A grammatically correct sentence that includes 1) two coordinate clauses conjoined with *and, but,* or *so* (two T-units); 2) an independent clause plus a subordinate cause conjoined with *because, since,* or *while;* 3) an independent clause with an embedded phrase with a secondary verb: gerund, infinitive, or participle; or 4) an independent clause with a compound verb phrase
- That night I dressed up as a witch too, but I was a lot uglier. [cc]
- When Ash got there, he ran into Johnny. [cc]
- Once there was a boy who got in an accident and couldn't go to school. [cc]
- We were glad to be rich. [cc]

Note: A developmental progression in this coding system would involve increasing frequency of sentences in the following sequence: [si], [sc], [ci], [cc]. [d] indicates dialect.

combine two independent clauses. For example, "He saw her/and then he decided to turn around" would be scored as two T-units but one complex correct [cc] sentence. "She putted the dog's collar on/but he shook it off" would be scored as two T-units, but one complex incorrect [ci] sentence. Although *so* generally acts as a coordinating conjunction (e.g., *He tried it so she did too*), it also can serve as a subordinating conjunction. The test for subordination is to ask whether the meaning is the same as *so that* or *so as* (e.g., *Jim tightened the rope so that the alien couldn't get away* [1 T-unit]). When students link more than two T-units with coordinating conjunctions, we code a run-on [ro] sentence at the beginning of the third independent clause. That T-unit, and any additional linked T-units, then are coded as either simple or complex sentences (correct or incorrect) depending on whether they stand alone or are conjoined. In other words, the run-on code does not affect other sentence codes, but is coded in addition to other codes.

A student's pattern of sentence production can be used to gauge maturity, as well as to provide qualitative information regarding the student's current challenges in the area of sentence formulation. Roth and Spekman (1989) analyzed the syntax of original spoken narratives produced by students with and without learning disabilities (ages 8 years to 13 years, 11 months) and found that the only syntactic difference was that students with learning disabilities used fewer complex correct sentences, although they attempted as many complex sentences. Scott and Windsor (2000) also found that students with LLDs produced significantly more grammatical errors in their written narrative and expository summaries than either their chronological age–matched or language age–matched peers.

Measures of specific error types, which justify [si] and [ci] sentence codes, also can help educators to understand an individual student's grammatical formulation difficulties and suggest a next step in intervention. Qualitative descriptions to consider include verb tense errors, pronoun errors, subject–verb agreement problems, word omissions, and word order confusions.

Qualitative analysis also can be performed to look for evidence of higher-level syntax attempts, even though some of these sentences may include elements that would be considered incorrect. Errors on attempts, in fact, might demonstrate a student's readiness to learn new forms (Weaver, 1982). Examples of sentence types that indicate higher levels of maturity in sentence production are presented in Table 15.8 (based on work by Scott, 1988a, and Scott & Stokes, 1995). Hughes and her colleagues (1997) suggested scanning a sample and documenting occurrences of these less-frequently occurring sentence constructions. A qualitative analysis also could include a more detailed look at the presence or quality of sentence elements that are not as complex as these, but represent more than simple syntax, such as elaborated noun and verb phrases and prepositional phrases. This finer focus on the qualitative features of sentence elements assists in identifying both strengths and needs present in a student's sentence-level skills.

Sentence Variability

Although not an error, some students show an overreliance on one or two sentence constructions in their compositions. Reduced sentence variability can interfere with story interest and limit the child's opportunity to focus on more complex relationships among ideas.

Counting occurrences of overused sentence forms can provide a baseline for sentence-level targets. An objective might be established, for example, to reduce the

Table 15.8. Later developing complex sentence structures

Structure	Examples
Complex noun phrases	One day there was a girl named Jeannie/and there was a boy named Nathan. [cc]
	The owner kicked the little girl out and told her she could not come back no [d] more. [ci]
	Everyone believed that if you own [v] a dragon, it will [v] make you healthy and have good luck. [ci]
	All of a sudden she saw a white dragon and a man wrestling and playing with each other. [ci]
	Then it stopped storming. [cc]
	Each morning they could find words written on the web. [cc]
Appositives	Ping, the man, could talk in Dragon. [sc]
Relative clauses	The boy heard a voice under the bed that said I am coming to get you. [cc]
	A long time ago there was a bull named Cool Dude, who always mind [v] [d] his own business. [ci]
Adverbials	By the time the police came, the woman and child was [v] [d] dead. [ci]
	When they were about to enter, they found an abandoned convertible and keys. [cc]
	Back in the cave where the man was, he started to think who she was [coh]. [ci]
	So when she heard what he said, she started screaming at him. [cc]
	Her father let Fern have the pig until it got big. [cc]
Coordinated noun or verb phrases	So the ambulance came and took the people. [cc]
Cleft constructions	It was 30 minutes later that she woke up wondering where she was. [cc]

Sources: Hughes et al. (1997); Roth and Spekman (1989); Scott (1988b); Scott and Stokes (1995).

Note: Narratives produced by third through fifth graders in our research. The [v] code was used to mark tense or agreement errors on verbs. If influenced by dialect, [d] was coded, too.

number of sentence run-ons, in which the child strings together multiple independent clauses. In this case, the instructor and child might set a goal during the revision of a story to use fewer *and then* connections. Scaffolding would focus on exploring alternative ways for relating ideas temporally with different words (e.g., *after, later, when*), and on helping the student consider whether relationships might be more than temporal, justifying a connector such as *because* or *if . . . then.*

Aaron, a third-grade student with LLDs, overused the word *then* to start a series of temporally linked sentences in the following excerpt from "Part two" of the "X-men has a battle with Dan and I." In this paragraph, Aaron began seven out of nine simple sentences with "then we . . ."

Then we ate pizza. Then we went to bed. Then we ate the rest of the pizza for breakfast. We were hungry. Then we went to the store. We stole 10,000 more pound of pizza. Then we had a battle with the X-men. Then we ran to the tractor. Then we got on the tractor.

Intervention with Aaron targeted sentence variability by counting with him the number of times he used the *then* construction and brainstorming other ways to connect ideas across sentences, such as using *because,* for more interest. In later revisions, Aaron replaced *then* with *later, the next day,* and *after that.* With scaffolding, he also attempted to combine some of his simple sentences into complex ones.

Subordination Index

Another measure of sentence development and complexity is the subordination index (e.g., Scott, 1988b). The degree of subordination is a measure of the average number of all clauses (independent and subordinate) per T-unit. To tally the subordination index, the examiner divides the total number of clauses by the total number of T-units. As writers become more mature in their use of written language, the number of subordinate clauses increases gradually. By seventh grade, students use more subordination in their written language than in their spoken speech (O'Donnell, Griffin, & Norris, 1967). Subordination also differs with level of performance. For example, Gutierrez-Clellen (1998) found that Spanish-speaking students who were low achieving retold book and film narratives using shorter T-units and fewer sentences with infinitives, nominal clauses, or relative clauses (resulting in lower subordination index score) than their average achieving Spanish-speaking peers. Scott and Windsor (2000) found that MLTU differentiated students with LLDs from age-matched peers but that the number of clauses per T-unit (i.e., subordination index) did not. Scott and Windsor hypothesized that the students with LLDs in their study might have used more early developing clauses, such as nominal infinitival complements (e.g., *He wanted to go back; The girl pretended to watch*), inflating their clause per T-unit scores and obscuring differences.

Arreyona wrote seven simple correct, two complex incorrect, and three complex correct sentences, including "I did not laf at him becuse if his teeth did not come out evry body would call him a baby/ and he is seven" (a very mature sentence). Verb-tense inconsistency (*He allways acks* [should have been *asked*] *his mother was his toeth loes*) and subject–verb agreement (*He know* [attributed to dialect] *how to count by 2s and tiye is shoes*) were responsible for the two sentences judged incorrect according to standard edited English. Goals were written for Arreyona to produce complex sentence constructions with particular attention to verb tense and agreement issues. At this point, we remind readers that 1) Arreyona was not found to have a disability; 2) all students can have individualized general education objectives, not just students with disabilities; and 3) learning to write using standard edited English is a goal of the general education curriculum.

Word-Level Analysis

Word choices greatly influence the quality and clarity of a written work. They add color, interest, and specificity. Some students work within the confines of a reduced vocabulary. Others have difficulty retrieving words with ease. Students whose spoken vocabulary appears more sophisticated than their written vocabulary may be limiting their word choices based on either word-retrieval limitations or spelling skills.

We address both word choice and spelling at the word level of analysis. Good spellers draw on at least three aspects of word knowledge (Treiman & Bourassa, 2000a):

- Phonology, which governs how sounds and sound sequence patterns are arranged to make words

- Morphology, which governs how word parts or morphemes are combined
- Visual orthographic memory, which supports recall of visual patterns of letter sequences

Questions that guide assessment at the word level include

- What type and variety of words does the student use in writing?
- Do word choices in writing parallel those in spoken communication?
- What do spelling error patterns tell us about the strategies the student brings to the spelling task?

Analyzing Word Choice Maturity and Diversity

The Word Level section of the Writing Process and Product Worksheet provides a framework for quantitative and qualitative measures that consider word choice and variability, developmental spelling stages, and strategies for analyzing spelling error patterns.

Higher-Level Word Choices

More mature vocabulary choices create meaning and interest. Some words get the job done in a clear and simple way, whereas others add deeper shades of meaning and entertainment. Valued word choices can be specific and unusual content words, as well as grammatical function words that bind together individual sentences and create linkages across sentences. Sometimes, words have individual impact; other times, as in the case of similes and metaphors, they team up in a special phrase (e.g., *He sang like a chicken*). As students move from an informal oral language style to a more formal literary style, they often discover the varied and powerful uses of words within and across sentences and within broader units of discourse.

To analyze skill level in written vocabulary, we observe the type and quality of word choices. At the most basic level, judgment can be made about whether the student's vocabulary choices adequately or appropriately convey the intended meaning. In the case of stories, this might mean the word choices allow the reader to comprehend the story elements. In expository text, it might mean that the content words are appropriate to establish and support the topic. Both narrative and expository text also require the use of relational vocabulary choices to connect ideas across text. Both also present opportunities to use content-specific vocabulary, such as might be drawn from the science or social studies curriculum, either in expository reports (e.g., to describe a natural phenomenon) or narratives (e.g., to set the scene for a world travel story).

Beyond asking whether words are chosen to adequately convey the message, attention can be directed to identifying mature, interesting, or unique words. Determining which words can be characterized as mature at any given grade level is always to some degree subjective, but we find that general agreement is fairly easy to achieve. There also are guidelines for recognizing mature word choices that can serve as benchmarks for indexing a student's growth in this area over time. One feature of mature word choice is word frequency. Words that are used less frequently tend to be more mature, although that is not always the case. To determine if a word has a low frequency of occurrence, choices can be compared with word lists available in books or computerized word banks (Fry, Kress, & Fountoukidis, 2000), although this approach may be too time consuming and cumbersome to be used in practical everyday settings.

A second strategy is to compare a student's word selections with those of his or her peers. When students write on the same topic, teachers can develop topic-specific indices for both content and relational word choices. Even when student writers select their own material across diverse topics, teachers may identify patterns in the type and quality of words used (e.g., high numbers of descriptive adjectives and adverbs).

A third strategy is to note the presence of figurative language and humor as indications of higher word-level skill. Students exploring the world of literary devices such as simile, metaphor, analogy, and alliteration show understanding of the many facets of word usage and an awareness of how to engage an audience. Movement from use of culturally common colloquial expressions to creation of original literary forms marks an important form of developmental progression.

Word Diversity Measures

Type–Token Ratio (TTR) is a traditional measure of vocabulary diversity. When Templin (1957) introduced it in her classic studies, she found TTR to be steady across the age range from 3 to 8 years. TTR is computed by dividing the number of different words (types) in a sample by the number of total words (tokens) in a sample. As a rule of thumb, a TTR of 0.5 is generally considered evidence of adequate vocabulary diversity. TTR, however, is problematic in that it depends on length of text. That is, short, immature texts might have only a few words, but if they are not repeated, the TTR will be inflated. For example, a story with only 40 words, 30 of which are different, will have a TTR of 0.75. Longer texts, conversely, are likely to have progressively lower TTRs because of increasing proportions of high-frequency function words (e.g., *is, was, the, and, of, to*). They may have TTRs below 0.5, even though they might be filled with interesting and unusual words. This leads to the conclusion that, unless the length of compositions is controlled, the TTR is a poor measure of vocabulary diversity, and controlling length of written samples is difficult, due to a wide range in story length, with some quite short.

Another way to document vocabulary diversity is to make a simple count of the number of different words (NDW) in the story. This method is recommended as preferable for judging developmental advances through the school-age years and distinguishing children with and without language disorders (Bennett, 1989; Watkins & DeThorne, 2000; Watkins et al., 1995). Scott and Windsor (2000) found that the NDW measure differentiated students with LLDs from typically developing peers in written narrative (but not expository) summaries. Their sampling context, in which the students watched narrative or expository films prior to summarizing them, may have influenced this result by supplying most of the vocabulary. The number of different words in an original story or report might be more discriminative, although more research is needed to test this hypothesis. Computer analysis programs, such as SALT (Miller & Chapman, 2000), make the process of computing NDW much easier than counting by hand. When children exhibit an overreliance on certain words (e.g., *this, that, stuff, thing, her, his, got, good, pretty*), however, engaging the student to count instances of such all-purpose words can help build ownership for an objective targeting the use of more varied and interesting vocabulary (see "retired" word minilesson in Chapter 4).

Word Usage Errors

Word choice quality needs to be viewed not only by looking at the characteristics of an individual word but also the context in which it occurs. Mature words used incorrectly in a given context may indicate confusion regarding the finer meanings of a word. Students who venture into using new and different words often recognize the power of words. Although they are not always successful in usage, these students may be actively attempting to build a new skill. Documenting occurrences of usage error patterns can assist teams to characterize initial levels of performance and suggest individual objectives.

Stories that contain a high number of words that are vague or lack specificity may suggest problems with word retrieval or an overreliance on familiar (and possibly easy to spell) words. Some additional probing of the student's vocabulary in spoken storytelling might help to clarify the nature of the problem. Students who produce more mature choices in spoken language may not recognize the importance of word choice in their written compositions until it is brought to their attention. Following some discussion on the power of word choice, these students can learn to take pride in selecting less common and more interesting words. Students who struggle in both spoken and written language need objectives that target vocabulary development and retrieval in both modalities.

Vocabulary Learning Evidence

The words students write derive from their spoken and written language experiences. Expository writing, in particular, offers an excellent opportunity to observe the information-gathering and note-taking processes and to assess students' reading comprehension as it relates to written expression. Some students interpret text in their own words, demonstrating that they have comprehended it, whereas others copy text without apparent concern for meaning or relevance to their chosen topic, demonstrating limited comprehension. Dynamic assessment probes of a student's understanding of the vocabulary contained in notetaking samples can assist in identifying when a student needs scaffolding to make sense of the new vocabulary. Scaffolding also may help such students find words they would like to use in their own writing without copying verbatim from a source.

Arreyona chose simple, relevant words to relate her story. With the exception of one verb-tense problem, she produced no word-usage errors. She did not, however, demonstrate any word choices or expressions that were particularly colorful, interesting, or mature. Next-step objectives for Arreyona targeted use of stronger verbs and descriptive words.

Spelling

Spelling errors are obvious to readers and influence audience perceptions of an author's maturity. Stories that contain numerous spelling errors, especially errors that are not closely related to their targets either phonetically or visually, can render a paper unreadable. An assessment of spelling could include a count of spelling errors divided by the total number of words (multiplied by 100 to convert to percentage correct). The percentage method is preferable to a raw count of misspelled words because students' written products often get longer as they learn to write better, and they may misspell more words in longer pieces, even though the proportion of misspelled words is decreasing.

Beyond computing percentage of errors, describing a developmental level or characterizing the qualitative nature of spelling errors is important. This step helps teams to illuminate what strategies a student is and is not bringing to the spelling process. Instructional targets and strategies grow out of this type of qualitative evaluation. For it to be useful, however, educators need a framework for judging developmental progression.

Developmental progressions for spelling have been described (e.g., Gentry, 1982; Rhodes & Dudley-Marling, 1988; Mather & Roberts, 1995). Although developmental scales are somewhat controversial (Treiman & Bourassa, 2000a, 2000b), we have found the progression presented in Table 15.9 to be useful for describing students' spelling capabilities and establishing intervention targets. This developmental progression captures the primary stages: scribble writing, prephonetic, semiphonetic, phonetic, transitional, and conventional. These stages are not discrete, and students may use strategies from more than one stage during the same piece of writing. They do, however, capture a gradual progression in a student's awareness of the linguistic features of words and how morphology (word parts) relates to orthography (spelling patterns). This knowledge builds over time into conventional spelling.

By observing a student's spelling pattern and comparing it with the requirements of conventional spelling, educators can identify the strategies that a student brings to the spelling process and target those not yet in use. When judging spelling, we make note of a student's successes (e.g., knows silent *e* rule, knows *-ight* word part), in addition to observing error patterns. To detect error patterns, we list several of the student's errors

Table 15.9.   Developmental spelling progression

Stage of spelling development	Description of students' abilities
Scribble	Produce letter-like sequences to convey meaning
Prephonetic stage	String unrelated letters together to convey meaning (e.g., "takyskp" for *My brother hit me.*)
	Understand that letters convey meaning, but not sound–symbol relationships (e.g., "i.i.tnp num." for *I like to play with some new friends.*)
Semiphonetic stage	String letters together to form words with only a few sounds represented, most often the first and last (e.g., "fid" for *friend*, "pwo" for *play*, "buud" for *brother*, "propm" for *policeman*)
	Write single letters to represent syllables or words (e.g. "ne" for *any*, "b" for *be*, "r" for *are*, "u" for *you*)
Phonetic stage	Use sound–symbol relationships to "sound out" words (e.g., "akros" for *across*, "bekoz" for *because*, "heer" for *here*, "lafin" for *laughing*)
	Attempt to correctly order sounds in a word (e.g., "deteshin" for *detention*, "uankt" for *yanked*, "frandshap" for *friendship*, "parelizd" for *paralyzed*, "jrownding" for *drowning*)
Transitional stage	Show awareness of morphologic endings (e.g., -ing, -ed, -able, –tion).
	Recall visual orthographic patterns, alternatively called "sight" words, word "families," and word "chunks."
Conventional spelling	Employ multiple strategies to spell
	Learn context dependent spelling (e.g., homophones—*their, there; to, two, too*)

Sources: Gentry (1982), Mather and Roberts (1995), and Rhodes and Dudley-Marling (1988).

next to the correct spelling (e.g., *laft/laughed*) directly on the worksheet or on the bottom of the sample transcription. This helps illuminate how closely they resemble target words in sound or visual appearance. In some instances, the pattern closely reflects one of the stages of spelling development illustrated in Table 15.9. In other instances, clear patterns are difficult to discern. In either case, objectives are established to target features not yet observed and skills needed to progress to the next level of development.

Students at the earliest stage of spelling, the scribble stage, produce letter-like sequences to convey meaning. As they learn to produce actual individual letters—at the prephonetic stage—they string unrelated letters together, demonstrating an understanding that letters are combined to spell words but not yet demonstrating sound–symbol relationships. For students in such early stages of development, students' story probes generally involve some dictation as well as student writing attempts. Scaffolding students to produce word attempts as independently as possible is important. With direct instruction, students at the semiphonetic stage should begin to make sound–symbol associations. At first, they only represent a few sounds in a word, then across syllables and words. As students move into the phonetic stage of spelling, they demonstrate strength in analyzing sound and syllable segments in a spoken word and translating them into written words with sound–symbol encoding skills. Their spelling errors resemble a word phonetically as in "sed" for *said*, "tuff" for *tough*, "takt" for *talked*. During this phase, students who speak a dialect or have articulation impairments may show spelling that mirrors their own articulation patterns.

To spell successfully, in addition to sound–letter correspondences, students must implement a strategy of writing word parts, in which they demonstrate their knowledge of spelling–meaning connections. Rather than relying solely on a strategy for sounding out words letter-by-letter (sound-by-sound), students need instruction and guidance to analyze words according to larger morphological units and to recognize and recall the orthographic patterns of word roots and affixes (Read, 1971, 1986; Templeton, 1992). The added knowledge allows them to progress to the transitional and conventional stages of spelling. Evidence of learning in this area includes preserved syllables, correct spelling for common root words and "word families," and correct spelling of affixes (e.g., *-ing, -ed, re-*). Inconsistent spelling of word roots and affixes suggests weakness in processing words at a morphological level. It also may reflect influence of spoken dialect on spelling. Goals in the area of spelling can be established for strengthening areas of literate word knowledge and for learning new strategies for spelling unfamiliar words.

Arreyona demonstrated spelling skills in the transitional stage of development. She showed strength for spelling high-frequency function words, including words with silent *e*, and the irregular form of *know*. Even her spelling errors showed strength in sound–letter correspondence. For example, *laughed* was spelled "laft." In this case, her phonetic representation of the final morpheme showed her oral language strength. To spell the word conventionally, however, Arreyona would have to represent the *-augh* orthographic pattern, as well as the past tense morpheme *-ed*. When Arreyona spelled the word *asks*, her spelling, "acks," matched her spoken language dialect. Arreyona also demonstrated her recognition of the orthographic pattern *ack* in the process.

Other spelling errors were characterized by incorrect double vowels or vowel combinations (e.g., "toeth" for *tooth*, "becase" for *because*) and missing letters. To promote growth in spelling, objectives and instruction for Arreyona focused on recognizing the linguistic meaning of the morpheme *-ed* and representing it consistently as *-ed* in spelling, as well as learning new families of root morphemes represented in her writing efforts.

Writing Conventions Analysis

Writing conventions assist readers to make sense of text by providing information in a standard way. The use of writing conventions is rule governed and requires practice for mastery. Although there are numerous rules for writing conventions and use, three primary types are reviewed in this section: capitalization, punctuation, and formatting. On the Writing Process and Product Worksheet, the Conventions Level section addresses both quantitative and qualitative aspects of writing conventions.

As with spelling, a clear model exists for judging what is correct and incorrect in standard use of writing conventions. A potential flaw, however, is that it can be tempting to judge a student's skill level by asking only the quantitative question, "How many times is a given convention present in an obligatory context?" Although the answer to this question can be informative, it is not enough, and it can even be misleading when students limit their use of conventions as a trade-off for generating text. Dan, for instance, omitted periods consistently, but when asked about the purpose of periods and where periods should go, he responded knowledgeably. Dan explained that he didn't have time to put them in now, but would add them at some later time. At a later point, he was scaffolded to value punctuating while writing.

In the area of capitalization, we have seen students whose inconsistent use of capital letters was related to lack of mastery of the mechanics of handwriting or using the shift key on the computer. Some students are unclear about the rules for capitalization. Differential diagnosis is important in deciding which intervention strategies to employ. Questions of a more qualitative nature can focus observations on students' meta-knowledge and awareness of written conventions. Such questions might include

- Is there a pattern of use or misuse of conventions?

- What do error patterns communicate about knowledge of sentence structure as well as conventions?

- What can students report about their use of writing conventions when asked?

Arreyona inconsistently marked sentence boundaries with periods and capitalization, showing partial skill in using sentence punctuation. A goal was established for her to recognize sentence boundaries and mark them with punctuation. Likewise, she did not indent to organize ideas into paragraphs. This became another writing conventions goal for her.

ASSESSING RELATED SPOKEN LANGUAGE ABILITIES

The relationship between spoken and written language has been described as dynamic and reciprocal (e.g., Catts & Kamhi, 1999). Chapter 2 describes many features that spoken and written language processes share, as well as important differences between them. The writing lab approach integrates opportunities for using conversational language in social interactions with peers and adults with opportunities for learning formal literate communication. The spoken language assessment process has two primary purposes. It is designed to

- Compare discourse-specific (e.g., narrative, persuasive, informational) spoken- and written-language skills in order to develop educational goals and instructional strategies

- Establish conversational-language goals that foster effective participation in the spoken-language contexts of the writing process approach.

Comparing Spoken and Written Language Skills

Written language has been described as more decontextualized than spoken language (see Chapter 2) in that writers must include enough information to communicate with an audience separated by time and space, whereas oral communicators share those dimensions and can rely more on nonverbal context to convey meaning. Overlaps exist, however, in style along the informal to literate language-use continuum. By comparing students' spoken to written communication skills within a genre, such as storytelling or information giving, educators can identify where students struggle in language use. As a result, they can identify objectives that address the area of need (Scott & Windsor, 2000).

Some students, particularly those with learning disabilities, show markedly higher-level skill in spoken than written language. Those skills can be tapped for scaffolding written language efforts. For example, Manuel was a fourth-grade boy with severely limited word decoding and encoding skills. Manuel generated stories using the printed words he could find in his environment. For example, one of his stories was about bulls and Chicago because of a baseball cap with a sport team logo that was handy. These stories demonstrated Manuel's resourcefulness, but they did not convey the narrative maturity of the spoken stories he generated without the constraints of limited spelling skills. Manuel's strengths were used to scaffold his weak areas when he was encouraged to tell his stories orally first, contributing to the creation of story-specific word banks, which remained available during drafting.

Other students, including some with LLDs, demonstrated improved spoken discourse after producing a written piece that allowed them to "see" their work and revise prior to presentation. For example, Sarah was a fifth-grade student whose oral communication was disorganized and difficult to follow. Sarah had a pattern of switching topics mid-sentence and rarely including clear referents for pronouns. For Sarah, working on planning and organizing her ideas in written language assisted her to organize herself better in spoken communication as well. Sarah's goals, and a story she wrote while working on them, are presented in Chapter 16.

Assessing Spoken Narrative Language

The same quantitative and qualitative measures described for analyzing written stories can be applied to assessing spoken language samples. That is, at each level of language processing (discourse, sentence, word), parallel data can be analyzed from a spoken language sample. We are not proposing that all evaluations routinely include in-depth analysis of both written and spoken language samples. Nor are the observations recommended here intended to replace a comprehensive spoken language evaluation that would address both receptive and expressive modalities. Instead, we suggest that the results of informal observations of skill in spoken language can be used to guide, direct, and maximize intervention in the varied contexts of the writing lab. Questions that may guide the gathering of spoken narrative information include

- Is there a difference between skill level in one modality that could be used to support development in the other?

- What similar language difficulties noted in both modalities might benefit from intervention in multiple contexts?

In some cases, spoken-narrative assessment goals require sample transcription and coding. At other times, observations of a more general nature provide adequate comparison data. Suggestions for formal coding of spoken discourse differ from guidelines for coding written stories only in a few ways: 1) do not count "maze" behaviors (Loban, 1963), such as fillers (*ah, um*), repeated words, false starts, revisions, self-corrections (e.g., *I mean*), or abandoned utterances; and 2) recognize that the use of *and* to connect ideas is not considered a run-on error in oral communication. Also be aware that several research teams have found that the syntax produced by school-age students in spoken-language narratives does not differ significantly from that in their written narratives (Gillam & Johnston, 1992; Scott & Windsor, 2000).

Spoken Language Contexts in the Writing Lab

The writing lab approach is rich with opportunities for developing conversational language skills in turn-taking, speaking in front of a small group, relating feelings and ideas, and practicing giving and receiving criticism. For example, peer conferencing, minilessons, and teacher conferencing all are essentially spoken communication contexts that can be scaffolded as language-learning opportunities addressing spoken language goals. Questions that guide the assessment of spoken language in writing process contexts include

- Does the student's level of interactive skill permit easy exchange of information?

- What linguistic and pragmatic skills influence success and failure in peer and adult–child discussions?

On the Writing Process and Product Worksheet, the "spoken contexts" portion is organized to allow for a quick yes/no inventory of behaviors in the areas of listening and comprehending, manner, topic maintenance, and linguistic skill. Qualitative description could define contexts further, as well as the specific behaviors observed. Individualized objectives for participation in spoken language contexts grow out of these observations of a student's interactive skills in interviews and peer conferencing, as well as in any of the other spoken language contexts of the writing process.

Arreyona enthusiastically shared her written work with peers, clearly articulating and using appropriate loudness and eye contact in both one-to-one and group interactions. Just as enthusiastically, she shared her opinions and insights with peers, although not always diplomatically. At times, she showed difficulty listening to work of peers without interrupting, especially with those outside of her immediate circle of friends. She was sensitive, however, to peer attention and perceived criticism when others asked questions regarding her work. Peer conferencing and author chair activities offered Arreyona opportunities to work on goals for listening, accepting constructive criticism, and taking the perspective of others.

SUMMARY

This chapter has presented methods for assessing samples of written language processes and products and for assessing spoken language in writing lab contexts. Writing-process instruction challenges students to integrate language knowledge across levels and modalities. Looking at abilities across language levels allows for a systematic analysis of linguistic skill and processing. Although each level can be characterized independently, in actuality, levels are interdependent on each other. For example, to successfully write a story that relates information causally, students need to be able to relate several pieces of information within and across sentences, choose relational words, construct complex sentences, and demonstrate ease in generating text (Berninger, 2000). In addition, world knowledge comes into play in that students need to relate information in ways that represent their world experience.

The assessment worksheets provided in this chapter are meant to serve as observation guides. They are detailed enough to support several lines of inquiry into a student's skill at each level—discourse, sentence, word, writing conventions, and spoken communication. They are not meant to imply that all assessments should include documented skill in each category. That is, we expect professionals to choose the measures that best match their own assessment purposes and to modify them as necessary to meet their needs. The result should be a set of objectives and some preliminary ideas about where to begin the process of intervention. This type of informal sample assessment is ideal for assisting the processes of dynamic assessment and for measuring progress over time for groups or individual students.

Appendix

Writing Assessment Forms

The first two forms in this appendix can be used to summarize data regarding a student's written and spoken language skills as demonstrated through a writing sample. The last form provides student writing samples coded in SALT and accompanying ratings and comments. Note that the mixed stories can be used to practice scoring using the levels listed in Table 15.3.

The contents of the appendix are

1. Writing Process and Product Worksheet

2. Writing Assessment Summary and Objectives Worksheet

3. Examples of narrative scoring

Writing Process and Product Worksheet

Student _____ Teacher _____ School _____ Grade _____ Observer _____ Birth date _____ Age _____

Date of sample _____ Sampling activity _____

Assessing writing processes

Planning and organizing
— Approaches writing tasks willingly
— Arrives at topic independently
— Picture
— Graphic organizer Type _____
— Notes
— Dictates

Drafting
— Refers to planning
— Proceeds quickly from start to finish
— Pauses periodically
— Revises —— changes spelling —— word choice
— Dependent on others for spelling

Revising and editing
— Rereads work   — Corrects grammar
— Adds information   — Corrects spelling
— Rewords ideas   — Corrects punctuation
— Clarifies references   — Edits
— Reorganizes content

Assessing written products

Discourse level
Fluency
— Total # words
— # words/T-unit

Structural Organization
— True to genre: _____
Maturity level:

Cohesion
— Clarity within sentences
— Clarity across text
— Pronoun reference cohesion
— Verb tense cohesion

Sense of audience
— Title —— End
— Creative and original
— Relevant information
— Adequate information
— Dialogue/Other literary devices

Sentence level
T-units
— Total # T-units
— # words/T-unit
— range of T-unit length

Types of sentences
— # Simple incorrect
— # Simple correct
— # Complex incorrect
— # Complex correct
— # Run-on clauses (after 2 coord.)

Variability
— Varied sentence types
— Overreliance on a particular
    construction

Word level
Word choice
— Mature and interesting choices
— Overreliance on particular words
— Usage errors

Spelling accuracy
— % incorrect

Spelling developmental stage   Examples:
— Prephonetic   _____
— Semiphonetic   _____
— Phonetic   _____
— Transitional   _____
— Conventional   _____

Conventions
Capitalization
— Initial letter of sentence
— Titles   — Proper nouns

End punctuation
— Periods   — Question marks

Commas
— Divide series   — Divide clauses

Apostrophes
— Contractions   — Possessives

Quotation marks
— Direct quotes

Formatting
— Paragraphs
— Poetry/other   _____

Assessing spoken language in writing process contexts

Manner
— Articulates clearly
— Speaks fluently
— Uses natural prosody
— Appropriate eye gaze
— Appropriate loudness

Listening and comprehension
— Makes eye contact with speaker
— Listens without interrupting
— Seeks clarification when needed
— Follows directions

Topic maintenance
— Situationally appropriate
— Provides adequate information
— Asks relevant questions
— Shares opinions
— Reflects on own work and others'
— Engages in conversational turn-taking

Linguistic skill
— Organizes ideas adequately
— Completes utterances
— Uses specific vocabulary

Copyright © 2001 Nelson, Van Meter, and Bahr.

Writing Assessment Summary and Objectives Worksheet

Student _____

Assessment sample _____

Grade _____

Genre _____

Teacher _____

Date _____

Observations and impressions	Goals and objectives
Writing processes	
Planning and organizing	
Drafting	
Revising and editing	
Written products	
Discourse level	
Sentence level	
Word level	
Conventions	
Oral language	
Writing process oral contexts	
Genre specific	

Copyight © 2001 Nelson, Van Meter, and Bahr.

Story using SALT	Rating and comments
- Zelda was so happy [sc]. - It was her birthday {.}[p]. - But her whole family was not there [cc]. - [ro] And that was a problem {.} because{Case}[sp] her family was always{alwase}[sp] there on her birthday [cc]. - So she call/ed everyone {.}[p]. - and they said they would be late [cc]. - [ro] and they all came [sc].	First-grade girl (7;6) End-of-year probe Abbreviated episode. Clearly stated problem. Planning implied but not explicit.
- One sunny morning when a unicorn was be/ing born the baby unicorn could walk [awk] [ci]! - This was strange [sc]. - All the other baby unicorn/s can't{cant}[sp] walk" said one unicorn,. - but the mother of the unicorn was proud of her baby [cc]. - Baby unicorn had white hair and a long tail[p] [sc]. - She want/ed *a tall horn too [si]. - But first{firt}[sp] she has[v] to prove that she is brave [ci] - After a few week/s the unicorn was older,. - and it was time [cc]. - She said goodbye{good by}[sp] to her mother, and succeeded [cc]. - And she got tall horn/s as she wish/ed [cc]. - {The end}.	First-grade girl (7;1) Mid-year probe Complete episode. Includes explicit goal ("she has to prove that she is brave"). One could argue for a rating of abbreviated episode because it is not completely clear that proving she was brave required leaving her mother. The rating is less important, however, than recognizing the opportunity to scaffold the student to tell readers what proving she was brave required.
- Once{Ouse}[sp] upon{apon}[sp] a time{tame}[sp] a bee came along{alone}[sp] and was look/ing{lookeing}[sp] for a hive [cc]. - It found{fond}[sp] my corner{cone}[sp] of our{are}[sp] garage{groge}[sp] [p] [cc]. - It start/*ed make/ing{makeing}[sp] a hive [ci]. - When I came out to the bus stop{stup}[sp] I saw{sow}[sp] it[p] [cc]. - I told my mom and when my dad got home he spray/ed{sprad}[sp] it[p] [cc]. - [ro] and the bee flew{fley}[sp] [v] away [si].	First-grade girl (6;10) End-of-year probe. Abbreviated episode. Although the solution comes after an explicit action by the main character ["I told my mom"], the goal setting is implied. The clear ending makes this almost a complete episode.
- Lacy love/ed her bear{bare}[sp] [p] [sc]. - But one day she lost{loste}[sp] her bear{bare}[sp] and could{cod}[sp] not find{finde}[sp] her[p] [cc]. - She look/ed{lookd}[sp] in her treasure{tresher}[sp] box. - and it was/n't{wasint}[sp] there[p] [cc]. - She look/ed{lookd}[sp] on her piano{peanow}[sp]. - and it was there [cc].	First-grade girl (6;9) Mid-year probe Abbreviated episode. "Looking" implies goal orientation, but she does not give her story a conclusion.

(continued)

413

(continued)

Text	Commentary
• I read the celery{cerey}[sp] stalk/3s at mid/night book [sc]. • It is scary{skaray}[sp] [sc]. • It is very funny [sc]. • I read it every{erv}[sp] week [sc]. • It is funny because the pet/s can talk [cc]. • Zavid and Zate were friend/s [sc].	Second-grade boy (7;6) Mid-year probe Isolated description. Not true to genre. Although there is one causally connected sentence, it does not characterize the discourse.
• "Look out"! said Zate to Zavid [cc]. • "Be quiet"! said Zavid [cc]. • "No"! said Zate [cc]. • Zavid got hit by a tree and died [cc]. • Zate was sad [sc]. • The end.	Second-grade boy (7;9) (same as previous) End-of-year probe Causal (reactive) sequence. Things just happen and there are reactions, but no goal-directed behavior or planning.
• My dad bought{bote}[sp] me a brand new {.}[p] videogame. • and this guy{gou}[sp] on it {.}[p] can make electric{elachitk}[sp] pole/s[awk] [p] [ci]. • it is{.}[p] nice. • and we all like it [cc]. • [ro] and I love my dad very much [sc].	Third-grade boy (8;11) Beginning-of-year probe Isolated description. Has the feel of a "what next?" writing strategy. Needs scaffolding to plan and to use story grammar structure.
• One day I saw a big fat dog[p] [sc]. • He was talk/ing to me. • and I was talk/ing to the fat dog[p] [cc]. • [ro] and the fat dog bit me. • and I call/ed the dog pound{pode}[sp] [p] [cc]. • [ro] and the{th}[sp] man took the fat dog to the dog pound{pode}. • and I went home[p] [cc]. • [ro] and I told my mom about the fat dog. • and she told me about her very, {very, very, very, very, very} bad day at work too{to}[sp][p] [cc]. • [ro] and she saw the very, {very, very, very} fat dog[p] [sc]. • {the end}.	Third-grade girl (9;0) End-of-year probe Abbreviated episode. This story provides opportunities to ask more about what happened and why. It also is a good example of run-on sentences. One could scaffold the student to consider which "ands" are necessary and to find word choices other than "very" to express her meanings.

414

Writing sample	Description
• Our family just got a new dog[p] [sc]. • it is a little puppy [sc]. • We bought everything{everithing}[sp] a dog could{cowd}[sp] want [cc]. • One day he got loose and trample/ed on the next door neighbor/z{neighbors}[sp] flower/s [cc]. • My mom and dad got a notice about the dog [sc]. • me and my sister said we don't want him to go [cc]. • We don't have enough money right now[p] [sc]. • We are try/ing to save for our new house [cc]. • So the problem was solve/ed by me and my sister get/ing a new job do/ing a paper route{rout}[sp] make/ing{makeing}[sp] 500 dollar/s a month. • and we save/ed up all our money together for a long time [cc]. • and my mom and dad save/ed up their{ther}[sp] money too [sc]. • and we move/ed to a new house. • and now our dog won't be put to sleep [cc].	Third-grade boy (8;9) End-of-year probe Complete episode. Story includes clear planning to reach a goal and resolution of the problem introduced in the beginning.
• One day four friend/s had meet [v] at a park [si]. • Their{there}[sp] name/s was[v] Kiaria, Alice, Bobby, and Timmy [si]. • One day the girl/s{grils}[sp] went to the store [sc]. • When they went to the store I[awk] saw my teacher Mrs P and her children Max, Martha [p] [ci]. • I ask/ed/ed{acked}[sp] my teacher if they[awk] can come to Kiaria/Z birthday [ci]. • When we left the store we saw the two boy/s [cc]. • They said hi [cc]. • When we went to Peter Piper Pizza [awk] [ci]. • The next day I went to my teacher/*Z house. • and we told my teacher that we had fun [ci]. • {the end}.	Third-grade girl (9;7) End-of-year probe Temporal sequence. The events are chained temporally, with no problem and no causal relationships.
• Stuff/ed{stuff}[sp] animal/s{anr}[sp] is[v] good[p] [si]. • I like pooh the best then[awk] all[p] [si]. • I got him for christmas[p] [sc]. • He is red and yellow[p] [sc]. • He them[awk] is cute{qute}[sp][p] [si]. • He can talk too{to}[sp][p] [sc]. • He say[v] I love honey[p] [ci]. • I do too{to}[sp] [sc]. • I don/'t{dont}[sp] like looke[p] [sc]. • I like pooh [sc].	Third-grade girl (8;6) Mid-year probe Isolated description. Written by the same girl who wrote the fat dog story (abbreviated episode) at the end of the year.

(continued)

(continued)

<table>
<tr>
<td>

- {The Boy Who Couldent Write} [t]
- Once upon a time there{their} [sp] was a boy.
- and his name was Nate[p] [cc].
- [ro] and he was a little lad[p] [sc].
- he was 8 just like I was.
- and he loved to play[p] [cc].
- he had the best friend/s in the world{.} [p].
- [ro] And he was the fast/est{fastes} [sp] run/er in class[p] [sc].
- he was brave but he could/n't{couldent} [sp] write[p] [cc].
- he always/s had speech/es but he did/n't{din't} [sp] write it down [cc].
- He was so sad.
- and he want/ed to know how to write [cc].
- Every time he heard{herd} [sp] write/ing{writeing} [sp] business{bisnass} [sp] he would look at a girl and consotrate {concentrate} [sp] on her[p] [cc].
- he wish/ed he was a normal kid{.} [p] Who would be able to write but he {but he} [awk] skip/ed{skiped} [sp] 1st grade[p] [ci].

</td>
<td>

Third-grade girl (9;1)
End-of-year probe

Abbreviated episode. Ending doesn't bring clear closure. Note on paper, however, indicated that her plan was longer than her final draft. She apparently ran out of time to complete the episode.

</td>
</tr>
<tr>
<td>

- Once there{their} [sp] was a dragon that had no friend/s[p] [cc].
- she try/ed to get some.
- but every time she try/ed they said no [cc].
- [ro] and once she saw a person that almost said yes.
- but she said no and said I have too many friend/s any{eney} [sp] way and walk/ed away[p] [cc].
- the dragon was sad and said I/'m gonna make a friend.
- and they will be nice to me[p] [cc].
- she went to her grandfather/Z house to get a potion{pochin} [sp] to make people her friend [cc].
- She drank the stuff that her grandfather gave her.
- and she said that she has friend/s now [cc].
- the dragon is a grown up now.
- and she has more friend/s [cc].
- [ro] and she has more friend/s than ever [sc].

</td>
<td>

Third-grade girl (8;5)
Beginning-of-year probe

Complete episode. Clear goal setting and intentional actions by main character. Ending brings closure to episode.

</td>
</tr>
<tr>
<td>

- {How my dog walke's} [t].
- My dog walk/3s{walke's} [sp] crook/ed{crecked} [sp] [sc].
- I play with my dog [sc].
- I love my dog [sc].

</td>
<td>

Third-grade girl (8;9)
Mid-year probe

Isolated description.

</td>
</tr>
</table>

416

• My family{famle} [sp] is go/ing to Florida{flode} [sp] . • [ro] and I am go/ing in the boat{dote} [sp] [cc] . • [ro] and we are go/ing in a plane{pian} [sp] . • [ro] and I get{git} [sp] to go swim/ing{swimen} [sp] [cc] . • [ro] and I get{git} *to sit in the hot tub{hotwptube} [sp] . • and I am go/ing to MichiganAdventure{meshign avnvher} [sp] [ci] . • [ro] and I am go/ing to PeterPiperPizza{pedrpteresu} [sp] . • and I am go/ing to PuttPuttGolf{pte pte golf} [sp] and{an} [sp] game/s{gams} [sp] [cc] . • and I am go/ing to play [cc] .	Third-grade boy (7;11) Beginning-of-year probe Isolated description. Similar to temporal sequence, but really no temporal sequential elements. Student had language learning disabilities.
• {My dogs} [t] . • I had 5 dog/s. • and they all died{did} [sp] [p] [cc] . • My first{frstd} [sp] dog/z name was rocket{roket} [sp] . • and he got ran over [cc] . • [ro]and I love[v] my dog [sc] . [8;3 third grade boy at mid-year probe]	Third-grade boy (8;3) Mid-year probe Causal (reactive) sequence. Same student with LLDs who wrote previous story. Although there are causal links, the episode is not fully developed. It has no goal setting.
• [pic] . • One day a girl name/ed kitty found a magic box {boox} [sp] [cc] . • She open/ed it [sc] . • Kitty made a wish on it [sc] . • Kitty wish/ed that she had a pink pony [cc] . • She wish/ed that her mother to come back to life [awk] [ci] . • Kitty/z mother came back to life [sc] . • Kitty went on a picnic {picc} [sp] with her mother [sc] . • She was so happy. • and they live/ed happily {happliey} [sp] ever after [cc] .	Second-grade girl (7;11) End-of-year probe Complete episode. Although the goal setting relied on magic, this qualifies as a complete episode.
• I like watch/s {wocis} [sp] [sc] . • They are cool [sc] . • They *are pretty {prirte} [sp] [sc] . • They are nice {nic} [sp] [sc] . • They tell {tall} [sp] time {tame} [sp] [sc] . • They could {caid} [sp] be different {difrt} [sp] color/s {calars} [sp] [sc] . • I am get/ing {giting} [sp] it{pro} tomorrow {to marrow} [sp] because {dcasza} [sp] I clean/ed {clainged} [sp] my room [ci] . • It is a PowerPuff Girl/z {paff gllies} [sp] watch [sc] . • {Good-bye} .	Second-grade girl (8;2) End-of-year probe Isolated description. Although there is one sentence with causal links, it does not characterize the majority of the story.

(continued)

- {the golden seed} [t].
- Once there was a princess{prinses} [sp] that was walk/ing in her garden.
- [ro] and she trip/ed{treped} [sp] over a seed [cc].
- [ro] and she turn/ed{terned} [sp] around{aroand} [sp] and saw a hole[p] [cc].
- she look/ed in the hole.
- and there was a golden seed [cc].
- [ro] and the girl just thought{thout} [sp] it was a pumpkin seed and plant/ed it [p] [cc].
- the next day she look/ed in her garden to see if the pumpkin had grown.
- and instead{instead} [sp] of see/ing a pumpkin she saw all her plant/s were{whre} [sp] gol-den{goldin} [cc].
- [ro] so she sent out guard/s{gards} [sp] to find another golden seed.
- but when they came back they{thay} [sp] said they{thay} could not find another golden seed [cc].
- [ro] so the princess{prenses} went off{of} [sp] look/ing for the golden seed[p] [cc].
- what the girl did/n't notice{notes} [sp] was one of her guard/s{gards} was miss/ing{mis-ing} [sp] [p] [cc].
- finally{finaly} [sp] she found{fownd} [sp] a golden seed.
- but she did not know that the one guy *had touch/ed{tuched} [sp] [v] the golden seed and turn/ed into{to} [sp] solid{salid} [sp] gold [ci].
- [ro] and the guard/s{gards} hid him in the bush/s{boashes} [sp] right{write} [sp] by the seed.
- so the princess{prenses} touch/ed the seed and turn/ed to solid{solad} gold [cc].
- [ro] so the rest of the guard/s{gards} live/ed sad/ly but happily{happy} [sp] ever after with{wath} [sp] a garden{gardin} that was solid gold [ci].
- {the end}.

- {About my dog} [t].
- My dog can eat fast[p] [sc].
- It can do front{frot} [sp] flip/s{fleps} [sp] and back flip/s{fleps} [p] [sp] [sc].
- It can walk on his{hes} [sp] front{frit} [sp] paw/*s{po} [sp] [si].
- He has alot of hair{hare} [sp] [p] [sc].
- His{hes} [sp] name is Eric[p] [sc].
- He has{hase} [sp] floppy{flape} [sp] ear/s{ers} [sp] [sc].
- He got hit{het} [sp] with a football.
- and he has{hase} [sp] a girlfriend{gril frind} [sp] [cc].
- He is 19.
- and the girl{gril} [sp] is 18 [cc].
- {The end}.

Third-grade girl (8;6)
Beginning-of-year probe

Complex multiple episode. This story includes deception and obstacles in the path. The prevalence of run-on sentences suggests an area for scaffolding, along with scaffolding of ortho-graphic–morphemic relationships.

Third grade boy (8;6)
Mid-year probe

Isolated description. The student who produced this was later identified with LLDs. There is a hint of a problem in the story when the dog got hit with a football, but it is not developed. No reaction is described, and no goal setting is implied or stated.

Using Goals, Objectives, and Benchmarks to Guide Instruction and Measure Change

In the writing lab approach, instructors encourage and support students to write about their ideas and to work on their language while creating published works for an audience of peers, teachers, parents, and others. This encouragement sets the context for developing and practicing thinking, language, and writing skills for the purpose of making meanings clear and interesting. It also provides opportunities to engage in purposeful social communication with peers.

Each student comes to the writing lab with a unique set of developmental strengths and needs. As described in Chapter 15, intervention begins with assessment of baseline levels across the language targets (originally described in Chapter 2). Then, goal areas and objectives are established to lead students to next higher levels of skills in each of those areas. The purpose of developing goals, objectives, and benchmarks is to provide a structure to guide instruction and measure change. This chapter discusses how to write objectives that identify specific targets and how to establish benchmarks for documenting change over time in relevant goal areas.

CONNECTING OBJECTIVES TO ASSESSMENT

Relevant goals and objectives should be connected to the writing and other language demands a student faces in real-life classroom and personal endeavors. Several questions guide the process of developing goals, objectives, and benchmarks that are relevant to individual students' needs:

- What does the student know?

- What does the student need to know to progress to the next step of maturity?

- What supports will the student need to reach that step?
- What measures will capture evidence of change?

The question of what the student already knows can be answered using assessment information derived from formal testing, interviews, and the informal assessment methods described in Chapter 15. What the student needs to know can be determined using description of the next level of maturity for a particular language target area. The supports a student needs to reach next higher levels for particular language targets are the topics of Chapters 4, 5, and 6. Chapter 15 addresses measures that can be used to capture evidence of change. This chapter adds information about instructional objectives and other methods for documenting change.

By answering such questions, teams can individualize intervention plans and design systems to monitor progress for particular students. The process starts with assessment of a student's current performance. That level provides the immediate baseline against which further progress is measured. For example, in the area of discourse, an appropriate objective for a student who currently is producing narratives at the level of temporal sequences would be to include causal elements in order to reach the next higher level of reactive sequences. In the area of sentence production, an appropriate objective for a student who currently is producing mostly simple incorrect sentences would be to increase (over baseline) the proportion of simple correct sentences and to begin to include complex sentence structures (both correct and incorrect at first). In the area of word production, an appropriate objective for a student who currently is producing invented spellings mostly at the phonetic level would be to produce spellings that demonstrate transitional-level knowledge, such as components of irregularly spelled words (e.g., "lagh" for *laugh*) and evidence of morphemic knowledge (e.g., *-ing, -ed*).

Delineating the next step in maturity for a student across domains of language targets (discourse level, sentence level, word level, writing conventions, spoken communication) helps teams visualize desired outcomes. Analysis of the knowledge, skills, and strategies a student needs to work on at each higher level leads the instructional team to make decisions about the types of instruction and experiences that will encourage advanced learning. Out of this process come the benchmarks that will allow the team to document change.

By addressing questions about the type and amount of support a student is likely to need to achieve an objective, teams collaborate in thinking specifically about designing a learning context and establishing conditions to encourage the shift toward higher levels of independence and competence. Two types of support are considered in these goal-setting discussions. The first is educator support in the form of instructional scaffolding. The second is learning supports such as word lists, story grammar prompts, and punctuation strategy lists. Chapters 4, 5, and 6 offer suggestions about such supports.

The decision about how many goal areas or objectives to target for an individual student varies with classroom situations and students' IEPs. In traditional language intervention on discrete skills in pull-out settings, it might be possible to target a maximum of three or four short-term objectives at once. In writing labs, it is possible to target many more objectives simultaneously. This is because objectives are addressed in an integrated fashion within the same activities, not as discrete targets. By using the framework proposed for assessment in Chapter 15, teams establish baseline information for each of the writing process stages and product levels, as well as for oral communication. Baseline levels and developmental sequences make it possible to establish benchmarks and to know which features to scaffold as children engage in writing lab activities. The multiple contexts of the writing lab offer opportunities for working on several objectives across consecutive days. Although not all targets are addressed daily, a comprehensive set of objectives allows for flexibility across contexts and student states of readiness, thus allowing educators to respond more easily to teachable moments.

COMPONENTS OF OBJECTIVES

Goals establish general areas of focus and set long-term targets in terms of higher levels of knowledge and performance. Objectives go a step beyond goals to specify contexts and criteria that indicate a successful outcome. According to IDEA 1997, students' IEP goals could be written with benchmarks as an alternative to short-term objectives. Benchmarks are operational definitions of points along the way toward a more far-reaching goal. They are more concise than fully elaborated short-term objectives and possibly are easier for a team to keep in mind during intervention. Thinking out the full components of short-term objectives, however, remains a useful planning tool. Quantified or qualitative descriptions of writing processes and products can then serve as benchmarks for progress reports.

The components of well-written performance objectives are familiar to practiced educators. They include

- What the student will do (an operational description of the new knowledge, skill, or strategy to be demonstrated)

- Under what conditions (the instructional or observational circumstances)

- How well (a criterion statement to specify skill level)

This section addresses guidelines for defining individualized goal areas and writing objectives that can be realized through the inclusive, computer-supported language-learning contexts of the writing lab approach.

The "Who" of Objectives

In special education, goals and benchmarks are important components of IEPs. A feature of the inclusive writing lab approach, however, is that the "who" of objectives should not be just students with disabilities. Rather, everyone should have goals.

It is important to convey the message that all people (both students and teachers) can benefit from setting and pursuing deliberate, intentional goals. It may take some discussion, and even a shifting of paradigms, to move beyond the notion that objectives are purely remedial. In one collaborative summer enrichment program, we were surprised when some teachers disagreed passionately with our recommendation to write abbreviated forms of students' summer program objectives on the back of all of the students' nametags, regardless of whether they were identified as having special needs.

These teachers expressed deep concerns that the written objectives would identify all students as "special ed."

Printing goals on name tags was a technique devised for short-term interventions. It had proved effective for helping students gain ownership for their short-term goals and assisting teams of professionals to direct their scaffolding toward specific targets. That summer we learned, however, that for some teachers and students, the idea of having individualized objectives had become a badge of special education.

We argued then, as we do now, that all learners (including adults) can benefit from individualized objectives to direct learning efforts and measure success. Drawing on the research principle, we solved the dispute that summer by agreeing to experiment with the technique and to discuss its success as the workshop progressed. As reflective practitioners, instructors wrote personal goals on the backs of their name tags as well, and we each kept journals related to our efforts to reach those goals. Flipping of name tags and sharing of personal goals and progress toward them became part of the culture in this writing lab experience. The conflict was resolved when the group used the research principle to examine the positive evidence of change.

An important aspect of developing individual ownership for goals and objectives is to involve students in writing their own goals. We have found that students who reflect on their goals and have copies written in simplified student versions (i.e., "kid language") are more motivated and directed in their learning efforts. Students who are aware of their objectives also can participate more actively in measuring and celebrating change. The case study included later in this chapter provides an example of how this is done.

The "What" of Objectives

One of the challenges in objective writing is to find a balance between targeting specific skills and focusing on the whole communication event. The informal assessment process described in Chapter 15 leads to a set of balanced goal areas that target 1) both processes and products and 2) both spoken and written language. It provides a road map for fostering change and scaffolding students to higher levels of knowledge, skills, and strategies.

Knowledge refers to what a student knows or thinks. Some students show surprising insights in that they can discuss metacognitively skills they have not yet been able to demonstrate in practice (McAlister et al., 1999). For example, some may be able to describe the revision process adequately but never use it spontaneously. Others may be able to state the rules of end punctuation but not use it as they write. Of course, there are times when students do not have the knowledge base to draw on, and in these cases, providing explicit instruction about the missing knowledge becomes a first priority.

Skills appear during performance of a planned, intentional function. They take practice to become automatic. An example of a skill is the ability to formulate complex sentences. Another skill is the ability to detect errors while editing. A challenge for the educator is to keep skill training anchored in relevant learning contexts to avoid fragmentation and to build automaticity.

Strategies are used to guide actions and solve problems in oral and written use. They imply executive control of writing processes and the use of intentional, deliberate decision processes for regulating actions in order to achieve immediate and long-term goals. Mnemonic devices, such as "*i* before *e* except after *c*," are strategies. Other strategies are to use graphic organizers for planning to include the parts of a story. Self-questions for judging whether meanings are communicated adequately also are strategies. As with all strategies, writing process strategies only work if used well. Targeting the use of strategies involves helping students to recognize the value of strategic, intentional approaches, as well as knowing when, where, and how they should be used.

Armed with strategies, skills, knowledge, and appropriate scaffolding supports to solve their individual writing problems, students experience more independence and the self-assurance that comes with success. In such cases, success breeds success. In the process, language and communication abilities grow in ways that support learning in other parts of the curriculum. No matter the level at which a student begins, significant improvements can be measured for each targeted area. These higher levels then become the new baseline against which next benchmarks are set.

The "Criteria" of Objectives

Two questions help instructors define the criteria or benchmarks for knowing when an objective has been met:

- What will change look like?

- How will I know that change has occurred?

Measures of change should be designed to answer these questions with both quantitative and qualitative data. The data might consist of evidence of new knowledge, skills, or strategies. Change also can be described in terms of increased degree of independence and reciprocal reduction in instructional supports needed to participate actively or complete a task.

Traditionally, ratios and percentiles have dominated as means of quantifying change. Part of the reason for the frequent use of percentages is that they lend an aura of ob-

Table 16.1. Examples of methods for quantifying writing processes and products

Example writing process targets	Example written product targets
Planning: Will generate topics, ideas, or details independently, during individual brainstorming.	Discourse-level: Will produce story or report with higher level of discourse maturity and increased number of words per story.
Organizing: Will use story mapping for planning, generating schema independently, and filling in each component.	Sentence-level: Will produce higher level sentence types along the progression, simple incorrect [si], simple correct [sc], complex incorrect [ci], complex correct [cc].
Drafting: Will draft independently for at least 10-minute periods with no adult support.	
Revising: Will reread and make revisions to improve discourse- or sentence-structure elements or add more interesting words.	Word-level: Will produce more different words, more words judged as interesting, and words spelled at least at the transitional level.
Editing: Will proofread and correct spelling or punctuation errors.	Spoken communication: Will contribute at least once to each group discussion and will look at partner and wait for turn when engaging in peer editing.
Publishing/presenting: Will finish in time to use special formatting and illustrating features on the computer prior to publishing deadline.	

jectivity to documentation. Another reason is that the number of occurrences of a behavior compared with the number of opportunities for some behaviors provides a reasonable way to measure change. Some behaviors, however, are not captured well with percentages, such as appropriate eye contact or use of story grammar elements. Table 16.1 provides several means for quantifying evidence of change in both writing processes and written products. Most assume reference to baseline performance using similar rating scales, checklists, and observational data within a limited period of time or within a specific context or condition.

STRATEGIES FOR ORGANIZING OBJECTIVES

Objectives can be written with subobjectives that further define the multiple steps and strategies involved in teaching a new knowledge, skill, or strategy. Subobjectives can be organized in two ways, using a vertical or horizontal strategy.

Vertical Objective Writing Strategy

A vertical strategy involves arranging the steps to meet a target in a hierarchical or sequential order, with each step a precursor to the next. That is, the second objective depends on accomplishing the first; the third on accomplishing the second; and so forth. The following is an example of an objective with vertically arranged subobjectives for learning to use sentence-level punctuation over a series of sessions.

The student will punctuate sentences by

1. Reading sentences aloud with moderate scaffolding, listening for pauses at the end of ideas, and identifying sentence boundaries

2. Adding end punctuation and capitals during editing with moderate scaffolding

3. Using both end punctuation and initial capital letters independently during drafting

Accomplishing the stages of this objective might require several weeks. Starting from a baseline frequency of 0 sentence markers for a story with 12 sentences, progress would be reported as actual data from the student's writing produced either as an assessment probe or curricular project. The benchmark of the first subobjective is the demonstration of the knowledge of sentence boundaries by pausing appropriately while rereading during revising and editing. Once the student can use the rereading strategy and demonstrate knowledge of sentence boundaries, the target switches to the twin skills of punctuation and capitalization. Then, progress is measured in written products as the number of sentences the student has punctuated correctly with moderate scaffolding. Finally, the objective is met when the student begins to use capitals and periods independently while drafting.

Horizontal Objective Writing Strategy

A horizontal subobjective strategy differs from a vertical one in that the subobjectives are targeted simultaneously instead of sequentially. It is a multipronged approach to meeting a broader objective with several components. Each subobjective targets a different but related strategy or skill the student needs to learn to accomplish a common language or communicative objective. The following is an example of an objective with horizontally arranged subobjectives for a student functioning at the transitional level who needs to move closer to conventional spelling.

The student will develop conventional spelling skills by

1. Producing multisyllabic words syllable-by-syllable and spelling at least one familiar word part correctly (root morphemes, e.g., *act, tele,* or bound morphemes, e.g., *-ing, un-, pre-, act, -tion, -ed*)

2. Showing knowledge of at least three new word families while drafting (e.g., *-ate, -ight, -ought*)

3. Spelling at least three new high-frequency "tricky" words consistently (e.g., *was, the, and*)

4. Using the computer-supported personal dictionary as a tool for spelling support during drafting

Summary for Objective Writing

Short-term objectives that are effective for guiding intervention and measuring change have three major components—a statement of 1) what the student will do, 2) under what conditions, and 3) how well. When designing intervention, it is helpful to think of objectives in both horizontal and vertical organization. Horizontally organized objectives address related but different targets simultaneously, either in the same activity or in temporal proximity. Vertically organized objectives address stages of development for essentially the same target sequentially, perhaps in increasing levels of maturity or independence. In vertical sequences, higher-level objectives only come into play when lower-level ones have been achieved, but horizontal objectives are addressed in tandem, integrated fashion. Comprehensive plans involve both types of organization. In this chapter, we also emphasize that objectives are not just for students with special needs. They are for everyone. This is a key element of making inclusive, integrated services work to help all children achieve higher levels of competence, no matter what their incoming proficiency levels are.

PLANNING OBJECTIVES ACROSS LANGUAGE TARGETS

When planning objectives, instructors can target writing processes and products as well as spoken and written language interactions.

Targeting Writing Processes and Products

As noted previously, one of the challenges in planning objectives is to use the balance principle to target specific skills within the context of integrated communication events. Balance also is needed for targeting language processes and products. Table 16.2

Table 16.2. Example objectives across language targets

Goal area	The student will
Writing processes	
Planning and organizing	1. Brainstorm topics prior to writing
	2. Use graphic organizers to plan and organize work before writing
	3. Complete discourse organization template prior to writing
	4. Conduct research and write notes for planning
	5. Put information from research sources in own words
	6. Outline story or report
	• With paper and pencil
	• Using computer software
	7. Tell story aloud before drafting
	8. Brainstorm alternative character responses and story endings
Drafting	1. Use planning sheets to guide writing
	2. Work independently for _____ minutes
	3. Integrate ideas from plan into well-constructed draft
	4. Draft with greater fluency, producing at least _____ new words per session
	5. Use _____ computer feature while drafting
	6. Insert punctuation on-line while drafting
	7. Show the confidence to use invented spelling while drafting rather than constantly asking for help
Revising and editing	1. Participate in revising and editing (daily, at prescribed intervals)
	2. Add information to increase ease of reading for audience
	3. Move information to increase organization
	4. Self-evaluate work using a personalized guide sheet for specific skills
	5. Read aloud slowly to monitor for missing or extra words and agreement problems
	6. Identify errors in syntax, word choice, spelling, and punctuation, and correct with _____ (heavy, moderate, or minimal) scaffolding
Publishing and presenting	1. Use computer software features to format and illustrate work prior to publishing
	2. Organize self and work schedule to allow time for final preparation of manuscript before publishing deadline
	3. Look at audience intermittently while presenting work, use a loud enough voice to be heard, and read with an appropriate rate
Written products	
Discourse level	1. Write a more mature story by adding _____ to reach _____ level of narrative maturity
	• Isolated description—character and/or setting described with words
	• Action sequence—at least two events connected temporally
	• Reactive sequence—major events connected causally
	• Abbreviated episode—problem stated and main character's intentions implied
	• Complete episode—clear planning to achieve goal
	• Complex/multiple episodes—obstacle in path, or more than one abbreviated or complete episode
	2. Add _____ (background, character, setting, description) to complete story
	3. Add title, conclusion, and ending to story
	4. Clarify pronoun reference

Goal area	The student will
	5. Write in a consistent point of view
	6. Write in a consistent verb tense
	7. Write an introductory sentence that grabs reader's attention
	8. Organize paragraph information moving from main idea to supporting details
	9. Refrain from including tangential or off-topic information
	10. Write _____ topically related sentences (number)
	11. Write paragraphs with _____ (temporally, causally, logically) related elements
Sentence level	1. Increase variety of sentence types
	2. Limit use of a particular (_____) structure
	3. Write simple sentences with all required elements
	4. Combine sentences using coordinating conjunctions (*and, but, or, so*)
	5. Expand sentences with prepositional phrases
	6. Combine sentences using subordinate clauses (joined with *because, after, since, while, if...then*)
	7. Code switch from "home language" to standard English ("book language")
Word level (spelling)	1. Demonstrate sound–symbol associations
	2. Use phoneme, syllable, and morpheme representation strategies during drafting
	3. Show knowledge of word families of increased numbers (_____) and types: _____
	4. Show knowledge of grammatical and other bound morphemes
	5. State and apply rules for adding morphemes
	6. Use a personal dictionary for assistance in spelling difficult high frequency words
	7. Distinguish multiple spellings for words that sound alike (homophones; e.g., *there/their, to/two/too*) and use the appropriate spelling for the context
	8. Use computer software spelling checker feature to identify problems and revise to correct spellings
Word level (word choice)	1. Change _____ words to more interesting choices
	2. Add _____ descriptive or other interesting words
	3. Use literary techniques of simile, metaphor, and other literary phrasing
	4. Use transitional phrasing in expository writing (e.g., *first, second, finally* in sequential writing; *similarly, in contrast, in comparison* in compare/contrast writing)
Spoken communication	1. Demonstrate attentive listening by • Refraining from interrupting • Refraining from distracting behaviors • Providing nonverbal listening and eye contact cues
	2. Demonstrate effective speech production by • Using a loud enough voice • Initiating and maintaining eye contact with group members • Using clear articulation • Speaking in complete sentences • Relating information in organized fashion • Supplying on-topic contributions in group settings • Using appropriate turn-taking behaviors

continued

Table 16.2.   *(continued)*

Goal area	The student will

	3. Participate actively by
	    • Contributing _____ comments per session
	    • Offering author group feedback related to story interest and clarity

Writing conventions	1. Identify sentence boundaries
	2. Use end punctuation while drafting
	3. Use capitalization to identify
	    • Proper nouns
	    • Initial letters of sentences
	    • Content words in a title
	4. Use punctuation and formatting conventions of dialogue
	5. Divide long text into paragraphs at appropriate points
	6. Use commas to
	    • Divide elements in a series
	    • Set off phrases

uses the system of language targets outlined in Chapter 2 (also discussed in Chapter 15) to suggest objectives across the five written-product goal areas (discourse level, sentence level, word level, spoken communication, and writing conventions). It also includes objectives for students during the areas of the writing process (planning and organizing, drafting, revising and editing, publishing and presenting). These objectives can be further individualized for specific students.

The general strategy is to select or write objectives that target next higher levels over current baseline levels within each domain. The following are examples of objectives that target combined processes and products. Note, as well, that any of the following example objectives could include a vertically organized subsequence that would target, first, performance with heavy scaffolding; second, performance with moderate scaffolding; and third, independent performance.

For a student whose baseline behavior includes a struggle to generate ideas independently, an objective might be "Will brainstorm multiple story ideas, creating a list of three or more." If a student has a baseline behavior tendency of avoiding planning, writing immediately, and producing stories at the level of temporal sequence, an objective might be "Will plan using story grammar supports, provided by a text-based graphic organizer, and produce a narrative that includes a causal relationship." Students whose baseline writings include a dominant use of simple sentences might have the objective "Will combine ideas into complex sentences with a variety of subordinate or relative clauses, using at least three different conjunctions (e.g., *if . . . then, because, although, when, where, after*) or relative pronouns (e.g., *who, which, that*). For a student who has been using an overabundance of pronouns with unclear referents and often leaving readers with inadequate information, the objective might be "Will use revision processes to yield discourse in which all pronoun references are clear and zero instances of inadequate information are left." Finally, a student who has often refused to take the author chair, whose reading decoding abilities are still emerging, and who tends to give minimal responses in spoken communication, might have as an objective "Will willingly take the author chair, read independently, and respond with substance to questions asked by peers about work."

Note that areas of overlap between language levels also can be addressed in objective writing. For instance, a discourse-level objective to include more description to meet audience needs might be accompanied by a sentence-level objective to include sentences with prepositional and adverbial phrases and a word-level objective to include adjectives, adverbs, and uncommon vocabulary. An example of such a horizontally organized objective might be

Will produce a story at least at the level of "reactive sequence"

- In which the characters and relationships are described with a majority of complex correct sentences

- Combined with at least three different conjunctions

- With at least five examples of high-level, unusual vocabulary (spelled independently at the transitional level)

Progress for any of these objectives would be documented with data gathered during observations of the student's writing processes and examples of increased performance in the student's successive written narratives.

Objectives derived within and across categories must be modified to achieve an appropriate balance between parts and wholes for individual students. For example, Dan was a student who experienced difficulty at the discourse level in his early writing lab experiences. His early story writing attempts were minimal, with few words per story. He initiated two stories, with 10 and 15 words respectively, while his peers (students with LLDs, like Dan) were producing an average of three- to four stories, with more than 50 words each. In addition to these observations, discussions with Dan and his mother revealed idea generation and discourse comprehension to be areas of major concern. Vertically organized objectives were established for Dan to increase his ease in generating story ideas and producing more mature and longer stories. It was decided that production fluency (measured as numbers of words per story), as well as story grammar levels, could serve as indicators for the second subobjective. Within the second subobjective is a vertical hierarchy sequence. Dan's objective read as follows.

Dan will show increased discourse-level skills by

1. Using brainstorming to generate multiple ideas while planning

2. Producing more mature stories, measured as

    Increased fluency in terms of numbers of words per story (more than the baseline of 12.5 words per story)

    Higher levels of story grammar maturity above his baseline level of "isolated description"

    - Temporal (action) sequence—with events arranged sequentially

    - Causal (reactive) sequence—with events described causally

    - Abbreviated episode—with a stated problem and implied goal direction

Joseph was another student with limited fluency. Although his first written story was only 15 words in length, Joseph told much longer and more detailed stories in spoken language. Joseph's greatest challenges were with spelling. His invented spellings were sometimes at prephonetic levels, and Joseph seemed to limit his word choices and written language formulation based on his uncertainty in how to spell. For Joseph, addressing his fluency problems meant starting at the word level, not the discourse level. Joseph's stronger spoken discourse skills were used to help him generate a greater variety of words at the same time his sound–symbol association and emerging orthographic skills (e.g., *-ed, -ing*) were targeted. This yielded an objective with horizontal organizational structure, except for subobjective sequences.

Joseph will show increased phonetic spelling abilities by

1. Producing stories with increased numbers of

    Total words over his baseline of 15

    Different words over his baseline of 8

2. Using increased phonetic-alphabetic (sound–symbol association) knowledge to spell novel words—with letters representing complete phonemic information (not necessarily conventional spelling) for all words in his stories, with

    Heavy scaffolding

    Moderate scaffolding

    Minimal scaffolding

    Independence

3. Developing emerging knowledge of morphologic-orthographic (word chunk to spelling pattern) associations as evident in spelling chunks of words (e.g., *-ing, -ed, un-*) with not more than moderate scaffolding

For Joseph, progress was measured by counting the total number of words and number of different words in his subsequent compositions. As noted in Chapter 15, the computer analysis program SALT (Miller & Chapman, 2000) offers a handy tool for performing such computations, but for short samples like Joseph's, the counts may be performed by hand. Joseph's SLP also analyzed the proportion of words he spelled phonetically and the proportion of times when he demonstrated emerging knowledge of morphemic and orthographic patterns in his spelling when opportunities presented themselves. Although we did not use this measure for Joseph, a standard word processing program also could have been used to tally the number of letters (characters) Joseph produced per word as a means of capturing his attempts to accurately spell higher-level, more phonemically complex words.

Targeting Spoken and Written Language Interactions

Language demands in the classroom involve reciprocal interactions between spoken and written language. Although most students show similar skills in both, many have some language skills that are relatively stronger in one modality or the other. For example a student who has difficulty at the discourse level while writing might demonstrate better discourse skills while telling stories in spoken language. This can serve as a starting place for building a bridge to more mature written language. Another student, who uses faulty sentence structure when speaking, might benefit from focusing on sentence-structure in its written form while drafting, rereading, and revising.

Colin, like Joseph, showed stronger oral storytelling skills than written ones, also related to his spelling weaknesses. A strategy for Colin was to use his oral story telling as a planning and organizing strategy and to provide written supports in the form of words from his spoken story as print support in a word bank that could remain on the side of his computer screen (Chapter 8 describes such features as supports for drafting). For Colin, the word bank was generated with paper and pencil, then entered into a software program that supported customized word banks. With this tool, Colin could easily access printed words during drafting. His integrated word and discourse level objective read as follows.

Colin will show increased discourse-level and word-level maturity by

1. Telling his story aloud to an educator during planning

2. Entering words from the paper-and-pencil version accurately into his computer-supported word bank

3. Using words from his personal word bank when drafting his story

Sarah, a fifth-grade student, showed a different pattern of strengths and needs (see Chapters 14 and 15). Sarah demonstrated disorganized discourse in both spoken and written domains, but she did not have the spelling difficulties exhibited by Joseph and Colin. Sarah's mother reported that she could not keep track of her daughter's conversations. Sarah's teacher observed similar difficulties when Sarah attempted to organize and sequence her ideas in written stories or when she tried to summarize her reading assignments using spoken language. In a baseline written story probe, Sarah wrote two disconnected sentences to produce a story attempt judged as isolated description. In a baseline spoken story probe, she shifted topic mid-sentence and reenacted her story as a drama, speaking in first person for her characters, rather than retelling it using narration. Sarah's contributions in author group often were tangential or lacked key information.

Sarah's discourse needs were addressed with relatively greater success using the more permanent structure of written language, which allowed Sarah time to review and revise her language in a more systematic and recursive manner than she could manage while speaking. Spoken language discourse also was targeted, but work on it was built into related activities drawing on her recent written-language experience. That is, Sarah's instructional objectives addressed the discourse level by focusing on written language partially as a support to spoken communication. Sarah's discourse objectives had three subobjectives (see also Box 16.1): Sarah will demonstrate discourse-level skills for staying on topic by

1. Writing a story

    Using written notes to organize and cue spoken narratives containing three temporally related pieces of information

    Writing a story with temporally and causally linked information

2. Participating actively in author group

    Writing three-point notes in preparation

Expressing herself in a clear, concise manner while explaining the focus of her topic

Making no inappropriate or off-topic responses during presentation and using her fingers to tick off main points

3. Commenting on or answering a question in each large group session while staying on topic

Aaron also was an elementary-school student participating in an after-school writing lab. Aaron's case example was introduced in Chapter 2 (Box 2.1). Like Sarah, Aaron's needs were clearly evident in his conversational spoken language as well as in his written language. There were differences, however. Whereas Sarah's spoken language was affected in the area of language use, involving pragmatics and discourse organization, Aaron's greatest difficulties were in the area of language form, involving phonology, morphology, and syntax. Most obvious were Aaron's confusions in articulating the phonemes /w/, /r/, and /l/. He confused these three liquid and glide phonemes consistently in both spoken and written forms. For example, Aaron's spelling errors paralleled his speech confusions, as seen in baseline story productions of "ras" for *was* and "sal" for *saw.*

Objectives for Aaron targeted parallel phonological developments in spoken and written language. Intervention was aimed at taking advantage of reciprocal relationships discussed in Chapter 2. Techniques included teaching phonemic awareness and discrimination while helping Aaron develop sound–symbol associations for sounding out words. Aaron also benefited from memorizing the spellings of certain frequently

---

Box 16.1.   Sarah's News Story

Sarah produced the following story for her class newspaper project while working on her three objectives.

Babysittng

Babysitting is fun and you get paid. It's fun because you get to know the kids. Here are some tips about babysitting and how it can be a lot of fun. Activities are a good thing to keep the kids occupied.

Practicing with your little brother is a good way to become a baby sitter. Now, here are some babysitting questions to ask parents. What to feed the kids and what don't to feed the kids like candy and pop. When do the kids go to bed?

I interviewed Mrs. Van Meter. She is a parent, and a expert about babysitters. She gave good advice about where you can get babysitters. Mrs. Van Meter said you can, ask your friends, and put up adds. She said what kind of babysitters are fun, and good. I think babysitting is fun and you get to know a lot.

used words, such as *all, saw, was, were,* and *are,* using a special minilesson page in his author notebook, which he learned to turn to independently as both a speaking and spelling reference. He commented that if he could spell a word, he could say it. Aaron's word-level objective read as follows.

Aaron will show improved production of the phonemes /w/, /r/, and /l/ in written and spoken words by

1. Producing accurate spellings of the words *all, saw, was, were,* and *are,* using

    Phonemic awareness and sound–symbol associations (with instructor scaffolding reducing vertically from heavy to light)

    Memorized patterns (starting with reference to written author notebook supports and transitioning to independent productions)

2. Producing accurate articulations for words, including the phonemes /w/, /r/, and /l/, by

    Referring to print supports and memorized spelling patterns

    Demonstrating phonemic awareness by articulating the correct phonemes in sequence

DOCUMENTING EVIDENCE OF CHANGE

The measurement strategies proposed here can be used to document higher quality, greater consistency, and more independent use over time. Several measurement strategies could be used to document change, for example:

- Repeat the baseline sampling procedure, and analyze resulting processes and products for targeted improvements.

- Chart daily growth in writing lab work, and keep a journal with descriptions of progress.

- Collect evidence from outside sources.

In addition to noting changes in specific objective areas, instructors should be vigilant for opportunities to document broader outcomes. Along the road to capable writing, we have observed turning points as students have developed new self-perceptions and independent risk taking that extend beyond task and curriculum. The case study for Spencer, which appears in Chapter 13, showed how this occurred for him.

Along with educators tracking change, students can participate actively in choosing targets and documenting new learning. Students are involved in constructing versions of their objectives to keep in their author notebooks. These are brought out frequently for reference and to support self-evaluation of students' own learning. This strategy is consistent with both the constructive learning and ownership principles and promotes student-directed learning.

Marcus was a fourth grader who was introduced in Chapter 1 (see Table 1.2 for a list of goals he kept in his author notebook). Most of his schoolwork was average, but he had difficulty completing it independently and staying on task. His mother attributed some reading comprehension difficulties to Marcus's not knowing all of the word meanings. His teacher also was concerned that Marcus rarely volunteered to contribute to classroom discussions. She described his listening comprehension as good "when we're reading stories out loud or we're reading social studies and science." She noted as well that when Marcus did volunteer, his answers were accurate; however, when he was asked to do an assignment, he procrastinated.

Marcus's teacher referred him for the after-school CREW lab held at his elementary school because she thought that writing with computers might encourage him to communicate more of his ideas. Marcus was well liked by both his teachers and peers. His mother described him as a compassionate child who might be afraid to raise his hand in formal class interactions, but who got along well with peers. This is indeed what was observed in the CREW lab. His mother and teacher both identified the most significant areas of need for Marcus as self-organization and independent goal-directed focus to stay on track and complete academic activities.

Baseline Sample: A Starting Place

Marcus wrote his baseline probe after being given directions designed to elicit expository discourse (see Chapter 14). That is, he was asked to think about a topic that was interesting to him and to plan and write a report about it. The techniques used to analyze the probe were those described in Chapter 15. The SLP graduate clinician who was working with Marcus produced the following summary of his probe.

Writing Processes—To plan his baseline sample, Marcus independently chose the topic of helicopters, which he introduced as a "choper." He used a semantic web to plan with words or phrases in each bubble. When drafting, Marcus incorporated the ideas from his plan by beginning with a topic sentence and following with supporting sentences. Marcus did not return to his draft to revise or edit when he was finished writing.

Written Product—In his baseline sample (Figure 16.1), Marcus formed 5 complex incorrect [ci] sentences, relying on the syntactic formula, "they used it for/when . . . " He has difficulty with prepositions and verb tense cohesion, resulting in several awkward sentences and one illogical sentence: "They used the choper for the museons if you dress up as a army man." His MLTU of 12.17 reflected his ability to combine several ideas in one sentence, but the high rate of syntactic difficulty reflected problems with the sentence combining process, as well as with the lack of review and revision. At the word level, he used some interesting words but overused many of the same words—producing 38 different words within 73 total words, 12 of which (16%) were misspelled. His spelling was judged to be at the conventional level.

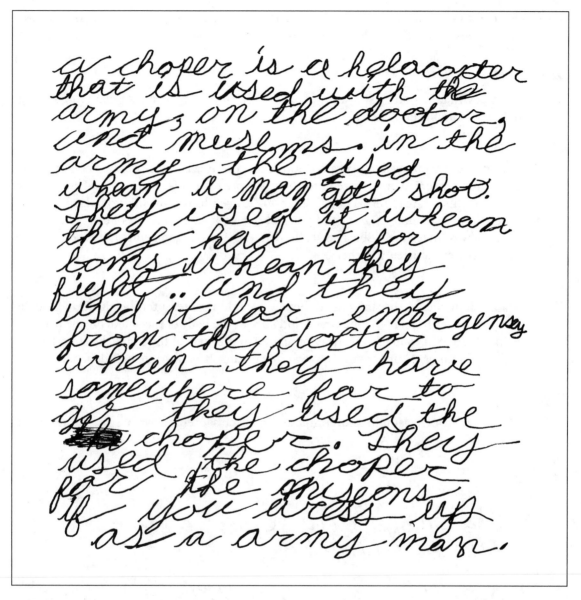

Figure 16.1. Marcus's helicopter story.

Goals, Objectives, and First Semester Progress

Marcus's goals and objectives were developed to take him beyond these baseline levels. The SLP graduate clinician and Marcus talked about the goals, and the clinician scaffolded Marcus to describe the goals using his own words. The goal page, which preceded the goals listed in Table 1.2, had a special place in Marcus's author notebook so he could refer to it during his two sessions per week. During the fall semester, the students in the CREW lab selected their own topics to research and write about. Marcus decided to write about snakes. Intervention techniques and progress for Marcus after 15 sessions during 3 months were reported for each objective.

Objective 1

Marcus will take notes using a numbering/bulleting form or other organizing strategy of his own on his chosen topic.

Intervention

Marcus was encouraged to read a portion of his resource book, close the book or darken the computer screen, and write notes on his topic using his own words. The clinician modeled this strategy for Marcus. She also showed him how she organized her own notes for her graduate courses and pointed out how each note was bulleted and each heading was underlined. She also scaffolded Marcus to organize his notes so that similar ideas were written together.

Progress

Marcus immediately began to use bullets while taking notes after the clinician modeled it. He told the clinician that he wrote notes about the body of the snake on one page (see Figure 16.2). If he found a new idea not related to the body of the snake, he started a new page in his notes. Marcus came up with this organizational strategy independently.

Objective 2

Marcus will form simple and compound correct sentences with scaffolding by the clinician.

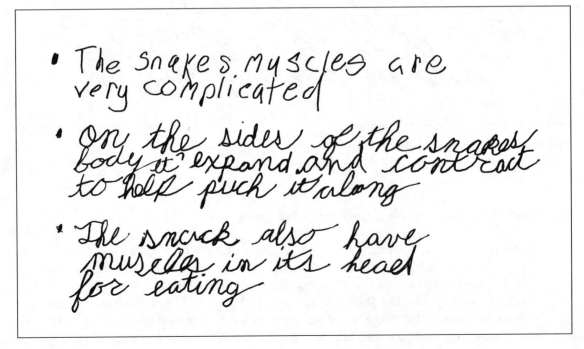

Figure 16.2. Marcus's notes about the body of the snake.

Intervention

Marcus was scaffolded to 1) read his sentences aloud to himself and check whether they made sense; 2) allow the clinician to read sentences and paragraphs to him, then judge whether they were correct; and 3) change or rewrite his sentences so that they were correct by adding or deleting words to make a sentence logical.

Progress

Marcus continued to have difficulty identifying a sentence as incorrect when he read it aloud for himself, although he generally could identify incorrect sentences when they were read aloud by the clinician. Occasionally, Marcus added missing elements while reading aloud without recognizing that the words were not present in his writing. This suggests that he needs additional practice reading and reflecting on what he has written, but that his oral language skills are relatively stronger. The clinician provided moderate scaffolding to help Marcus correct all of his sentences for the published draft of his article.

Objective 3

Marcus will revise and edit his work by

1. Checking that a variety of sentence types appear

2. Moving ideas or sentences around to make the best organization

3. Using the spelling checker to identify and correct spelling errors

4. Checking that all words and concepts that might be unfamiliar to a reader are explained in the written piece

5. Checking that sentences have capital letters and periods in the right places

Intervention

Scaffolding was used to encourage Marcus to cross out and revise first on paper, due to limited computer time (see Figure 16.3), then to transfer these changes to the computer, where the clinician showed him how to use the cut-and-paste features. During drafting, the clinician encouraged Marcus to use his best independent spelling and scaffolded him to say words slowly in syllables when he was unsure of them to hear the sounds in sequence. The spelling checker feature was introduced during revising with scaffolding whether to "accept" or "reject" suggested spellings. A self-questioning strategy was taught to remind him to ask himself how to begin and end sentences and whether his meaning would be clear for his audience.

Progress

In his final draft, Marcus revised his sentences (with scaffolding) to make his paragraphs clear and concise. He used the spelling checker first with some scaffolding and then independently. He capitalized the beginning letter of each sentence in his final draft. Marcus used computer-supported revising features by blocking and deleting text and placing the cursor in the correct place to add text. His published product appears in Figure 16.4.

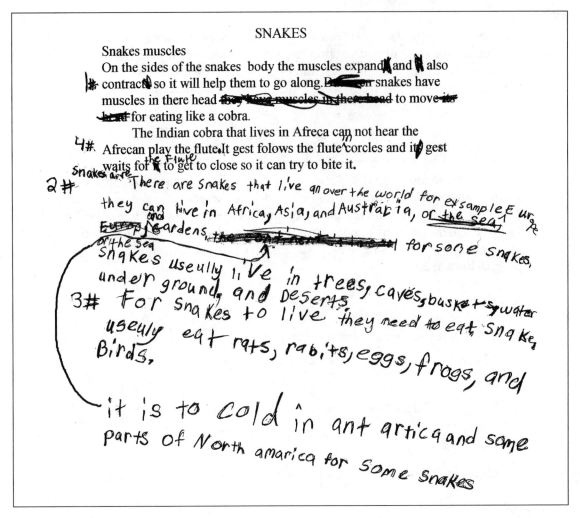

Figure 16.3. Marcus's revisions on paper.

Second Probe: Establishing New Objectives

Marcus wrote his second probe following the same directions for expository discourse samples used for the baseline probe. This time, he chose to write about tigers. His clinician's analysis, using the techniques described in Chapter 15, yielded the following evidence of growth and continued needs.

> Writing Processes—Marcus had difficulty choosing a topic for this sample and also required scaffolding (e.g., "What do tigers look like?") to formulate supporting information for his topic. After he got started, he created a semantic map with a single-level hierarchy (Figure 16.5), which he referred to often as he drafted his story. Marcus stated that the concept map made writing easier. He used the ideas on the map but also added details as he drafted. He made one capitalization and one spelling revision while drafting but did not revise or edit after drafting, even when prompted by the clinician.

SNAKES

Snakes muscles

On the sides of the snakes body the muscles expand and also contract so it will help them to go along. Snakes have muscles in their head to move for eating like a cobra.

The Indian cobra that lives in Africa can not hear the African play the flute. It just follows the flute circles and its just waits for it to get too close so it can try to bite it.

Where snakes live

There are snakes that live all over the world for example they can live in Africa, Asia, and Australia, or Europe. They also live in the sea, and gardens. It is too cold in Antarctica and some parts of North America for some snakes. Snakes usually live in trees, caves, baskets, water, underground, and deserts. For snakes to live they need to eat. Snakes usually eat rats, rabbits, eggs, frogs, and birds.

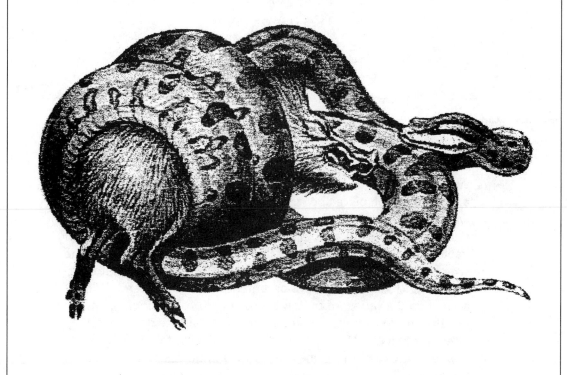

Figure 16.4. Marcus's snake story.

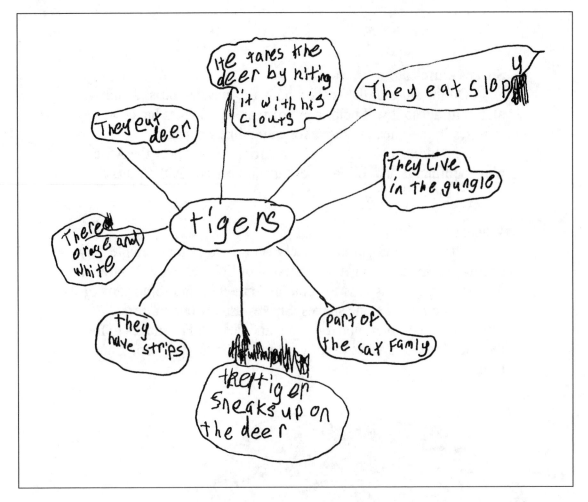

Figure 16.5.   Marcus's semantic map for his tiger story.

Written Product—In his second probe (Figure 16.6), Marcus produced a two-paragraph piece about tigers. At the discourse level, his report was creative and original. He used a conversational style and sense of humor. Marcus clustered ideas into subtopics (e.g., description, eating habits), but each paragraph contained three different topics, and he switched topics abruptly without transition. He did not use introductory or concluding paragraphs or sentences. At the sentence level, Marcus used a variety of sentence structures, producing six simple correct [sc] and four complex correct sentences [cc], one demonstrating attention to logic, "There [they're] part of the cat family so if someone from the cat family comes up they won't hert each other." Although he did not use all capitalization and punctuation conventions correctly, when he did use periods, he followed them with capital letters in the next sentence. At the word level, he used interesting and mature word choices (e.g., *sneaks, intelligent*). He misspelled 13 of 85

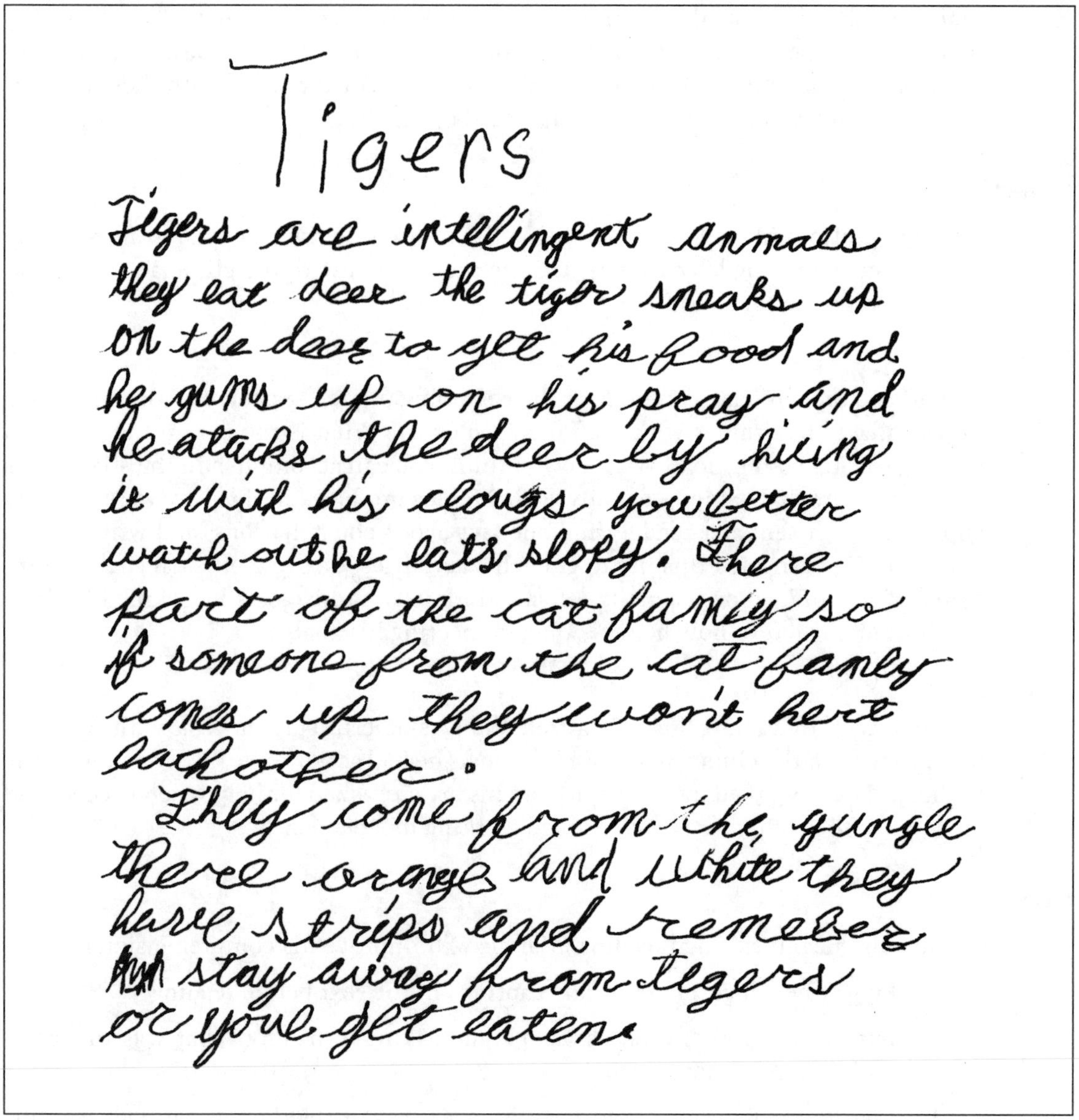
Tigers

Tigers are intelingent anmals
they eat deer the tiger sneaks up
on the deer to get his food and
he gums up on his pray and
he atacks the deer by hiting
it with his clougs you better
watch out he eats slopy. There
part of the cat famly so
if someone from the cat famly
comes up they won't hert
eachother.
They come from the gungle
there orange and white they
have strips and remeber
stay away from tigers
or youl get eaten.

Figure 16.6. Marcus's tiger story.

total words (15%), and misspellings were phonetically and/or visually (orthographically) similar to the target words.

Goals, Objectives, and Second Semester Progress

For the second semester, the planning team decided to have the students select their topics around the theme of outer space. A field trip to the local planetarium was planned to help the students build interest and world knowledge in potential subtopics. During the next 3 months, Marcus attended 19 sessions in which he worked on his goals and objectives while planning, researching, and writing a report on constellations. At the conclusion of this semester, Marcus's SLP (another graduate student clinician) reported the following progress on the goals that corresponded with those on Marcus's personal goal page shown in Chapter 1 (Figure 1.2).

Objective 1

Self-organization: Marcus will establish a list of three to five personal goals to be accomplished in writing lab each day, writing them down with the clinician and checking them off as he finishes them.

Intervention

Marcus and the clinician conferred at the beginning of each session. He formulated his list of three to five things with scaffolding, such as "What is the next thing you need to do in writing your article? What do you think you can accomplish in the 30 minutes we have to work?" Examples of daily goals Marcus produced in this way were: 1) write an introduction sentence; and 2) find one fact about constellations, and write it on a note card. He then used this list to guide his activities, crossing off each goal as completed. The clinician occasionally refocused Marcus on his goals by asking him how much time was left or how he was doing in meeting his goals.

Progress

As Marcus drafted and edited his article, he was able to stay on task with minimal prompting from the clinician. He used the goals he had set to guide his work during the session. Marcus worked independently on his article, asked for help when needed, and returned to the computer and continued working independently.

Objective 2

Reading for meaning: When reading, Marcus will improve his comprehension by

1. Looking at headings, pictures, and captions in the text before reading

2. Stopping at the end of each paragraph and asking himself, "What was this paragraph about? What did I learn?"

3. Writing down a few key words or a sentence on a note card to use later when drafting his article

Intervention

The clinician used a personal minilesson to introduce Marcus to the strategy of looking at headings, pictures, and captions before reading the text, using several sources available in the library to model the process. She also taught him to stop at the ends of paragraphs for self-questioning and scaffolded him to practice the notetaking strategy he had learned the first semester.

Progress

At the end of the semester, as Marcus referred to books for information, he looked at pictures, headings, and captions in order to help him locate specific information in the text prior to reading. While reading, he continued to require cues to stop at the end of each paragraph but showed improving skills in recalling and understanding what he read in his paraphrases of the material for notetaking. He occasionally referred back to the text to remind himself of content.

Objective 3

Oral communication: During author group, Marcus will

1. Maintain eye contact with his conversational partners while they are speaking to improve his listening and his comprehension

2. Provide the peer author with one positive comment

3. Provide the peer author with one suggestion that could improve his or her work

Intervention

Because Marcus often fidgeted or manipulated objects during listening tasks, the clinician was not sure he was listening and comprehending, especially when he could not answer questions or give feedback about what was said. He was scaffolded to look at the speaker and to provide appropriate feedback to his peers regarding their work (e.g., "Could you tell Jonathan something you liked about his article? Could you suggest something he could add or change?")

Progress

During the last sessions of writing lab, Marcus recalled what it took to be a good listener by checking his author notebook minilesson materials. He maintained eye contact with the speaker and provided feedback with substantive information ("I liked when you said it would take 10 trillion years to get to the Big Dipper"). Prior to the publishing party, Marcus watched himself on videotape and determined independently that he needed to look at his audience during the presentation of his article. He decided to "read until there is one word before the period, then remember it and look up, then say the word." He used this strategy to maintain eye contact with his audience during the presentation of his article at the publishing party.

Objective 4

Writing: Marcus will improve his discourse organization, spelling, and use of writing conventions while drafting, revising, and editing, by using

1. A topic sentence, as least three supporting ideas, and a summary sentence in each paragraph

2. Capitalization and punctuation to mark sentence boundaries

3. Spelling checker to identify and correct spelling errors with clinician scaffolding

Intervention

While researching his topic, Marcus was given note cards and scaffolded to put one idea on each card so that he could group them into "facts that go together." When necessary, a feedback scaffold was used (e.g., "Do these two facts go together? Let's read them and see if they talk about the same topic?") Next, Marcus was guided to label each group with a phrase telling why they go together. These labels formed the basis for his introductory sentences, given the scaffold to think, "What is this paragraph going to be about?" To encourage the use of writing conventions to mark off sentences, Marcus was taught to use self-talk to prompt himself to remember writing conventions and to become aware of natural breaks where they belonged. When Marcus paused after typing an idea, for example, the clinician asked him, "Is that the end of one idea or one of your thoughts? What should you be reminding yourself just now?" The clinician also scaffolded Marcus to make thoughtful decisions as he practiced using the spelling-checker feature.

Progress

In his final article (see Figure 16.7), Marcus used the spelling checker as well as his resources to correct spelling (e.g., when he could not remember how to spell the name of a specific star, he independently went to the library shelves and looked in a book where he had found the information). He marked all sentence boundaries with minimal cues from his peers and clinician. He was able to use his organization strategies with minimal scaffolding to produce a three-paragraph article. He required prompting to indent his paragraphs. Each paragraph contained an introductory sentence and three facts from his note cards. When asked "Why was it so easy for you to keep working on your article by yourself and not get distracted?" Marcus replied, "Because . . . I'm so organized!"

ENGAGING STUDENTS IN MEASURING CHANGE

With our colleagues, we have developed a number of tools to support the process of helping students develop ownership for their goals. Figure 16.8 illustrates the "What I Did Today" tool introduced in Figure 4.4 for keeping track of the stages of the writing process. Marcus and his instructor used this form to record his daily activities and communicate specifically about the steps he was taking to improve his writing processes and products.

It has been our practice in recent writing lab experiences to take story-writing probes three times per school year—once in September, once in January or February, and once in April or May. During one inclusive writing lab, we decided that it would nice for our third-grade students, as well as their teachers, to see the evidence of their progress. We developed the student self-evaluation tool that appears in the Chapter 4 appendix. An example of how this form was completed by Randy (who was introduced in Box 6.2) appears in Figure 16.9. The wonderful thing about this particular illustration is that Randy, who had started the school year as a reluctant writer, found joy in writing by mid-year. By the end of the school year, Randy initiated the request to use the form to evaluate his third probe in comparison to his second.

Both of these examples are important to convey the value of engaging students in evaluating their own progress. The more students can become aware of the specific standards for writing processes and products, the more they can play the central role in directing the change process in their own lives.

CONSTELLATIONS

CONSTELLATION

This paragraph is about history of constellations. In the 16 century explorers went to the southern seas and mapped the southern sky. That means they wrote down the stars. They went to the sea and saw the stars that nobody knew about and the map became ancient. The men had a long piece of paper and put down the stars and saw things like animals and traced them the men named the 88 constellations so they could remember them. Constellations have been developed as early as 4,000 B.C almost 6,000 years ago.

This paragraph is about describing constellation. There are 1,300 bright stars in the constellations. When you look at the constellations you can see bright stars and dull ones. It's harder to find the rest of the bare constellation because the stars are dull and more spread out than the big dipper. There are 88 constellations in the sky they move every month and they are very far away.

Leo the lion is a constellation. Leo the lion has 15 stars in its body there is a big star in the lions foot. Leo the lion's hart is a star called Regales. The best time to see him is April. I picked Leo the lion because he is one of my favorite animals.

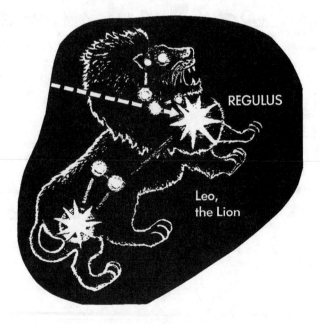

REGULUS

Leo,
the Lion

Figure 16.7. Marcus's constellation story.

What I Did Today...

Circle one.
Monday/Wednesday
Oct. 22, 1997
Month   Day,   Year

Topic **Snakes**

Circle all you did today.
Researching & Planning   Dráfting   Revising

My Comments: garden snakes dont bight

Teacher's Comments We worked on note-taking & searching
on computer. CMB

Circle one.
Monday/Wednesday
H   3   91
Month   Day,   Year

Topic **Snakes**

Circle all you did today.
Researching & Planning   **Drafting**   Revising

My Comments: next time we are going to use the computer

Teacher's Comments Marcus worked very hard today learning
how to organize notes.

Circle one.
Monday/Wednesday
1/10/97
Month   Day,   Year

Topic Snakes

Circle all you did today.
Researching & Planning   **Drafting**   Revising

My Comments: working on computers

Teacher's Comments Marcus put his notes into the computer—
need to move to paragraphs

Circle one.
Monday/Wednesday
1/17/97
Month   Day,   Year

Topic Snakes

Circle all you did today.
Researching & Planning   Drafting   Revising

My Comments: Goal: 2 paragraphs

Teacher's Comments didn+ get to youse the
computer that much

Figure 16.8.   What I Did Today tool completed by Marcus.

Student Self-Evaluation

About my story	First story	Second story
	Number of sentences: 3	Number of sentences: 19
	Number of words: 27	Number of words: 215
Setting	Where? none When? none Who? none Main Characters: none Others:	Where? home When? one day Who? me mom dad Main Characters: Others:
What was the problem?	I don't have any-thing Todo	My dad smoking and Driking beer
How was it solved? How did it end?	name People that Went to my Pird	I Sad if you don't Stop smoking you can't go to my birthday Pirty
Special words and facts that made my story interesting:		My birthday

Figure 16.9. Student self-evaluation tool completed by Randy.

SUMMARY

In this chapter, we have described the process of writing goals, short-term objectives, and benchmarks as one that is both comprehensive and flexible. In this way, it exemplifies both the balance principle and the dynamic principle. We also have reiterated the importance of the constructive learning and ownership principles, by showing how students can be involved in writing versions of their goals for inclusion in their author notebooks and in analyzing their own written language samples.

Both writing process and language product targets can be used to provide organizing schemas for instructional objectives. In most cases, the integrated activities of the writing lab approach call for combined objectives targeting integrated knowledge, skills, and strategies. Subobjectives can be arranged with either a vertical (sequential) or horizontal (simultaneous) pattern. Vertical patterns work best for moving through writing process stages and for gradually withdrawing scaffolding support and targeting increased independence. Horizontal patterns work best when students need to learn multiple, strategic approaches to complete a process, such as several approaches to planning or to spelling unknown words.

Chapter 16 ends with the case example of Marcus, which illustrates these principles and procedures for writing objectives and documenting progress. It leads naturally into the final chapter of the book, which presents evidence of change of two types—group data demonstrating quantitative evidence of change and individual stories of change demonstrating both quantitative and qualitative evidence that the writing lab approach can make a difference in students' lives.

17

Evidence of Change

Is there evidence to support that a writing lab approach works to enhance the language and learning of students in inclusive settings? To answer this question, it is necessary to show that all students benefit. First, one must show that the approach results in success for students with language disorders and other special education needs. For these students, success can be measured as achievement of the outcomes targeted by students' IEPs, enriched by indicators of growth in broader academic and social arenas.

Second, it is necessary to demonstrate that the inclusive, collaborative efforts of the team result in success for the *other* students who participate in the writing lab activities—ranging from students with literate language learning risks to students with unusually strong academic and literate language learning abilities. In Chapter 13, we provide evidence from teacher interviews to respond to the fear of many general educators that the writing lab approach will add on activities that take them outside of their regular curriculum, but it is not enough simply to show that including students with special needs does not distract from addressing general education goals. An inclusive program cannot be considered successful, and it is not likely to be adopted, unless success can be demonstrated for all students in a classroom, across a broad range of ability levels.

In this chapter, we offer qualitative and quantitative, individual and group evidence that positive growth does occur for all students in a writing lab approach. Quantitative data are summarized for three probes gathered for a group of elementary school students in three third-grade inner-city classrooms across a school year. Interwoven with the group data are seven individual case studies for students with identified special education needs who were included in those classrooms during writing lab activities. Finally, to demonstrate the potential for growth among secondary as well as elementary school students, the chapter ends with a case study for an eighth-grade student with learning disabilities who participated in an after-school computer-supported writing lab experience.

USING A CASE STUDY FORMAT TO DOCUMENT CHANGE

In addition to providing evidence of change, the case study format used in this chapter can serve as a model for making periodic reports to those immediately interested in a particular student's progress. We have found this format preferable to much longer reports, both for those who have to write the reports (e.g., the report card timed feedback on progress required for compliance with IDEA), and for those who read them. This format also helps teams organize information and think about individualizing instruction for particular students. Although detailed case studies are constructed primarily for students with special language-learning needs, all students (and their instructors) can benefit from goal-directed learning to reach new heights of success and to mark and celebrate progress along the way. Learning the format becomes a way of thinking about students that can be applied for keeping track of all students' needs and for planning appropriate levels and methods of challenge and support. It also can help teams implement the research principle by reflecting on their own skills and ways they can improve the team's performance and student outcomes.

Over the years during which we have developed this abbreviated case study format, we have used it to report on student progress to students, parents, teachers, and school administrators, as well as to broader audiences interested in learning about the writing lab approach. The format draws on data gathered and summarized using the procedures and tools presented in Chapters 15 and 16. The case study format has four parts: 1) baseline description of a student at the start of a reporting period, 2) goals and benchmarks, 3) instructional strategies, and 4) evidence of change at the end of the reporting period. In addition to using descriptive and quantitative data to provide evidence of change, actual samples of the student's work (both probes and portfolio samples, including works in progress) are used to provide concrete, and often the most compelling, evidence of change. Boxes 17.1 through 17.4 provide examples of how varied the descriptions can be, depending on the focus at a particular stage in a student's development.

Baseline Description

The baseline description should provide a snapshot of the student at the beginning of a reporting period. In addition to personal descriptors, such as gender, age, grade, and any special education diagnosis, the baseline description should summarize the student's primary strengths and needs. It also should include key data points from the writing sample assessment worksheet (e.g., numbers of words and types of sentences produced in probes, examples of spelling patterns). These can serve as starting points for establishing benchmarks that will move the student toward improved written and spoken language outcomes.

Box 17.1. Case Study for Natividad

At the beginning of the school year, Natividad was a third grader (chronological age 8;10) with speech-language impairments, who was learning English as a second language to her family's native Spanish. Natividad displayed the following behavior:

- Avoided writing by shuffling papers, looking down at the floor, putting a finger in her mouth
- Provided minimal responses to questions and scaffolding
- Used limited vocabulary in written and spoken expression

In her initial probe (see Figure 17.1), she produced

- A concrete topic organized as an isolated description
- Spelling skills at the conventional level
- A mismatch between her planning and her first draft, with inadequate cohesion and information for audience (e.g., never mentioned *sister* as referent for *she* in first draft, although *sister* was in the plan).
- An overreliance on a single syntactic pattern, but at the [cc] level.

Goals and benchmarks were established for Natividad to

- Initiate interaction and respond appropriately in groups
- Demonstrate increased self-confidence by being willing to participant in formal presentations and peer group interactions
- Use more varied and specific vocabulary, including action verbs, other specific vocabulary, and correct verb tense (from IEP goals).

Instructional strategies and supports for Natividad were designed to

- Modify the environment (e.g., by helping Natividad find a quiet place during drafting so that she could concentrate; bringing in a special, small audience of selected family and friends when Natividad was unable to present her poetry to the larger group assembly).
- Demonstrate patience to wait for Natividad to initiate ideas and respond to questions during scaffolding.
- Expand vocabulary through interest in culturally and personally relevant authentic material (e.g., she blossomed when writing a story about a trip back to Central America and when she could share vocabulary and experiences with her interested classmates).
- Hold Natividad accountable for increasing independence (e.g., teacher scaffolding, "I'm going to check back with you.")

Natividad, at the end of the school year (see Figure 17.2), displayed

- Increased confidence (willing to share work from author chair)
- Increased genre repertoire (e.g., poetry) and use of story grammar web for planning

(continued)

Box 17.1.   *(continued)*

- Expanded vocabulary (e.g., *characters, setting, drinking fountain, pushed*)
- Increased fluency (length in words during 1-hour probe)
- Attempts at complex sentences and irregular past tense verbs
- Increased sense of self as a full member of the class as indicated by social involvement of friends in problem solving

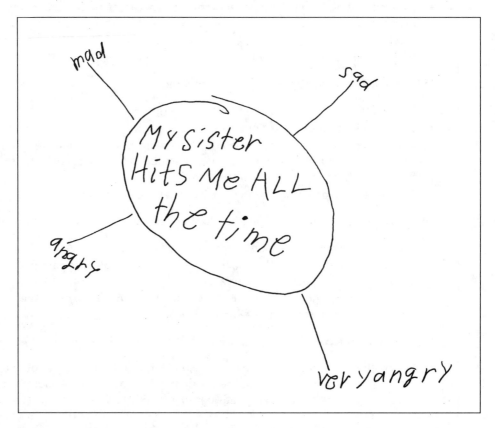

Figure 17.1.   Natividad's initial graphic and written plan and drafted probe.

(continued)

Goals and Benchmarks

The goals and benchmarks in these case study profiles often are cryptic versions of targets that would be presented in greater detail in more formal documents. They are similar to the goals that we recommend writing in collaboration with students in their author notebooks. These goals should reflect IEP goals for students who have them, but they are specific to writing lab language-learning opportunities and the outcomes that can result from them, essentially acting as subobjectives from the more formal plans. As a reminder, writing lab goals might include any spoken or written language objective that could be targeted in other contexts. Examples include contributions to oral

Box 17.1. *(continued)*

My sister is very hice to Me and MY nom is haveing a baby and it's in october 6d 1999.

It makes mae sad when she hits me.
It makes me mad when she hits mes
It malkes me angry when she hits me.
It makes m very mad when she hits me.

(continued)

Box 17.1.   *(continued)*

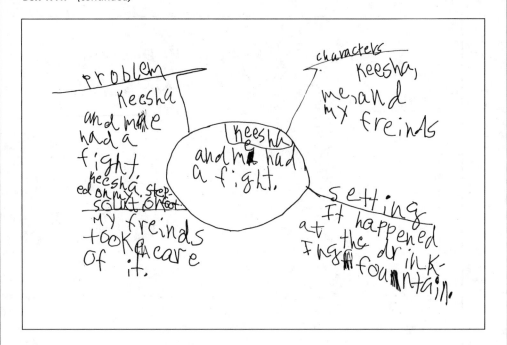

problem
Keesha
and me
had a
fight,
keesha step-
ed on my
foot
my freinds
took care
of it.

characters
keesha,
me, and
my freinds

keesha
and me had
a fight.

setting
It happened
at the drink-
ing fountain.

keesha and me had
a fight and keesha
steped on my foot and
keesha pushed
me and hited me.
It happened at the
drinking fountian.
and my freinds
took care of it
and they ~~took~~ talkod
to her.
the end.

Figure 17.2.   Natividad's end-of-year plan and probe.

class discussions or being accepted into small-group peer conversations in the classroom or on the playground. The case studies in this chapter provide other examples.

Instructional Strategies

The bulleted points that outline instructional strategies should describe both scaffolding techniques and other supports. They might include computer software supports for any aspect of the writing process (as discussed in Section II), or other classroom or author notebook supports (see Chapter 4).

Evidence of Change at End of Reporting Period

The final section of the case study is a set of points that connect back to the established goals and benchmarks, providing data and examples to document change in the targeted areas. Any evidence of broader outcomes should be documented at this point as well. This process provides an opportunity for an instructional team to think about next steps. In other words, a student's accomplishments at the end of one reporting period become the baseline for the following stage of instruction and intervention.

Samples of the Student's Work

Perhaps the most effective data for documenting a student's status at any point along a continuum are samples of the student's actual written work. These could include planning and edited drafts constructed as part of periodic written-language probes, as well as curriculum-based works in progress produced during implementation of the writing lab. To keep those portfolios current, we have found it helpful to have ready access to a copy machine, as well as an adjustable stamp for documenting the date when particular drafts were produced. It is also helpful to add notes to the photocopied samples when appropriate to document the degree of scaffolding that went into a polished final product. We keep file folder portfolios for students with disabilities together with portfolios of work for typically developing students in the same class. These written products provide a major source of data for analyzing change and for comparing a student's performance with an appropriate peer group. The primary sources of qualitative data for writing processes and spoken communication are the journals we (and our graduate students) keep of what students say and do while engaged in writing lab activities. During writing lab activities, we keep our spiral notebook journals handy and, as much as possible, try to capture important events as they occur or immediately thereafter.

EVIDENCE OF LANGUAGE GROWTH

Evidence of language growth for students engaged in the writing lab approach comes both from our research and the work of others. We start by reviewing the work of others.

Box 17.2.   Case Study for Steven

Steven at the beginning of the school year was a third-grade student (chronological age 8;4) with special education needs related to speech-language delay and developmental disability. He had emergent-level reading and writing skills, including sound–symbol association difficulties and scribble-level mixed with prephonetic but alphabetic writing skills. In his first probe, he wrote, "sunent steru tith," and told an adult that it said, "I missed you." By covering his work with his body, he also showed concern that peers and adults would notice his inability to read or write. He spoke softly and rapidly, affecting intelligibility.

Steven dictated his first probe, and demonstrated problems organizing discourse and making sense to his listeners, but he had some knowledge of literary style. The dictation discourse went as follows: "I'm get a friend who be nice," whereupon the adult asked, "Were you telling me about a friend on the playground?" Then, Steven dictated, "Days later in the cave. There was a friend of mine in the cave," after which he announced, "That's it." When the adult scaffolded, "What was the problem?" Steven continued, "He's gonna be in the cave gettin' drinkin' water from the fountain. He went to me. Mike in a cave."

Goals and benchmarks were established for Steven to

- Display emergent-level reading and writing skills, including sound–symbol associations and the ability to read and spell an increasing number of words independently
- Organize discourse sequentially around a theme and include a problem and increasing elements of story grammar structure, such as causality
- Produce sensible, grammatically well-formed utterances in both spoken and written (dictated) communication
- Demonstrate increased confidence in speaking to peers and increased loudness and clarity so that his speech is intelligible to them

Instructional strategies and supports for Steven included

- Scaffolding of sound–symbol relationships and phonemic awareness, including work in his special education classroom, with assistance from the SLP to clarify his articulation of single phonemes, syllables, and words while working on his dictation and spelling
- Providing personal word banks to support independent spelling, by discussing first what Steven planned to write and including words on the paper that would be useful in his story. This and the shared pencil technique were used to support Steven in producing his second probe (see Figure 17.3)
- Scaffolding supports from peers, particularly Steven's table mate, Randy, who encouraged Steven to accept adult assistance and to move beyond his small set of limited topics to work on curriculum-related projects with classmates
- Providing support in the author chair to "read" his work with increasing independence, first from a trusted adult; then, from one particular peer; and finally, from a variety of peers

Steven at the end of the school year had the ability to read many of the words in his own work with increasing independence. For example, a videotape made at the end

(continued)

Box 17.2. *(continued)*

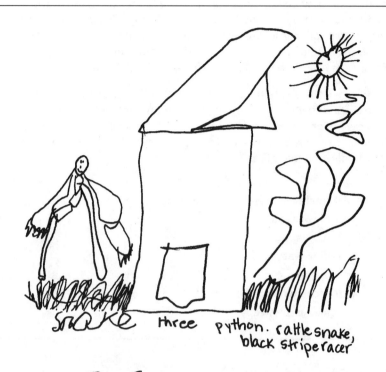

snake   three   python. rattlesnake,
                              black striperacer

The snake was in the tree. The snake was running through the woods. The snake went somewhere and ate a snake. The snake ate a pit and he ate a snake. Went out in the woods and going and drinking some water and eating a toad. It a te a deffrent snake. . . .

Figure 17.3. Steven's mid-year plan and probe using the shared pen technique.

(continued)

Box 17.2. *(continued)*

of the year showed Randy standing by the author chair, but Steven did not need Randy's help. "He's reading it!" Randy exclaimed, as Steven beamed. Steven also had increased phonemic awareness and the ability to generate spellings at the phonetic level. For example, toward the end of the semester, Steven wrote about one of his favorite teachers, "Miss. Hill is bwtfl [beautiful]."

He also had the ability to generate cohesive discourse and sensible sentences organized around themes that extended beyond his earlier repetitive themes of snakes and caves. For example, toward the end of the school year, Steven generated the following "five-senses" poem about watching television that showed his growing ability to reflect on himself and his environment.

> It smells like dust blowing around.
> It blows around.
> I sit on a rug.
> I drink water.
> I hear music.
> Watching movies on TV
> It makes me sleepy.

Evidence From Other Research

Evidence regarding the effectiveness of a writing process approach can be found in the work of several other research teams. The data are limited, and it is difficult to conduct highly controlled "clinical trials" in natural educational environments. Nevertheless, the evidence collected thus far is encouraging.

In 1996, the National Center for Educational Statistics in the U.S. Department of Education, Office of Educational Research and Improvement, reviewed data for fourth-, eighth-, and twelfth-grade students from the 1992 National Assessment of Educational Progress (NAEP) and concluded that the evidence supported the effectiveness of process writing approaches for general education students. In particular, they found that students who reported having teachers who always asked them to plan and do prewriting, to define their purpose and audience, and to produce more than one draft, had the highest average writing scores. Those who did prewriting on the actual national writing sample also had higher average proficiency scores but only if they used lists, outlines, or diagrams. Students who used unrelated notes or drawings on the NAEP test, or who wrote different versions or first drafts, performed about the same as those who did no prewriting (U.S. Department of Education, 1996).

MacArthur, Schwartz, and Graham (1991b) and MacArthur and colleagues (1993) also published evaluation results from their 2-year project on computers and writing instruction. This team conducted the workshops in 18 self-contained classrooms for students with learning disabilities ($N = 180$) at elementary- through middle-school levels. The results from the experimental classrooms were compared with those from 15 control classrooms (*N* = 125). A summary of positive outcomes from their computer-supported writing process approach included

- Significant improvements in overall quality of narrative and informative writing
- Longer compositions
- Fewer misspelled words
- Fewer mechanical errors

Evidence From a Year of Writing Lab Implementation

To provide evidence of the computer-supported writing lab approach in inclusive classrooms, our own research efforts have centered on use of the story-writing probe described in Chapter 14, analyzed with techniques described in Chapter 15. As readers will recall, the essence of this probe involves asking students at the beginning, midpoint, and end of the school year to: "Write a story. Your story can have a problem and what happened. It can be real or imaginary."

In this chapter, we review data for one of the school years during which we conducted a writing lab. During that year, we were working in an inner-city school in a moderate-sized Midwestern city. The school had a freshly outfitted computer lab, as well as multiple computer stations in the school's library. These technological supports, the presence of students with special education needs, and the school's new mission to implement writing process instruction made it ideal for a computer-supported team effort.

The school at that point faced many of the same challenges that typically face inner-city school programs. For example, the school was housed in an old two-story building with high ceilings and wooden floors (i.e., poor acoustics) that was situated in a low-income neighborhood. The families of students in the school were affected by many of the problems associated with poverty, such as substance abuse, crime, and insecure housing arrangements, as well as other forms of instability, and many of the students had emotional and behavioral issues. The population of the school was enriched, however, by its cultural diversity, with high proportions of students from African American, Hispanic, and immigrant families (see Figure 17.4). Also positive was the fact that we were welcomed by the building principal and her staff, the school's general- and special education teachers, the SLP, and the language-arts specialist.

The data reported in this chapter are based on evidence for 53 third-grade students from three third-grade classrooms who completed all three probes. These students were involved in writing lab activities 3 days per week across the school year. Typically, 2 of these days were spent in their third-grade classrooms, and 1 was in one of the school's two computer lab facilities. Children who spent the majority of their instructional time in the special-education classroom were included for all writing lab activities. The school's SLP addressed many of her student's IEP goals as part of writing lab instruction, and she addressed others in collaboration with the special-education teacher in that classroom. Although the special education teacher could not arrange her schedule to be in the general-education classrooms during writing lab activities, she supported the work by helping her students make the transition to general educa-

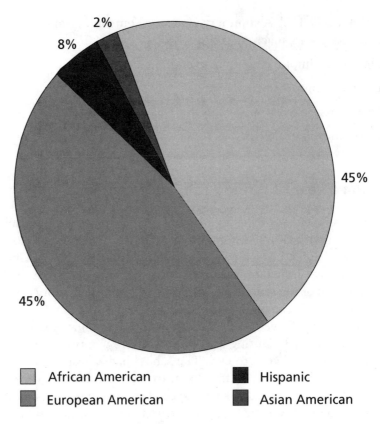

Figure 17.4. Race and ethnicity of third-grade sample.

tion rooms during writing lab times and by encouraging writing in her classroom on similar projects or the same projects. The team used the students' author notebooks to transport materials and works in progress back and forth between the two rooms (see Chapter 13 for a description). The SLP also assisted by facilitating communication across settings.

Two of us (Nickola Wolf Nelson and Adelia M. Van Meter) and two graduate students were present for writing lab activities on a staggered schedule. This generally ensured the presence of one or two extra adults beyond the classroom teacher to scaffold students' written and spoken communication and work toward instructional objectives during writing lab activities. The team met biweekly to plan, either after school or during the lunch period. Early in the school year, these meetings focused on projects, minilessons, and activities. Later in the school year, they focused on meeting the needs of individual students.

Of the 53 students completing all probes, 24 students (45%) were African American, 24 (45%) were European American, 4 (8%) were Hispanic, and 1 (2%) was Asian American (see Figure 17.4). Forty of the third graders (75.5%) were typically developing, but many of these students faced high educational risks due to economic disadvantage. Of the other 25%, 4 (7.5%) met criteria as having speech-language impairment but no other special education eligibility; 5 (9.5%) met criteria for a special education diagnosis (e.g., emotional impairment, learning disability, autism, educable

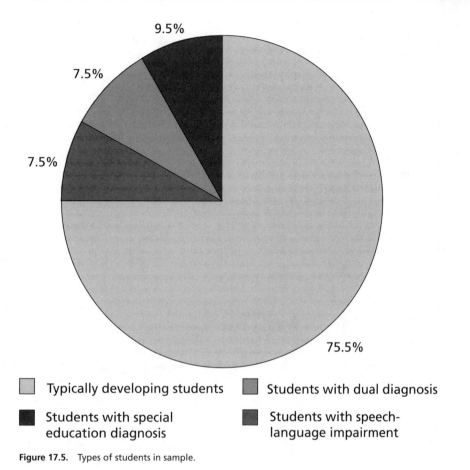

Figure 17.5. Types of students in sample.

mental impairment) other than speech-language impairment; and 4 (7.5%) met criteria for a dual diagnosis. These data are represented graphically in Figure 17.5.

Evidence From Case Studies of Students with Disabilities

Data for seven students with special needs are woven throughout this chapter. The students are Natividad, Nino, and Rose, who were placed in one set of team-taught classrooms, and Steven, Randy, Tamika, and Lonnie, who were placed in a separate third-grade room. More complete case studies are presented for Natividad, Steven, and Lonnie in Boxes 17.1–17.3. Natividad, Randy, and Lonnie received speech-language intervention services (Lonnie was dismissed from intervention during the school year, and Randy was added). Nino, Rose, Steven, and Tamika received services in the lower elementary special-education classroom for part of the day. Steven, Rose, and Tamika all had dual identification, receiving both speech-language and special-education services through their IEPs. Although the school district's cognitive referencing policy prohibited Nino from being labeled with speech-language impairment (i.e., there was not enough discrepancy between his low cognitive and low language abilities), the school's SLP was able to work with him both in writing lab activities and when she went into the special

Box 17.3.   Case Study for Lonnie

At the beginning of the school year Lonnie was a third-grade student (chronological age 8;3) with a speech-language impairment that was mostly resolved by the time he began participating in the writing lab. He had ongoing issues with written language expression characterized by avoidance behaviors and limited production. His baseline sample was at the level of reactive sequence, with 4 utterances, 24 total words, and 16 different words. Lonnie misspelled one third of the words, attempting phonetic strategies, but demonstrating underdeveloped phonemic awareness of characteristics of words (e.g., *fet/fell*), word boundaries (e.g., *branobick/brand new bike*), and orthographic patterns (e.g., *rod/rode*). Figure 17.6 shows Lonnie's initial probe.

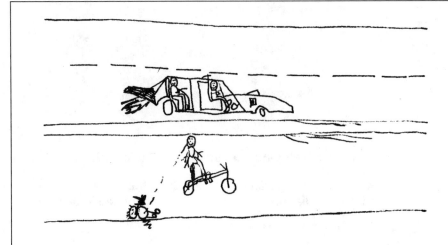

Figure 17.6.   Lonnie's initial plan and probe.

Goals and benchmarks were established for Lonnie to

- Generate story ideas and begin writing independently
- Produce stories with clear goals and planning (level of the complete episode)

- Demonstrate increased phonemic and orthographic awareness in independent spelling attempts
- Interact successfully with peers in conferencing and author chair experiences

Instructional strategies and supports for Lonnie included use of the authentic audience principle, with team members commenting on Lonnie's good ideas and drawing skill and scaffolding him to put those ideas into words in peer conferencing and author chair experiences. As Lonnie began to experience success in drawing "word

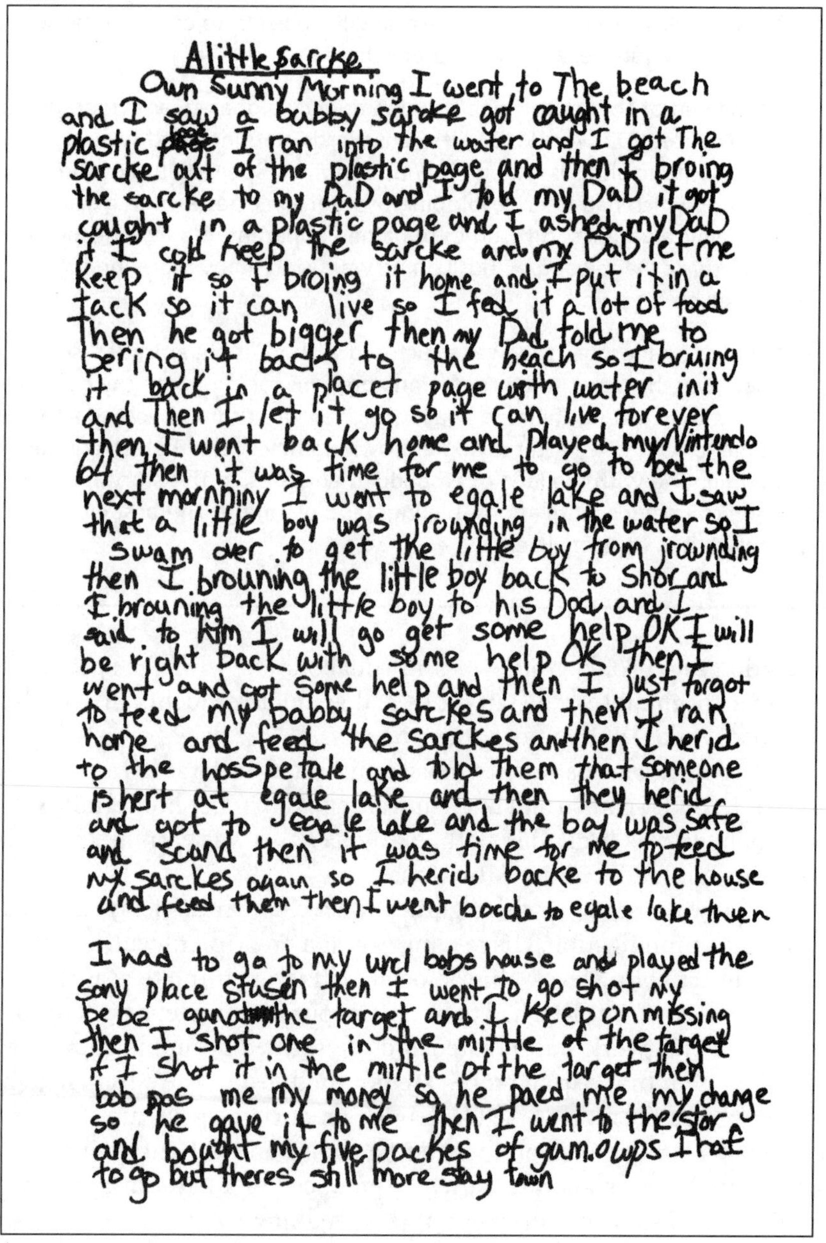

Figure 17.7.   Lonnie's final probe story.

(continued)

Box 17.3. *(continued)*

pictures" as well as graphic ones, his ownership of goals to write more took hold, and his interest in and attention to writing grew. This technique also involved scaffolding during drafting and revising activities, expressing interest in learning more about Lonnie's characters and their motivations and other logical and causal relationships among events that Lonnie seemed to have in his head, but that he did not always include in his writing.

To support higher level spelling skills, the team scaffolded Lonnie to recognize familiar word parts, to pronounce words slowly, to listen to and feel the sounds in his mouth in sequence, and to represent them in his spelling.

At the end of the school year, Lonnie's fluency bloomed, as evident in his final probe. He produced 377 words (122 different words) and included several interesting words and idiomatic phrases (e.g., *safe and sound*). He spelled 89% of the words correctly, some of which had later developing orthographic patterns (e.g., *caught, said*). Phonemic awareness difficulties remained apparent in a few misspellings (e.g., *sarke/shark, page/baggie*), but Lonnie was using many more independent strategies to spell on his own.

Lonnie's final probe story was structured with multiple episodes (see Figure 17.7). There was, however some confusion about his taking home the baby sharks he found, then letting them go again at his father's urging because later he hurried home to feed them after saving a drowning boy. Nevertheless, Lonnie clearly was experimenting with the idea of embedded episodes. In this story, he also described his main character's motivations, feelings, and planning. The best evidence for Lonnie's growth is in his story itself.

---

education room to do group work in collaboration with the special education teacher. Members of the research staff (SLPs and graduate students in speech-language pathology) also worked with all of these students.

Natividad was a student whose family had emigrated from Central America (see Box 17.1). Both Spanish and English were spoken in her home, but Natividad's language development was limited in both. Natividad also was extremely shy and had difficulty speaking out loud in group situations.

Nino was a student with significant developmental delays across domains, including oral communication. His reading was at a preprimer level, and his writing was at an emergent scribbling level. Nino's social skills were immature as well—so much so that in early sessions, he often had to be coaxed out from under a desk to participate. Because Nino's written work was dictated and transcribed by an instructor or a peer, quantitative data from his writing probes are not included in the summaries presented next.

Rose had been diagnosed as having an autism spectrum disorder. She communicated with both spoken and written language and delighted in entertaining her peers with sound effects and dramatically produced elements in her stories, but Rose had needs related to social interaction (e.g., making eye contact, joining groups) and abstract reasoning (e.g., inferential, higher-order thinking) typical of high-functioning students with autism spectrum disorders.

In the other classroom was Steven (see Box 17.2), whose speech and language skills had been dramatically delayed as a preschooler. Now, as a third grader, he could speak, but his phonology and prosody remained affected. He spoke rapidly and quietly with impaired phonological representation of words that made him difficult to understand. Steven had some emerging knowledge about print, but his spelling was mostly pre-phonetic. Steven was sensitive about his difficulties. For example, in early writing labs, he tended to produce letter strings and other scribble shapes (pretend writing), but he would cover his paper with his body so that no one else could see it. Data from Steven's probes are not included in the group reports because of his high reliance on dictation, which diminished as the year progressed. Steven's table mate was Randy. Randy had language-learning difficulties along with emotional issues, but he took on the role of mentoring Steven and helped him to become part of the class.

Tamika was a student with learning disabilities whose problems primarily involved reading decoding and written spelling difficulties. Tamika also spoke quietly and hesitated to participate in group discussions.

Finally, Lonnie had a history of speech-language impairment, but was functioning currently close to grade level (see Box 17.3). Lonnie avoided written expression. He filled pages during planning and writing time with elaborate drawings but few words.

Coding and Analysis Procedures

Prior to conducting the group data analyses, each probe in the set of third-grade samples was transcribed and coded using SALT (Miller & Chapman, 2000). Software coding strategies, which were similar to those described in Chapter 15, are reviewed in the following sections. The data from the coded samples then were compared statistically using the software program SPSS (SPSS Inc., 1999). Graduate research assistants entered the transcripts, dividing them into T-units, and coding them for errors of spelling, punctuation, and word use, as well as sentence complexity and correctness.

Reliability of transcription was computed as percentage of agreement for number of words (99%), number of different words (99%), and T-unit divisions (93%) for 10 randomly selected samples transcribed independently by two research assistants, with word and utterance (T-unit) counts performed by the SALT software. Reliability for coding was measured with one of us, who also checked all of the coded samples and made corrections as necessary. Reliability quotients for coding, computed by dividing the number of coding agreements by the total number of codes, ranged from 86% to 98% agreement for different sample sets. In early coding, we found reliability problems related to trying to code grammatical errors at a level that was too fine. We resolved this problem by using the code [awk] when a sentence violated rules of SAE syntax but the coder was not sure how to gloss the student's intended meaning and several alternatives were possible. The occurrence of an [awk] code led to coding the sentence as either [si] or [ci], depending on its structure. Cohesion [coh] problems involving ambiguous pronoun reference also led to judgments of sentence structures as incorrect.

Story scores were assigned to each narrative attempt consistent with the guidelines in Table 15.3, and reliability was measured by comparing our independent ratings. Agreement for story ratings on sets of stories ranged from 77% to 94%, with an average of 88%. Any disagreements were no more than one point apart, and these often occurred for stories with qualities of ratings at two levels. Any such discrepancies were resolved through discussion.

The results for the analysis of this group of written samples are reported by using the language levels we have used throughout this book. That is, changes are reported at the discourse level, sentence level, and word level. Although writing conventions (such as punctuation) often are targeted in instruction, and they do represent language knowledge, they are difficult to code reliably, particularly on photocopied transcripts where periods and commas may be difficult to identify. Also, capitalization is affected by punctuation, so coding for punctuation and capitalization are confounded. For these reasons, we have found that changes in punctuation and other writing conventions are better analyzed for individual students, but less meaningful for whole classes. Similarly, writing processes and spoken communication cannot be documented based on written product samples (except for some indirect evidence of planning and editing). Data on these elements are documented more effectively from the journal data kept for individual students, and their outcomes are represented better with the case study format than with analysis of group data.

Growth at the Discourse Level

At the discourse level, we analyzed probe samples for the presence of narrative story grammar features, using procedures described in Chapter 15 (Hedberg & Westby, 1993; Hughes et al., 1997; Stein & Glenn, 1982). Scores were assigned from 1 to 7 as follows:

1. Isolated descriptions—when students only described isolated people, places, or events

2. Temporal sequences—when students connected events temporally but without conveying cause–effect relationships

3. Causal (reactive) sequences—when students expressed cause–effect relationships but did not indicate a problem or imply that their characters had goals

4. Abbreviated episodes—when a story revolved around a clearly stated problem and the aims or attentions of major characters were implied

5. Complete episodes—when students stated clearly their characters' plans to achieve goals related to the problem and provided an ending to bring closure

6. Complex/multiple episodes—when students added obstacles in the goal path or wrote more than one abbreviated or complete episode

7. Interactive episodes—when a story included two major characters with separate goals and perspectives working at cross purposes

A multivariate repeated measures analysis of variance was used to analyze the change in story scores from the beginning, mid-year, and year-end probes for the four groups of children, based on disability (i.e., typically developing children, children with speech-language impairments, children with special education diagnosis, or children with dual diagnosis). Analysis using this statistical model of three within-subject probes multiplied by four between-group effects showed that story scores increased significantly as a function of time ($F = 28.455$; df = 2, 72; $p < 0.0001$), and that the groups were significantly different from one another (F = 3.517; df = 3, 36; p < 0.025), but there was no significant story-by-group interaction. The mean difference of +1.31 from the first to second story (SD = 1.18) yielded an effect size of 1.10 for the change from the beginning to the middle of the year. The mean increase of +0.48 from second to third probe (SD = 1.25) yielded an effect size of 0.38. The significant effect was an indicator that significant growth occurred for all students, regardless of special education needs. Results for the four groups are illustrated in Figure 17.8.

One caution is that, without a control group, we cannot with complete confidence attribute the growth to the treatment alone, as we do not know how much growth would have occurred due to maturation effects. More research is being planned to answer that question. In the meantime, these results contrast with the expectation that without intervention (and even with it), children with special needs usually fall further and further behind their general education peers (Stanovich, 1986). Evidence that they are keeping up, and even gaining ground, provides support for the effectiveness of the writing lab approach.

Among the students with disabilities across the three probes, Tamika's stories increased from an isolated description (score 1), to temporal sequence (score 2), to abbreviated episode (score 4). Natividad's three probes were rated as isolated description (score 1), abbreviated episode (score 4), and reactive sequence (score 3). Steven's narrative level was rated on his first probe as isolated description (score 1; mostly dictated)

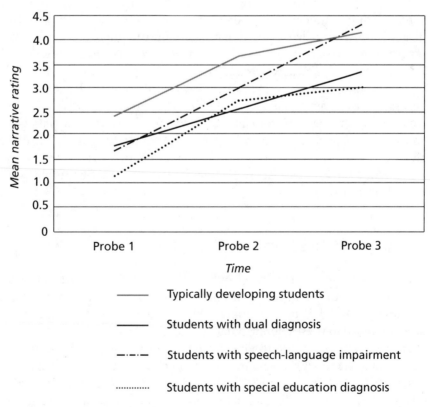

Figure 17.8. Story score growth by group.

and temporal sequence (score 2; dictated with some words written by Steven) on his second. Steven's third probe was missing from the data set. Randy produced temporal sequences (score 2) on both first and second probes, but a complete episode (score 5) on his third. Rose produced a reactive sequence (score 3) on her first probe, and abbreviated episodes (score 4) on her second and third. Lonnie produced a reactive sequence (score 3) on his initial probe, a temporal sequence (score 2) on his second, and a full narrative with complex/multiple episodes (score 6) on his third.

As a second measure of change at the discourse level across the school year, we measured fluency as the total number of words produced during the 1-hour samples. Word production fluency in written samples is a measure that others have shown to be valid and reliable for elementary school students (Hunt, 1965; Scott & Windsor, 2000). Paired t-tests showed significant growth for all students between the first and second probes ($t = 6.437$; $p < 0.0001$), and second and third probes ($t = 2.156$; $p < 0.037$). We note that because of the multiple t-tests run on those data, significance of tests with alpha levels greater than 0.001 are suspect. In cases of paired t-tests, effect sizes were computed by dividing the differences between means at each point in time, by the standard deviation for the whole group. An effect size of 0.91 was computed for the change from the beginning to mid-year probes in word production fluency, and an effect size of 0.33 was computed for change during the second half of the school year. The mean numbers of words produced in the 1-hour written samples for each of these three probes grew from 37.3 to 87.4 to 119.2 for these 53 third graders.

Word production fluency also was a major area of growth for most of the students with disabilities, whose average story length went from 33.3 to 56.7 to 191.2 words across the three probes. These averages were influenced by three of the students with disabilities who made remarkable progress on this measure. Rose's work increased in length from 44 to 83 to 292 words; Lonnie's increased from 24 to 64 to 377 words; and Randy's fluency increased from 53 to 208 on first to third probes (after dropping to 29 words on the middle probe). Natividad's word productivity remained about the same across the three probes (33 to 42 to 37). Her first story was an isolated description (score 1), but her second story (abbreviated episode; score 4) was judged better than her third (reactive sequence; score 3) on both discourse measures. Tamika's word productivity varied widely (17 to 71 to 43 words), but in Tamika's case, the 71-word second story was a temporal sequence (score 2), whereas the 43-word final probe was an abbreviated episode (score 4).

Growth at the Sentence Level

Two methods were used to assess advancing syntactic maturity. One involved dividing samples into "minimal terminal units" or T-units (Hunt, 1965, 1970), as described in Chapter 15. In addition, incomplete but stand-alone communication units (C-units) were included in these counts, but story titles and closings (e.g., *the end*) were not. This permitted us to compute the mean number of words per T/C-unit, another accepted method for measuring advancing syntactic complexity for school-age students (Hunt, 1965, 1970, 1977; Scott, 1988, 1994, 1999; Scott & Windsor, 2000). Mean length measures, when analyzed with paired t-tests, showed significant growth ($t = 3.085$; $p < 0.003$) from the first probe (MLTU = 7.05) to the second probe (MLTU = 8.56), but no significant change from the second to third probe (MLTU = 7.72). The effect size computed for the significant growth in MLTU during the first half of the school year was .44. The average numbers of T/C-units produced by the five students with disabilities for whom written data are available grew from 5 to 9 to 20, with mean lengths remaining around 6 or 7 words per T/C-unit (7.01 to 7.39 to 7.04 MLTU), yielding scores on the second and third probes similar to the average for their classmates.

Sentence-Level Coding

The second sentence-level coding method was designed to capture growth by coding sentences as correct or incorrect, based on standard edited English (a goal of the general education curriculum), and simple or complex, based on whether sentences include more than one finite or nonfinite verb phrase. We expected that as students matured and developed proficiency with standard edited English, they would produce fewer incorrect and more complex sentences along the continuum: simple incorrect [si], simple correct [sc], complex incorrect [ci], and complex correct [cc]. As a reminder of this coding scheme (see Chapter 15), a maximum of two independent clauses per compound sentence is allowed. Any additional conjoined independent clause is coded as a run-on [ro], but it is also coded as either [si] or [sc], depending on its form. If a run-on clause is made complex through embedding or subordination, or if it is connected to another T-unit with a coordinating conjunction, it is coded [cc] or [ci]. (Examples produced by this coding procedure can be found in the appendix to Chapter 15.)

Figure 17.9 shows students produced relatively few [si] sentences across any of the probes (no significant differences), but as they began to take more risks, they produced significantly more [ci] sentences at the second probe ($t = 3.624$, $p < 0.001$); then, they leveled off from the second to third probe (no significant difference) in [ci] sentence production. On the second probe, they also produced significantly more [ro] sentences ($t = 2.46$; $p < 0.017$), and they produced significantly more [sc] and [cc] sentences at mid-year and year-end probes ($t = 2.777$; $p < .008$; $t = 3.339$; $p < 0.002$) and ($t = 5.428$; $p < 0.0001$; $t = 2.242$; $p < 0.03$). The effect size for the increase in complex correct sentences from probe one to two was 0.77. The change from probe two to three had an effect size of 0.35. In other words, while they were becoming more fluent, students also were becoming better at producing well-formed, complex sentences, sprinkled appropriately with simple correct sentences.

Patterns of sentence-structure change for the group of students with disabilities mirrored that of their typically developing classmates, as [si] sentences almost disappeared, and both [sc] and [cc] sentences increased in frequency across the three probes (means per story of 2.13 to 2.15 to 4.17 for [sc]; and 1.13 to 3.5 to 5.8 for [cc]). The only major difference was a big increase in [ci] sentences in probe three (0.5 to 0.63 to 3.67 for [ci]), due mostly to Rose's experimenting with a variety of new sentence types and her frequent use of the African American Vernacular English features of her oral home language (e.g., "They mom say no. They beg they mom until they say yes and when they mom say yes they be so happy" [spelling corrected, but grammar as written]).

Dialectal Concerns and Sentence Coding

We are aware that the practice of counting sentences with dialectal features as "incorrect" is controversial, and we labored over it. We often marked dialectal forms sepa-

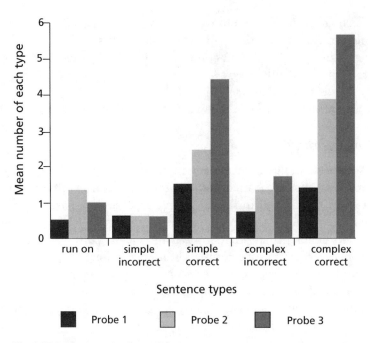

Figure 17.9. Sentence-level growth by type.

rately (with a [d] code) when analyzing individualized assessments, and we would never count dialectal forms as errors for purposes of determining disability (Espin et al., 2000). We think the decision to treat standard edited grammar as "correct" is warranted, however, when monitoring progress toward the general education goal of literate language use, especially when standard edited English is the explicit standard established by the students' school district as it was in this case.

We also believe that this decision appropriately addresses criticism by African American scholar, Lisa Delpit (1995), who disdained the tendency of well-meaning (but she claimed overly liberal) educators to view whatever children wrote during writing process instruction as acceptable. As noted in Chapter 2, Delpit emphasized that holding different standards for different students was a discriminatory practice and not in the best interests of students with different home dialects. Still, the issues are controversial, and we recommend that professionals resolve similar conflicts within their own home communities. Regardless, we remind readers of the importance of welcoming more complex grammatical attempts as signs of growth, even if all adult standards for "correctness" are not met (Weaver, 1982).

Growth at the Word Level

Word-level growth includes the previously reported increase in word-production fluency. In addition, students were using more different words as the school year progressed. Significant increases ($t = 6.910$; $p < 0.0001$; with an effect size of 0.97) in the number of different words were observed from the first probe (Mean = 24.0; $SD = 11.5$) to the second probe (Mean = 45.3; $SD = 21.9$) for the students who completed both probes. In a separate analysis, significant increases (t = 2.398; p < 0.021; with an effect size of 0.37) were found when comparing the second probe (Mean = 47.5; SD = 20.6) with the third probe (Mean = 60.1; SD = 33.8) for students who had completed both probes. Growth also occurred for the five students with disabilities who produced measurable written language. Their different-word average grew from 22.4 to 29.7 to 76.2 different words across the three probes. In addition, Steven grew from writing only his name independently in the first probe (other words were dictated), to writing two words (*snake* and *Samuel*) independently in the second, to writing whole pieces with only moderate scaffolding by the end of the school year, and reading them independently.

Word-level changes also were measured as improved spelling accuracy, as others have done (Deno, Marston, & Mirkin, 1982; MacArthur et al., 1993; MacArthur, Schwartz, & Graham, 1991a). Although the proportion of words spelled correctly by all students in the first probe (80.6%) did not grow significantly by the second probe (81.6%), it did grow significantly by the third probe (85.4%) when analyzed with paired t-tests (t = 3.134; p < 0.003; with an effect size of 0.49). In other words, students in the writing lab were able to demonstrate the production of higher numbers of different words and to spell a higher proportion of total words correctly by the year-end. Changes at the word level are shown in Figure 17.10.

The students with disabilities showed individual patterns of change in spelling. Randy, Tamika, and Natividad were relatively good spellers from the beginning of the year, with Randy consistently spelling 92%–94% of his words correctly, and Tamika and Natividad spelling around 85% of their words correctly across the school year. For them, growth came as they risked attempts to spell more different words. For Steven, spelling grew from his preliterate "scribble" writing attempts at the beginning of the school year, to producing words with phonetic-stage spelling by the year's end. For example, he wrote about one of his teachers, "Miss. Hill is bwtfl [beautiful]." Once Rose became confident enough to participate in writing and sharing stories, her difficulty in spelling was a prominent feature. Although she continued to spell high proportions of words incorrectly, she started to use more phonetic strategies by the third probe (e.g., "thay" for *they*; "ples" for *police*) and showed emerging awareness of orthographic patterns (e.g., *store* and *now*). Lonnie made the most dramatic progress in spelling, advancing from 67% to 78%, to 89% of his words spelled correctly, at the same time increasing his production of different words from 16 in his first and second probes to 122 different words in his third probe.

Growth for an Eighth Grader

Josh was referred to the after-school writing lab by his middle school special-education teacher. His grandfather transported him, and he participated after school 2 days per week throughout his eighth-grade year. Prior to entering the program, Josh produced a baseline story in response to a picture probe showing cave men and mammoths on the *Test of Written Language–2nd Edition* (Hammill & Larsen, 1991). Here is the sample, reproduced exactly as Josh spelled it:

> The cave men fited of the grat mamist. They trow spears at the
> mamist. They cepe coming. They wanead food. More cave men come

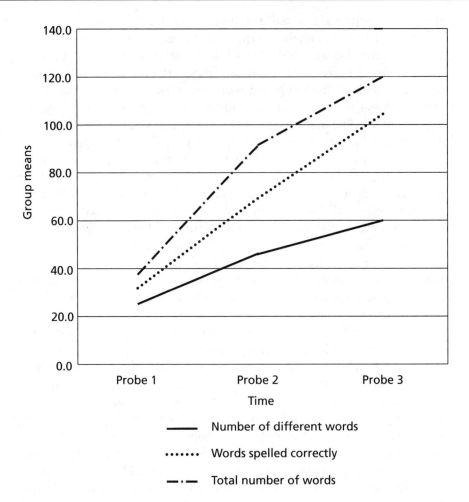

Figure 17.10. Word-level growth by measure.

and fit them off but they unsixses fil. The the trow rock and stowns
and they won the batil but not the wore betwen man and beast.
They ma come back or not but they will be retey.

This sample demonstrated his relatively strong discourse abilities, with characteristics of an abbreviated episode, but it also included a high proportion of spelling
that was difficult to decipher. In this initial probe, Josh spelled only 72% of the words
correctly, and he demonstrated some confusion about word boundaries and bound morphemes when he spelled *unsuccessful* as "unsixses fil." The sample included 59 words
(34 different word roots), divided into 11 T-units, yielding an MLTU score of 5.36
words. Josh showed glimmers of creative and higher-level thinking by commenting on
the war between man and beast, and he attempted a few more interesting words, but
he also showed some difficulty with cohesion. In particular, the reader is uncertain
whether the word *they* refers to the cave men or the mammoths at several points in the
story. The story included sentences of the following types: 2 [si], 1 [sc], 4 [ci], and 0 [cc].

Box 17.4.   Case Study for Josh

Josh at the beginning of the school year was an eighth grader (chronological age 13;7) diagnosed with a learning disability, particularly in written language. He had typical spoken communication and strong social skills. A cautious writer, Josh took few risks. He had many spelling errors, characterized by limited representation of morpho-orthographic patterns and inaccurate phonetic information.

Goals and benchmarks for Josh included

- Generate story topics (beyond dogs and horses) independently and write stories with higher levels of narrative maturity (complete and complex episodes)
- Incorporate interesting and unusual words in place of overused words, such as *very* and *nice*
- Use a higher proportion of complex sentences (at least two to three per story)
- Spell words correctly during revising, with instructor scaffolding as needed
- Show leadership by helping or encouraging members of his author's group at least three times per lab session
- Evaluate and revise at least two aspects of each story during every session (this objective was added toward the end of the school year)

Instructional strategies and supports for Josh included scaffolding self-questioning strategies to generate story ideas and using computer software supports for all stages of the writing process (picture supports and text-based organizers to assist story idea generation and planning; tools for inserting elaborated text during drafting and revising; keyboarding related to sound–symbol associations and orthographic pattern recognition; synthetic speech features to support new vocabulary identification; and using a spelling checker). In addition, audience feedback scaffolds could be used to assist Josh to work on improved cohesion, more complex sentence production, and the inclusion of more interesting vocabulary.

Josh also could receive instruction in independent spelling, such as saying words slowly in syllables to construct initial spellings (good phonetic equivalents) during drafting and using other word sources, including word banks and computer software features. Later, he could use spelling checker functions to edit spelling during revision with moderate-to-minimal scaffolding from the instructor.

Another goal was to scaffold Josh's leadership, story reflection and evaluation, and peer support discourse during author group meetings, held at the beginning and end of most lab sessions.

Although Josh continued to have some difficulty spelling, at the end of the school year, he improved to a transitional level and adopted a variety of compensatory strategies. Josh mastered use of the spelling checker option in two different software programs. When the spelling checker could not find an alternative spelling, he benefited from scaffolding to produce close phonetic equivalents that could be recognized by the computer.

Josh had no difficulty generating story ideas at the end of the school year. He mixed his interest in nature with experimentation in mystery writing, producing stories titled "Nature Nightmare" and "On the Edge of Extinction."

(continued)

Box 17.1. *(continued)*

In Josh's final story about a planet called *Zooms*, he worked both independently and with the instructor to produce six complex sentences. Two sentences he generated independently were, "The planet was on the verge of a war the planets first one," and "While we were rebuilding, the pirates attack the planet." With minimal scaffolding, Josh produced, "Some people wanted to leave it alone, but the environment was hurting so most of the counsel wonted to change their ways."

Most of Josh's sentences were grammatically correct and utilized appropriate writing conventions. Although he omitted some commas and apostrophes in obligatory contexts, he inserted them when scaffolded by the instructor.

Josh's mother commented at her final conference that his English grades had improved steadily over his eighth-grade school year. His teachers at school also had commented specifically on the improvement in Josh's writing since the beginning of the school year.

The goals and benchmarks established for Josh are shown in Box 17.4. During the fall session, Josh produced an early story in the lab using a computerized prompted story-writing template (see Chapter 7) to plan and write "Duke the Dog." The published version of this story, which Josh typed in all capital letters, but with scaffolded spelling, read as follows:

ONE MORNING DUKE WOKE ME UP. WE PLAYED WITH HIS CHEWY TOY. I THREW IT UP AND HE CAUGHT IT. WE DID IT A COUPLE OF TIMES. THEN WE ATE BREAKFAST. WE PLAYED SOME MORE. I LET HIM STAY OUT SIDE. IT WAS RAINING OUT. HE DIDN'T STAY OUT VERY LONG. HE WAS HYPER. BUT HE SETTLED DOWN. HE WENT TO SLEEP FOR A WHILE. THEN HE MESSED WITH THE CAT. THE CAT WAS NOT HAPPY. THE CAT RAN, THE DOG RAN AFTER IT. HE BARKED THEN HE STOPPED. IT WAS NO FUN ANY MORE. I PLAYED WITH HIM HE WAS HAPPY NOW.

This was a safe little story, organized as a temporal sequence, with no real problem, and hence, not much of a high point. In fact, early in this intervention, most of Josh's stories were nonfiction accounts of personal experiences. Discourse scaffolds for Josh at this point consisted of asking him to think about how a problem might lead his characters to have to respond in more interesting ways. Self-questioning was modeled as a strategy for generating story ideas (e.g., "Has something interesting happened to me or someone I know? Has something happened that I wish would have turned out differently?")

Also, about this time, Josh was introduced to the computer software *Once Upon a Time* (Compu-Teach), which provided scene creation tools, leading him to think about story topics beyond his immediate experience. He also used this tool to assist with adding more interesting vocabulary and spelling it correctly. For example, when working on one story, Josh was uncertain how to spell *astronaut*. He stopped writing, referred to the scene creation tool that listed available items, found the word *astronaut*, and wrote it on a piece of scrap paper. Then, he returned to his text, typing the word while checking his written note. Josh also used this strategy to spell *alien*. The software indirectly supported text elaboration as well. When one word wrapped onto the next page, beyond the scene he had created, Josh commented, "That word looks stupid there all by itself," then continued to type, doubling the length of his story. The final product was:

ONCE UPON A TIME THERE WAS AN ENCOUNTER IN SPACE. THE ALIENS WERE NOT HAPPY. THE ASTRONAUTS WERE TRESPASSING ON THE ALIENS LAND, BUT THE ALIENS WERE FRIENDLY. [page 1]
     THE ALIENS LET THE ASTRONAUTS EXPLORE THEIR LAND. THE ASTRONAUTS MADE A DEAL THEY COULD EXPLORE IF THEY KEPT QUIET. THEN THEY ALL GOT ALONG. [page 2]

Now Josh was on a roll, producing a complete episode, and experiencing positive feedback from instructors and peers about his interesting word choices. He still had some cohesion problems with the pronoun *they*. His T-units remained mostly simple, but he produced one complex sentence with the subordinate conjunction, *if*, in this story. The occasion for this sentence arose when his characters needed to resolve the conflict by setting conditions for co-existence of astronauts and aliens.

When Josh returned to the writing lab in January following the holiday break, he continued to work on complex sentence production, benefiting from scaffolding both at his computer and in author groups. For example, in his story, "On the Trail," Josh wrote, "The horses didn't act up at all. The horses spooked." When reading aloud to an instructor, however, he orally inserted the word, *until*, between these two sentences. The instructor responded, "Wow, Josh, *until* is an excellent connector word. It really helps me see what happened. But you know what? It isn't on the screen." That was all it took for Josh to reach for the keyboard and make the revision. This teachable moment, and similar experiences in which Josh's peers learned to ask him to explain his characters' motives, helped Josh begin to use more complex syntax to explain the more complex relationships that soon were characterizing his stories. During the period from February through April, Josh wrote and published four stories on varied topics, starting with "Nature Nightmare" and "On the Trail," then writing a story about "Josh," a park ranger, who stopped a poacher who was killing bald eagles, in a mystery called "On the Edge of Extinction." The last story Josh produced during the winter session was a complete episode. It included 188 total words, 100 different word roots, and 23 T-units, with an MLTU of 9.35 words, and sentences of the following types: 1 [si], 11 [sc], 1 [ci], and 7 [cc]. The published story read as follows:

Flight 101

It started off in space. I'm Tom and here is my band of misfits. We're
to protect the colony of Z-6. The colony is pretty peaceful. Sometimes

we help other colonies with their troubles. We fly a Mustang xl 117. Sometimes we engaged the enemy in battle at the very ends of the universe. One morning my squad found some pirates firing on a smaller colony. We fired on them. Before they left we got five of them, but this time they fired back, so we attacked them. They lost 11 of the 12 ships; we lost 2 of the 10. We let the one get away to tell the pirates. That day the colony of Z-6 was sad for the men that died that morning. The colony replaced the men and ship with new recruits and with the new Mustang xl 117. The next day we cleaned our Mustang xl 117s until they shined, loaded them up with fuel and ammo. The pirates attacked the colony so we scrambled the Mustang xl 117. Our squad took the pirates apart. The pirates never messed with the colony of Z-6 or any other colonies again.

THE
END

During the spring session that followed (during the final 2 months of the school year), Josh continued to work on his goals of sentence combining, spelling independently, revising and editing, and showing social leadership skills in his author group. His final story continued his "space pirates" theme, combined with his earlier environmental interests. It also was judged to be a complete episode. Although Josh's references still were not always completely clear, in this story he emphasized the landscape of consciousness by talking about the plans of the council (spelled "counsel") in addressing the planet's difficulties, leading it to be rated as a complete episode (with some characteristics of a complex/multiple episode story). This story included 128 total words, 77 different word roots, and 13 T-units, with an MLTU of 9.14 words, and sentences of the following types: 0 [si], 7 [sc] (including several with later-developing phrase elaboration), 1 [ci], and 5 [cc]. His final published story read as follows:

The Space Pirates are Back

This starts out at the edge of the universe. Our squadron flies Mustangs X L 117 to protect this world of Zooms. The planet was in the verge of a war the planets first one. The representatives were arguing about the natural resources and how they were being used in a bad way. It was hurting the environment and the animals. We were also having problems in the hanger at our base. Some people wanted to leave it alone, but the environment was hurting so most of the counsel wonted to change their ways. We had our Civil War. The representatives got their way. While we were rebuilding, the pirates attack the planet. My squadron forced them back for the day. One more battle and the pirates were no more.

THE
END

BROADER IMPLICATIONS OF CHANGE

Quantitative evidence of whole-group change is important. Administrative support and teacher volunteers are far more likely to be made available for language intervention approaches that can be shown to be good for all children. We believe that the evidence reported here of growth of key literacy skills at the word, sentence, and discourse levels is compelling.

Equally important are the less quantifiable changes in many of the students' views of themselves as literate communicators. The case studies for the students with disabilities, in particular, reflect their growing status as full members and "residents" of their third-grade classrooms (as discussed in Chapter 13). They became desirable communicative partners and students willing to take turns in group discussions and presentations. All of the students with disabilities in this intervention achieved measurable growth in their IEP objectives and in the general education curriculum. Josh achieved successful outcomes in his secondary school experiences, as well. The broader outcomes of increased abilities to interact socially with students in their classrooms extended to changes in the internal stories of self-efficacy and future possibilities that these students learned to tell themselves—one of the most important among the unlimited possibilities of the writing lab approach.

References

Adams, M.J., & Henry, M.K. (1997). Myths and realities about words and literacy. *School Psychology Review, 26,* 425–436.

Anderson, C. (2000). *How's it going? A practical guide to conferring with student writers.* Portsmouth, NH: Heinemann.

Anderson, G.L., Herr, K., & Nihlen, A.S. (1994). *Studying your own school: An educator's guide to qualitative practitioner research.* Thousand Oaks, CA: Corwin Press.

Apel, K., & Swank, L.K. (1999). Second chances: Improving decoding skills in the older student. *Language, Speech, and Hearing Services in Schools, 30,* 231–242.

Applebee, A.N. (1978). *The child's concept of story: Ages two to seventeen.* Chicago: University of Chicago Press.

Applebee, A.N., & Langer, J.A. (1983). Instructional scaffolding: Reading and writing and natural language activities. *Language Arts, 60,* 168–175.

Aram, D.M., Ekelman, B.L., & Nation, J.E. (1984). Preschoolers with language impairments: 10 years later. *Journal of Speech and Hearing Research, 27,* 232–244.

Areglado, N., & Dill, M. (1997). *Let's write: A practical guide to teaching writing in the early grades.* New York: Scholastic Professional Books.

Astington, J.W. (1990). Narrative and the child's theory of mind. In B.K. Britton & A.D. Pelligrini (Eds.), *Narrative thought and narrative language* (pp. 151–171). Mahwah, NJ: Lawrence Erlbaum Associates.

Atwell, N. (1987). *In the middle: Writing, reading, and learning with adolescents.* Portsmouth, NH: Heinemann.

Atwell, N. (Ed.). (1990). *Coming to know: Writing to learn in the intermediate grades.* Portsmouth, NH: Heinemann.

Bahr, C.M., Nelson, N.W., & Van Meter, A.M. (1996). The effects of text-based and graphics-based software tools on planning and organizing of stories. *Journal of Learning Disabilities, 29,* 355–370.

Bahr, C.M., Nelson, N.W., Van Meter, A.M., & Yanna, J.V. (1996). Children's use of desktop publishing features: Process and product. *Journal of Computing in Childhood Education, 7(3/4),* 149–177.

Bailet, L.L. (2001). Written language test reviews. In A.M. Bain, L.L. Bailet, & L. Moats (Eds.), *Written language disorders: Assessment into practice* (pp. 221–248). Austin, TX: PRO-ED.

Balajthy, E. (1988). Keyboarding, language arts, and the elementary school child. *The Computing Teacher, 15(5),* 40–43.

Ball, E.W., & Blachman, B.A. (1988). Phoneme segmentation training: Effect on reading readiness. *Annals of Dyslexia, 38,* 208–224.

Bangert-Drowns, R.L. (1993). The word processor as an instructional tool: A meta-analysis of word processing in writing instruction. *Review of Educational Research, 63,* 69–93.

Barenbaum, E., Newcomer, P., & Nodine, B. (1987). Children's ability to write stories as a function of variation in task, age, and developmental level. *Learning Disability Quarterly, 7,* 175–188.

Barnhart, J.E. (1990). Differences in story retelling behaviors and their relation to reading comprehension in second graders. In J. Zutell & S. McCormick (Eds.), *Literacy theory and research: Analyses from multiple paradigms* (pp. 257–266). Chicago: National Reading Conference.

Bartholome, L.W. (2002). *Typewriting/keyboarding instruction in elementary schools.* Retrieved December 11, 2002, from http://www.usoe.k12.ut.us/ate/keyboarding/Articles/Bartholome.htm

Bashir, A.S., Conte, B.M., & Heerde, S.M. (1998). Language and school success: Collaborative challenges and choices. In D.D. Merritt & B. Culatta (Eds.), *Language intervention in the classroom* (pp. 1–36). San Diego: Singular Publishing Group.

Batshaw, M.L. (Ed.). (2002). *Children with disabilities* (5th ed.). Baltimore: Paul H. Brookes Publishing Co.

Bear, L., Invernizzi, M., Templeton, S., & Johnson, F. (2000). *Words their way: Word study for phonics, spelling, and vocabulary development* (2nd ed.). Upper Saddle River, NJ: Prentice Hall Press.

Becker, H.J. (1985). The computer and the elementary school. *Principal, 65*(5), 32–34.

Bedore, L.M., & Leonard, L.B. (2001). Grammatical morphology deficits in Spanish-speaking children with specific language impairment. *Journal of Speech, Language, and Hearing Research, 44,* 905–924.

Belavitch, K. (1997). Ring the bell and run. In D. Barnes, K. Morgan, & K. Weinhold (Eds.), *Writing process revisited: Sharing our stories* (pp. 32–51). Urbana, IL: National Council of Teachers of English.

Bennett, C.W. (1989). *Referential semantic analysis* [Computer program]. Woodstock, VA: Teaching Texts.

Bereiter, C., & Scardamalia, M. (1987). *The psychology of written composition.* Mahwah, NJ: Lawrence Erlbaum Associates.

Berninger, V.W. (2000). Development of language by hand and its connections with language by ear, mouth, and eye. *Topics in Language Disorders, 20*(4), 65–84.

Beukelman, D.R., & Mirenda, P. (1998). *Augmentative and alternative communication: Management of severe communication disorders in children and adults* (2nd ed.). Baltimore: Paul H. Brookes Publishing Co.

Beukelman, D.R., & Mirenda, P. (with J. Sturm). (1998). Literacy development of AAC users. In D.R. Beukelman & P. Mirenda, *Augmentative and alternative communication: Management of severe communication disorders in children and adults* (2nd ed., pp. 355–390). Baltimore: Paul H. Brookes Publishing Co.

Blachman, B.A. (1994). Early literacy acquisition: The role of phonological awareness. In G.P. Wallach & K.G. Butler (Eds.), *Language learning disabilities in school-age children and adolescents* (pp. 253–274). Boston: Allyn & Bacon.

Blachman, B. (Ed.). (1997). *Foundations of reading acquisition and dyslexia: Implications for early intervention.* Mahwah, NJ: Lawrence Erlbaum Associates.

Blalock, J., & Johnson, D. (1987). *Adults with learning disabilities: Clinical studies.* New York: Grune & Stratton.

Bland, L.E., & Prelock, P.A. (1996). Effects of collaboration on language performance. *Journal of Children's Communication Development, 17*(2), 31–37.

Blischak, D.M. (1995). Thomas the writer: Case study of a child with severe physical, speech, and visual impairments. *Language, Speech, and Hearing Services in Schools, 26,* 11–20.

Boder, E., & Jarrico, S. (1982). *Boder Test of Reading–Spelling Patterns.* San Antonio, TX: The Psychological Corporation.

Bos, C.S. (1988). Process-oriented writing: Instructional implications for mildly handicapped students. *Exceptional Children, 54,* 521–527.

Botvin, G., & Sutton-Smith, B. (1977). The development of structural complexity in children's fantasy narrative. *Developmental Psychology, 13,* 377–388.

Bradley, L., & Bryant, P. (1983). Categorizing sounds and learning to read: A causal connection. *Nature, 301,* 419–421.

Bradley, L., & Bryant, P. (1985). *Rhyme and reason in reading and spelling.* Ann Arbor: University of Michigan Press.

Branscombe, N.A., Goswami, D., & Schwartz, J. (Eds.). (1992). *Students teaching, teachers learning.* Portsmouth, NH: Boynton Cook.

Bridges, L. (1997). *Writing as a way of knowing.* Portland, ME: Stenhouse Publishers.

Britton, J.N. (1979). Learning to use language in two modes. In N.R. Smith & M.B. Franklin (Eds.), *Symbolic functioning in childhood.* Mahwah, NJ: Lawrence Erlbaum Associates.

Brown, A.L., Campione, J.C., & Day, J.D. (1981). Learning to learn: On training students to learn from texts. *Educational Researcher, 10,* 14–21.

Bruner, J. (1975). The ontogenesis of speech acts. *Journal of Child Language, 2,* 1–19.

Bruner, J. (1977). Early social interaction and language acquisition. In R. Shaffer (Ed.), *Studies in mother–infant interaction* (pp. 271–289). San Diego: Academic Press.

Bruner, J. (1986). *Actual minds, possible worlds.* Cambridge, MA: Harvard University Press.

Bruner, J. (1990). *Acts of meaning.* Cambridge, MA: Harvard University Press.

Bryson, M., & Scardamalia, M. (1991). Teaching writing to students at risk for academic failure (Report No. UD 028 249). In *Teaching advanced skills to educationally disadvantaged students.* (ERIC Document Reproduction Service No. 338 725)

Butler, K.G. (1999). From oracy to literacy: Changing clinical perceptions. *Topics in Language Disorders, 20*(1), 14–32.

Calkins, L. (1983). *Lessons from a child: On the teaching and learning of writing.* Portsmouth, NH: Heinemann.

Calkins, L. (1986). *The art of teaching writing.* Portsmouth, NH: Heinemann.

Calkins, L. (1990). *Living between the lines.* Portsmouth, NH: Heinemann.

Calkins, L. (1994). *The art of teaching writing* (2nd ed.). Portsmouth, NH: Heinemann.

Carrow-Woolfolk, E. (1996). *Oral Written Language Skills.* Circle Pines, MN: American Guidance Service.

Catts, H. (1991). Early identification of dyslexia: Evidence of a follow-up study of speech and language impaired children. *Annals of Dyslexia, 41,* 163–176.

Catts, H.W. (1993). The relationship between speech-language impairments and reading disabilities. *Journal of Speech and Hearing Research, 36,* 948–958.

Catts, H.W., & Fey, M.E. (2001, November). *Causal and correlative links between spoken and written language difficulties in children.* Paper presented at the meeting of the American Speech-Language-Hearing Association, New Orleans.

Catts, H.W., Fey, M.E., Zhang, X., & Tomblin, J.B. (2001). Estimating the risk of future reading difficulties in kindergarten children: A research-based model and its clinical implementation. *Language, Speech, and Hearing Services in Schools, 32,* 38–50.

Catts, H.W., Hu, C.F., Larrivee, L., & Swank, L. (1994). Early identification of reading disabilities in children with speech-language impairments. In S.F Warren & J. Reichle (Series Eds.) & R.V. Watkins & M.L. Rice (Vol. Eds.), *Communication and language intervention series: Vol. 4. Specific language impairments in children* (pp. 145–160). Baltimore: Paul H. Brookes Publishing Co.

Catts, H.W., & Kamhi, A.G. (1999). *Language and reading disabilities.* Boston: Allyn & Bacon.

Cazden, C. (1988). *Classroom discourse.* Portsmouth, NH: Heinemann.

Chomsky, N. (1980). *Rules and representations.* New York: Columbia University Press.

Chomsky, N. (1981). *Lectures on government and binding.* Dordrecht, Holland: Foris.

Christenson, S.L., Thurlow, M.L., Ysseldyke, J.E., & McVicar, R. (1989). Written language instruction for students with mild handicaps: Is there enough quantity to ensure quality? *Learning Disability Quarterly, 12,* 219–229.

Clarke, L.K. (1988). Invented versus traditional spelling in first graders' writings: Effects on learning to read and spell. *Research in the Teaching of English, 22,* 281–309.

Cochran-Smith, M., & Lytle, S.L. (1993). *Inside-outside: Teacher research and knowledge.* New York: Teachers College Press.

Cochran-Smith, M., & Lytle, S.L. (1999). Relationships of knowledge and practice: Teacher learning in communities. In A. Iran-Nejad & P.D. Pearson (Eds.), *Review of research in education* (Vol. 24, pp. 249–305). Washington, DC: American Educational Research Association.

Cole, K.N., Coggins, T.E., & Vanderstoep, C. (1999). The influence of language/cognitive profile on discourse intervention outcome. *Language, Speech, and Hearing Services in Schools, 30,* 61–67.

Cole, K.N., & Harris, S.R. (1992). Instability of the intelligence quotient–motor quotient relationship. *Developmental Medicine and Child Neurology, 34,* 633–641.

Constable, C.M. (1987). Talking with teachers: Increasing our relevance as language interventionists in the schools. *Seminars in Speech and Language, 8*(4), 345–356.

Cooper, C.R., & Odell, L. (Eds.). (1977). *Evaluating writing: Describing, measuring, judging.* Urbana, IL: National Council of Teachers of English.

Cosden, M.A., Goldman, S.R., & Hine, M.S. (1990). Learning handicapped students' interactions during a microcomputer-based group writing activity. *Journal of Special Education Technology, 10,* 220–232.

Craig, H.K., & Washington, J.A. (1993). Access behaviors of children with specific language impairment. *Journal of Speech and Hearing Research, 36,* 322–337.

Creaghead, N.A., & Tattershall, S.S. (1985). Observation and assessment of classroom pragmatic skills. In C.S. Simon (Ed.), *Communication skills and classroom success: Assessment of language-learning disabled students* (pp. 105–131). San Diego: College Hill Press.

Cummins, J. (1984). *Bilingualism and special education: Issues in assessment and pedagogy.* Austin, TX: PRO-ED.

Daiute, C. (1985). *Writing and computers.* Boston: Addison Wesley Higher Education Group.

Daiute, C. (1989). Research currents: Play and learning to write. *Language Arts, 66,* 656–664.

Daiute, C. (1990). The role of play in writing development. *Research in the Teaching of English, 24,* 4–47.

Daiute, C. (1992). Multimedia composing: Extending the resources of kindergarten to writers across the grades. *Language Arts, 69,* 250–260.

Daiute, C., & Dalton, B. (1993). Collaboration between children learning to write: Can novices be masters? *Cognition and Instruction, 10,* 281–330.

Daiute, C., & Morse, F. (1994). Access to knowledge and expression: Multimedia writing tools for students with diverse needs and strengths. *Journal of Special Education Technology, 12,* 221–256.

Danoff, B., Harris, K.R., & Graham, S. (1993). Incorporating strategy instruction within the writing process in the regular classroom. *Journal of Reading Behavior, 25,* 295–322.

Delpit, L. (1995). *Other people's children: Cultural conflict in the classroom.* New York: New Press.

Denckla, M.B. (1994). Measurement of executive function. In G.R. Lyon (Ed.), *Frames of reference for the assessment of learning disabilities: New views on measurement issues* (pp. 117–142). Baltimore: Paul H. Brookes Publishing Co.

Denckla, M.B., & Rudel, R. (1976). Naming of object drawings by dyslexic and other learning-disabled boys. *Brain and Language, 3,* 1–15.

Deno, S.L. (1989). Curriculum-based measurement and special education services: A fundamental and direct relationship. In M.R. Shinn (Ed.), *Curriculum-based measurement: Assessing special children* (pp. 1–17). New York: Guilford Press.

Deno, S.L., Marston, D., & Mirkin, P.L. (1982). Valid measurement procedures for continuous development of written expression. *Exceptional Children, 48,* 368–371.

Diaz, R.M., & Berk, L.E. (1992). *Private speech: From social interaction to self-regulation.* Mahwah, NJ: Lawrence Erlbaum Associates.

Donahue, M.L., Hartas, D., & Cole, D. (1999). Research on interactions among oral language and emotional/behavioral disorders. In D. Rogers-Adkinson & P. Griffith (Eds.), *Communication disorders and children with psychiatric and behavioral disorders* (pp. 69–97). San Diego: Singular Publishing Group.

Donahue, M.L., Szymanski, C.M., & Flores, C.W. (1999). When "Emily Dickinson" met "Steven Spielberg": Assessing social information processing in literacy contexts. *Language, Speech, and Hearing Services in Schools, 30,* 274–284.

Duchan, J.F. (1986). Learning to describe events. *Topics in Language Disorders, 6*(4), 27–36.

Ebert, K.A., & Prelock, P.A. (1994). Teachers' perceptions of their students with communication disorders. *Language, Speech, and Hearing Services in Schools, 25,* 211–214.

Ehri, L.C. (1986). Sources of difficulty in learning to read and spell. In M.L. Wolraich & D. Routh (Eds.), *Advances in developmental and behavioral pediatrics* (Vol. 7, pp. 121–195). Greenwich, CT: JAI Press.

Ehri, L.C. (2000). Learning to read and learning to spell: Two sides of a coin. *Topics in Language Disorders, 20*(3), 19–36.

Elksnin, L.K., & Elksnin, N. (1995). *Assessment and instruction of social skills* (2nd ed.). San Diego: Singular Publishing Group.

Ely, D.P. (1993). Computers in schools and universities in the United States of America. *Educational Technology, 33*(9), 53–57.

Emig, J. (1971). *The composing processes of twelfth graders* (Research Report No. 13). Urbana, IL: National Council of Teachers of English.

Emig, J. (1977). Writing as a mode of learning. *College Composition and Communication, 28,* 122–127.

Englert, C.S. (1992). Writing instruction from a sociocultural perspective: The holistic, dialogic, and social enterprise of writing. *Journal of Learning Disabilities, 25*(3), 153–172.

Englert, C.S., & Palincsar, A.S. (1991). Reconsidering instructional research in literacy from a sociocultural perspective. *Learning Disabilities Research and Practice, 6,* 225–229.

Englert, C.S., Raphael, T.E., Anderson, L.M., Anthony, H.M., Stevens, D., & Fear, K. (1991). Making writing strategies and self-talk visible: Cognitive strategy instruction in writing in regular and special education classrooms. *American Educational Research Journal, 28,* 337–373.

Englert, C.S., Raphael, T.E., Anderson, L.M., Gregg, S.L., & Anthony, H.M. (1989). Exposition: Reading, writing, and the metacognitive knowledge of learning disabled students. *Learning Disabilities Research, 5,* 5–24.

Englert, C.S., Raphael, T.E., Fear, K.L., & Anderson, L.M. (1988). Students' metacognitive knowledge about how to write informational texts. *Learning Disability Quarterly, 11,* 18–46.

Erickson, B.J. (1992). A synthesis of studies on computer-supported composition, revision, and quality. *Journal of Research on Computing in Education, 25,* 172–186.

Erickson, K.A., & Koppenhaver, D.A. (1995). Developing a literacy program for children with severe disabilities. *The Reading Teacher, 48,* 676–684.

Espin, C., Shin, J., Deno, S.L., Skare, S., Robinson, S., & Benner, B. (2000). Identifying indicators of written expression proficiency for middle school students. *Journal of Special Education, 34,* 140–153.

Feuerstein, R. (1979). *The dynamic assessment of retarded performers.* Baltimore: University Park Press.

Fey, M.E., Long, S.H., & Cleave, P.L. (1994). Reconsideration of IQ criteria in the definition of specific language impairment. In S.F. Warren & J. Reichle (Series Eds.) & R.V. Watkins & M.L. Rice (Vol. Eds.), *Communication and language intervention series: Vol. 4. Specific language impairments in children* (pp. 161–178). Baltimore: Paul H. Brookes Publishing Co.

Fiderer, A. (1993). *Teaching writing: A workshop approach.* New York: Scholastic Professional Books.

Follansbee, B. (1999). *Understanding Dragon Dictate for Windows: Speaking to write project.* Retrieved from http://www.edc.org/spk2wrt/

Follansbee, B. (2001). *Update on speech recognition.* National Center to Improve Practice in Special Education Through Technology, Media, and Materials. Retrieved December 15, 2002, from http://www2.edc.org/NCIP/vr/VR_Bob.html

Francis, D.J., Fletcher, J.M., Shaywitz, B.A., Shaywitz, S.E., & Rourke, B.P. (1996). Defining learning and language disabilities: Conceptual and psychometric issues with the use of IQ tests. *Language, Speech, and Hearing Services in Schools, 27,* 132–143.

Friel-Patti, S. (1999). Specific language impairment: Continuing clinical concerns. *Topics in Language Disorders, 20*(1), 1–13.

Fry, E.B., Kress, J.E., & Fountoukidis, D.L. (2000). *The reading teacher's book of lists* (4th ed.). Upper Saddle River, NJ: Prentice Hall.

Fujiki, M., & Brinton, B. (1994). Social competence and language impairment in children. In S.F. Warren & J. Reichle (Series Eds.) & R.V. Watkins & M.L. Rice (Vol. Eds.), *Communication and language intervention series: Vol. 4. Specific language impairments in children* (pp. 123–144). Baltimore: Paul H. Brookes Publishing Co.

Fujiki, M., Brinton, B., Isaacson, T., & Summers, C. (2001). Social behaviors of children with language impairment on the playground: A pilot study. *Language, Speech, and Hearing Services in Schools, 32,* 101–113.

Fujiki, M., Brinton, B., Morgan, M., & Hart, C.H. (1999). Withdrawn and sociable behavior of children with language impairment. *Language, Speech, & Hearing Services in Schools, 30,* 183–195.

Gaffney, J.S., & Anderson, R.C. (1991). *Two-tiered scaffolding: Congruent processes of teaching and learning.* (Technical Report No. 523.) Champaign, IL: University of Illinois at Urbana-Champaign: Center for the Study of Reading.

Gallagher, T.M. (1991). *Pragmatics of language: Clinical practice issues.* San Diego: Singular Publishing Group.

Gee, J. (1990). *Sociolinguistics and literacies: Ideologies and discourses.* New York: Falmer Press.

Gentry, J.R. (1982). An analysis of developmental spelling in GNYS AT WRK. *The Reading Teacher, 36,* 192–200.

Gerber, A. (1993). *Language-related learning disabilities: Their nature and treatment.* Baltimore: Paul H. Brookes Publishing Co.

German, D.J. (1979). Word finding skills in children with learning disabilities. *Journal of Learning Disabilities, 12*(3), 43–48.

German, D.J. (1993). *Word finding intervention program.* Austin, TX: PRO-ED.

German, D.J. (1994). Word-finding difficulties in children and adolescents. In G.P. Wallach & K.G. Butler (Eds.), *Language learning disabilities in school-age children and adolescents* (pp. 323–347). Boston: Allyn & Bacon.

Gertner, B.L., Rice, M.L., & Hadley, P.A. (1994). Influence of communicative competence on peer preferences in a preschool classroom. *Journal of Speech and Hearing Research, 34,* 1308–1317.

Gillam, R.B., & Carlile, R.M. (1997). Oral reading and story retelling of students with specific language impairment. *Language, Speech, and Hearing Services in Schools, 28,* 30–42.

Gillam, R.B., & Johnston, J.R. (1992). Spoken and written language relationships in language/learning-impaired and normally achieving school-aged children. *Journal of Speech and Hearing Research, 35,* 1303–1315.

Gillam, R., McFadden, T.U., & van Kleeck, A. (1995). Improving narrative abilities: Whole language and language skills approaches. In S.F. Warren & J. Reichle (Series Eds.) & M.E. Fey, J. Windsor, & S.F. Warren (Vol. Eds.), *Communication and language intervention series: Vol. 5. Language intervention: Preschool through the elementary years* (pp. 145–182). Baltimore: Paul H. Brookes Publishing Co.

Gillam, R.B., Peña, E.D., & Miller, L. (1999). Dynamic assessment of narrative and expository discourse. *Topics in Language Disorders, 20*(1), 33–47.

Glenn, C.G., & Stein, N. (1980). *Syntactic structures and real world themes in stories generated by children.* Urbana: University of Illinois Center for the Study of Reading.

Goodman, K.S. (1969). Analysis of oral reading miscues: Applied psycholinguistics. In F. Smith (Ed.), *Psycholinguistics and reading* (pp. 21–27). New York: Holt, Rinehart, & Winston.

Graham, S. (1990). The role of production factors in learning disabled students' compositions. *Journal of Education Psychology, 82,* 781–791.

Graham, S., Berninger, V.W., Abbott, R.D., Abbott, S.P., & Whitaker, D. (1997). Role of mechanics in composing of elementary school students: A new methodological approach. *Journal of Educational Psychology, 89,* 170–182.

Graham, S., & Harris, K.R. (1989). Component analysis of cognitive strategy instruction: Effects on learning disabled students' compositions and self-efficacy. *Journal of Educational Psychology, 81,* 353–361.

Graham, S., & Harris, K.R. (1994). Implications of constructivism for teaching writing to students with special needs. *Journal of Special Education, 28,* 275–289.

Graham, S., & Harris, K.R. (1997). It can be taught, but it does not develop naturally: Myths and realities in writing instruction. *School Psychology Review, 26,* 414–424.

Graham, S., & Harris, K.R. (1999). Assessment and intervention in overcoming writing difficulties: An illustration from the self-regulated strategy development model. *Language, Speech, & Hearing Services in Schools, 30,* 255–264.

Graham, S., Harris, K., MacArthur, C.A., & Schwartz, S.S. (1991). Writing and writing instruction with students with learning disabilities: A review of a program of research. *Learning Disability Quarterly, 14,* 89–114.

Graham, S., Harris, K.R., & Troia, G.A. (2000). Self-regulated strategy development revisited: Teaching writing strategies to struggling writers. *Topics in Language Disorders, 20*(4), 1–14.

Graham, S., & MacArthur, C. (1988). Improving learning disabled students' skills at revising essays produced on a word processor: Self-instructional strategy training. *Journal of Special Education, 22,* 132–152.

Graham, S., Schwartz, S.S., & MacArthur, C. (1993). Knowledge of writing and the composing process, attitudes toward writing, and self-efficacy for students with and without learning disabilities. *Journal of Learning Disabilities, 26,* 237–249.

Graves, A., & Montague, M. (1991). Using story grammar cueing to improve the writing of students with learning disabilities. *Learning Disabilities Research & Practice, 6,* 246–250.

Graves, D.H. (1983). *Writing: Teachers and children at work.* Portsmouth, NH: Heinemann.

Graves, D.H. (1991). *Build a literate classroom.* Portsmouth, NH: Heinemann.

Graves, D.H. (1994). *A fresh look at writing.* Portsmouth, NH: Heinemann.

Greenhalgh, K.S., & Strong, C.J. (2001). Literate language features in spoken narratives of children with typical language and children with language impairments. *Language, Speech, and Hearing Services in Schools, 32,* 114–125.

Greenspan, S.I. (1997). *The growth of the mind.* Reading, MA: Perseus Publishing.

Grice, H.P. (1975). Logic and conversation. In P. Cole & J.L. Morgan (Eds.), *Syntax and semantics 3: Speech acts* (pp. 41–58). San Diego: Academic Press.

Gummersall, D.M., & Strong, C.J. (1999). Assessment of complex sentence production in a narrative context. *Language, Speech, and Hearing Services in Schools, 30,* 152–164.

Guralnick, M.J. (1992). A hierarchical model for understanding children's peer-related social competence. In S.L. Odom, S.R. McConnell, & M.A. McEvoy (Eds.), *Social competence in young children with disabilities: Issues and strategies for intervention* (pp. 37–64). Baltimore: Paul H. Brookes Publishing Co.

Gutierrez-Clellen, V.F. (1995). Narrative development and disorders in Spanish-speaking children: Implications for the bilingual interventionist. In H. Kayser (Ed.), *Bilingual speech pathology: An Hispanic focus* (pp. 97–127). San Diego: Singular Publishing Group.

Gutierrez-Clellen, V.F. (1998). Syntactic skills of Spanish-speaking children with low school achievement. *Language, Speech, and Hearing Services in Schools, 29,* 207–215.

Gutierrez-Clellen, V.F. (1999). Mediating literacy skills in Spanish-speaking children with special needs. *Language, Speech, and Hearing Services in Schools, 30,* 285–292.

Gutierrez-Clellen, V.F. (2000). Dynamic assessment: An approach to assessing children's language-learning potential. *Seminars in Speech and Language, 21,* 215–222.

Gutierrez-Clellen, V.F., & Quinn, R. (1993). Assessing narratives of children from diverse cultural/linguistic groups. *Language, Speech, and Hearing Services in Schools, 24,* 2–9.

Gutierrez-Clellen, V.F., Restrepo, M.A., Bedore, L., Pena, E., & Anderson, R. (2000). Language sample analysis in Spanish-speaking children: Methodological considerations. *Language, Speech, and Hearing Services in Schools, 31,* 88–98.

Hall, P., Jordan, L.S., & Robin, D.A. (1993). *Developmental apraxia of speech.* Austin, TX: PRO-ED.

Hammill, D.D., Brown, V.L., Larsen, S.C., & Wiederholt, J.L. (1994). *Test of Adolescent and Adult Language–Third edition (TOAL-3).* Austin, TX: PRO-ED.

Hammill, D.D., & Larsen, S.C. (1991). *Test of Written Language–2nd Ed. (TOWL-2).* Austin, TX: PRO-ED.

Hammill, D.D., & Larsen, S.C. (1996). *Test of Written Language–3rd Ed. (TOWL-3).* Austin, TX: PRO-ED.

Harbers, H.M., Paden, E.P., & Halle, J.W. (1999). Phonological awareness and production: Changes during intervention. *Language, Speech, and Hearing Services in Schools, 30,* 50–60.

Harris, K.R., & Graham, S. (1996). *Making the writing process work: Strategies for composition and self-regulation.* Cambridge, MA: Brookline Books.

Hayes, J., & Flower, L. (1980). Identifying the organization of the writing process. In L.W. Gregg & E.R. Steinberg (Eds.), *Cognitive processes in writing* (pp. 3–10). Mahwah, NJ: Lawrence Erlbaum Associates.

Heath, S.B. (1983). *Ways with words: Language and work in communities and classrooms.* Cambridge, England: Cambridge University Press.

Heath, S.B. (1986). Taking a cross-cultural look at narratives. *Topics in Language Disorders, 7*(1), 84–94.

Hedberg, N.L., & Stoel-Gammon, C. (1986). Narrative analysis: Clinical procedures. *Topics in Language Disorders, 7*(1), 58–69.

Hedberg, N.L., & Westby, C.E. (1993). *Analyzing story telling skills: Theory to practice.* Austin, TX: PRO-ED.

Hester, E.J. (1996). Narratives of young African American children. In A.G. Kamhi, K.E. Pollock, & J.L. Harris (Eds.), *Communication development and disorders in African American children: Research, assessment, and intervention* (pp. 227–245). Baltimore: Paul H. Brookes Publishing Co.

Hewitt, L.E. (1994). Narrative comprehension: The importance of subjectivity. In J.F. Duchan, L.E. Hewitt, & R.M. Sonnenmeier (Eds.), *Pragmatics: From theory to practice* (pp. 88–104). Upper Saddle River, NJ: Prentice Hall.

Higgins, E.L., & Raskind, M.H. (1995). Compensatory effectiveness of speech recognition on the written composition performance of postsecondary students with learning disabilities. *Learning Disability Quarterly, 18,* 159–174.

Higgins, E.L., & Raskind, M.H. (2000). Speaking to read: The effects of continuous vs. discrete speech recognition systems on the reading and spelling of children with learning disabilities. *Journal of Special Education Technology, 15*(1), 19–30.

Hine, M.S., Goldman, S.R., & Cosden, M.A. (1990). Error monitoring by learning handicapped students engaged in collaborative microcomputer-based writing. *Journal of Special Education, 23,* 407–422.

Hogan, K., & Pressley, M. (1997). *Scaffolding student learning: Instructional approaches and issues.* Cambridge, MA: Brookline Books.

Hopkins, G. (1998). *Keyboarding skills: When should they be taught?* Retrieved from http://www.education-world.com/a_curr/curr076.shtml

Hoyt, L. (2000). *Snapshots: Literacy minilessons up close.* Portsmouth, NH: Heinemann.

Hresko, W.P., Herron, S.R., & Peak, P.K. (1996). *Test of Early Written Language–Second Edition (TEWL–2).* Austin, TX: PRO-ED.

Hubbard, R.S., & Power, B.M. (1993). *The art of classroom inquiry: A handbook for teacher-researchers.* Portsmouth, NH: Heinemann.

Hughes, D., McGillivray, L., & Schmidek, M. (1997). *Guide to narrative language.* Eau Claire, WI: Thinking Publications.

Hunt, K.W. (1965). *Grammatical structures written at three grade levels.* Urbana, IL: National Council of Teachers of English.

Hunt, K.W. (1970). Syntactic maturity in school children and adults. *Monographs of the Society for Research in Child Development*(No. 134).

Hunt, K.W. (1977). Early blooming and late blooming syntactic structures. In C.R. Cooper & L. Odell (Eds.), *Evaluating writing: Describing, measuring, judging* (pp. 91–106). Urbana, IL: National Council of Teachers of English.

Hunt-Berg, M., Rankin, J., & Beukelman, D. (1994). Ponder the possibilities: Computer-supported writing for struggling writers. *Learning Disabilities Research and Practice, 9*(3), 169–178.

Hyter, Y.D., & Westby, C.E. (1996). Using oral narratives to assess communicative competence. In A.G. Kamhi, K.E. Pollock, & J.L. Harris (Eds.), *Communication development and disorders in African American children: Research, assessment, and intervention* (pp. 247–285). Baltimore: Paul H. Brookes Publishing Co.

Individuals with Disabilities Education Act Amendments of 1997, PL 105-17, 20 U.S.C. §§ 1400 *et seq.*

Isaacson, S. (1989). Role of secretary vs. author: Resolving the conflict in writing instruction. *Learning Disability Quarterly, 12,* 209–218.

Isaacson, S. (1991). Assessing written language skills. In C.S. Simon (Ed.), *Communication skills and classroom success* (pp. 224–237). Eau Claire, WI: Thinking Publications. (Original work published 1985)

Isaacson, S., & Gleason, M.M. (1997). Mechanical obstacles to writing: What can teachers do to help students with learning problems? *Learning Disabilities Research and Practice, 12,* 188–194.

Jackson, T., & Berg, D. (1986). Elementary keyboarding—Is it important? *The Computing Teacher, 13*(6), 8, 10–11.

Johnson, D.J., & Grant, J.O. (1989). Written narratives of normal and learning disabled children. *Annals of Dyslexia, 39*, 140–158.

Juel, C. (1988). Learning to read and write: A longitudinal study of 54 children from first through fourth grades. *Journal of Educational Psychology, 80*, 437–447.

Kaderavek, J.N., & Sulzby, E. (2000). Narrative production by children with and without specific language impairment: Oral narratives and emergent reading. *Journal of Speech, Language, and Hearing Research, 43*, 34–49.

Kail, R., & Leonard, L.B. (1986). Word-finding abilities in language-impaired children. *ASHA Monographs* (No. 25). Rockville, MD: American Speech-Language-Hearing Associations.

Kamhi, A.G., & Catts, H.W. (1999a). Language and reading: Convergences and divergences. In H.W. Catts & A.G. Kamhi (Eds.), *Language and reading disabilities* (pp. 1–24). Boston: Allyn & Bacon.

Kamhi, A.G., & Catts, H.W. (1999b). Reading development. In H.W. Catts & A.G. Kamhi (Eds.), *Language and reading disabilities* (pp. 25–49). Boston: Allyn & Bacon.

Kamhi, A.G., & Hinton, L.N. (2000). Explaining individual differences in spelling ability. *Topics in Language Disorders, 20*(3), 37–49.

Kaufman, S.S., Prelock, P.A., Weiler, E.M., Creaghead, N.A., & Donnelly, C.A. (1994). Metapragmatic awareness of explanation adequacy: Developing skills for academic success from a collaborative communication skills unit. *Language, Speech, and Hearing Services in Schools, 25*, 174–180.

Kemper, S., & Edwards, L. (1986). Children's expression of causality and their construction of narratives. *Topics in Language Disorders, 7*(1), 11–20.

Keogh, B.K. (1993). Linking purpose and practice: Social-political and developmental perspectives on classification. In G.R. Lyon, D.B. Gray, J.F. Kavanagh, & N.A. Krasegnor (Eds.), *Better understanding learning disabilities: New views from research and their implication for education and public policies* (pp. 311–324). Baltimore: Paul H. Brookes Publishing Co.

Kinnucan-Welsch, K. (2000, June). *Action research.* Presentation at the second summer institute for the Writing Lab Outreach Project, Western Michigan University, Kalamazoo.

Klecan-Acker, J.S., & Hedrick, L.D. (1985). A study of the syntactic language skills of normal school-age children. *Language, Speech, and Hearing Services in Schools, 16*, 187–198.

Klee, T. (1992). Developmental and diagnostic characteristics of quantitative measures of children's language production. *Topics in Language Disorders, 12*(2), 28–41.

Koegel, R.L., & Koegel, L.K. (1995). *Teaching children with autism: Strategies for initiating positive interactions and improving learning opportunities.* Baltimore: Paul H. Brookes Publishing Co.

Koppenhaver, D.A., Coleman, P.P., Kalman, S.L., & Yoder, D.E. (1991). The implications of emergent literacy research for children with developmental disabilities. *American Journal of Speech-Language Pathology, 1*, 38–44.

Koppenhaver, D.A., & Yoder, D.E. (1992). Literacy issues in persons with severe physical and speech impairments. In R. Gaylord-Ross (Ed.), *Issues and research in special education* (pp. 156–201). New York: Teachers College Press.

Koppenhaver, D.A., & Yoder, D.E. (1993). Classroom literacy instruction for children with severe speech and physical impairments (SSPI): What is and what might be. *Topics in Language Disorders, 13*(2), 1–15.

Labov, W. (1972). *Language in the inner city.* Philadelphia: University of Pennsylvania Press.

Leonard, L.B. (1998). *Children with specific language impairment.* Cambridge: MIT Press.

Leonard, L.B., & Bartolini, U. (1998). Grammatical morphology and the role of weak syllables in the speech of Italian-speaking children with specific language impairment. *Journal of Speech, Language, and Hearing Research, 41*, 1363–1374.

Lewis, B.A., Freebairn, L.A., & Taylor, H.G. (2000). Follow-up of children with early expressive phonology disorders. *Journal of Learning Disabilities, 33*, 433–444.

Lewis, R.B., Ashton, T.M., Haapa, B., Kieley, C.L., & Fielden, C. (1999). Improving the writing skills of students with learning disabilities: Are word processors with spelling and grammar checkers useful? *Learning Disabilities, 9*(3), 87–98.

Lidz, C.S., & Peña, E.D. (1996). Dynamic assessment: The model, its relevance as a nonbiased approach, and its application to Latino American preschool children. *Language, Speech, and Hearing Services in Schools, 27*, 367–372.

Light, J., & McNaughton, D. (1993). Literacy and augmentative and alternative communication (AAC): The expectations and priorities of parents and teachers. *Topics in Language Disorders, 13*(2), 33–46.

Loban, W.D. (1963). *The language of elementary school children.* (NCTE Research Report No. 1). Urbana, IL: National Council of Teachers of English.

Loban, W. (1976). *Language development: Kindergarten through grade twelve* (Research Report No. 18). Champaign, IL: National Council of Teachers of English.

Long, L. (1988). *Introduction to computers and information processing* (2nd ed.). Upper Saddle River, NJ: Prentice Hall.

Luckner, J.L. (1996). Written-language assessment and intervention: Links to literacy. *The Volta Review, 98*(1) [monograph], v–vi.

Lund, N.J. (2000). Assessment of language structure: From syntax to event-based analysis. *Seminars in Speech and Language, 21,* 267–274.

Lyon, G.R. (1995). Toward a definition of dyslexia. *Annals of Dyslexia, 45,* 3–27.

Lyon, G.R., Gray, D.B., Kavanagh, J.F., & Krasnegor, N.A. (Eds.). (1993). *Better understanding learning disabilities: New views from research and their implications for education and public policies.* Baltimore: Paul H. Brookes Publishing Co.

MacArthur, C.A. (1996). Using technology to enhance the writing processes of students with learning disabilities. *Journal of Learning Disabilities, 29,* 344–354.

MacArthur, C.A. (1998). Word processing with speech synthesis and word prediction: Effects on the dialogue journal writing of students with learning disabilities. *Learning Disability Quarterly, 22,* 158–172.

MacArthur, C.A. (1999). Word prediction for students with severe spelling problems. *Learning Disability Quarterly, 22,* 158–172.

MacArthur, C.A. (2000). New tools for writing: Assistive technology for students with writing difficulties. *Topics in Language Disorders, 20(4),* 85–100.

MacArthur, C.A., & Graham, S. (1987). Learning disabled students composing under three methods of text production: Handwriting, word processing, and dictation. *Journal of Special Education, 21,* 22–42.

MacArthur, C., Graham, S., Haynes, J.B., & DeLaPaz, S. (1996). Spelling checkers and students with learning disabilities: Performance comparisons and impact on spelling. *Journal of Special Education, 30*(1), 35–57.

MacArthur, C.A., Graham, S., & Schwartz, S. (1991). Knowledge of revision and revising behavior among students with learning disabilities. *Learning Disability Quarterly, 14*(1), 61–73.

MacArthur, C.A., Graham, S., & Schwartz, S.S. (1993). Integrating strategy instruction and word processing into a process approach to writing instruction. *School Psychology Review, 22,* 671–681.

MacArthur, C.A., Schwartz, S.S., & Graham, S. (1991a). Effects of a reciprocal peer revision strategy in special education classrooms. *Learning Disabilities Research and Practice, 6,* 201–210.

MacArthur, C.A., Schwartz, S.S., & Graham, S. (1991b). A model for writing instruction: Integrating word processing and strategy instruction into a process approach to writing. *Learning Disabilities Research and Practice, 6,* 230–236.

Maddux, C.D., Johnson, D.L., & Willis, J.W. (1997). *Educational computing: Learning with tomorrow's technologies* (2nd ed.). Boston: Allyn & Bacon.

Mandell, C.J., & Mandell, S.L. (1989). *Computers in education today.* St. Paul, MN: West.

Mandler, J. (1982). Some uses and abuses of a story grammar. *Discourse Processes, 5,* 305–318.

Mandler, J., & Johnson, N. (1977). Remembrance of things parsed: Story structure and recall. *Cognitive Psychology, 9,* 111–151.

Masterson, J.J., & Apel, K. (2000). Spelling assessment: Charting a path to optimal intervention. *Topics in Language Disorders, 20*(3), 50–65.

Mather, N., & Roberts, R. (1995). *Informal assessment and instruction in written language.* Brandon, VT: Clinical Psychology Publishing Co.

Mather, N., & Woodcock, R.W. (1997). *Mather-Woodcock Group Writing Tests* (GWT). Itasca, IL: Riverside Publishing.

McAlister, K. (1995). *The attitudes of children with specialized language-learning needs toward process writing.* Unpublished master's thesis, Western Michigan University, Kalamazoo.

McAlister, K.M., Nelson, N.W., & Bahr, C.M. (1999). Perceptions of students with language-learning disabilities about writing process instruction. *Learning Disabilities Research and Practice, 14*(3), 159–172.

McCabe, A., & Peterson, C. (1984). What makes a good story? *Journal of Psycholinguistic Research, 13,* 457–480.

McCabe, A., & Peterson, C. (Eds.). (1991). *Developing narrative structure.* Upper Saddle River, NJ: Lawrence Erlbaum Associates.

McCabe, A., & Rollins, P.R. (1994). Assessment of preschool narrative skills. *American Journal of Speech-Language Pathology, 3*(1), 45–56.

McGhee, R., Bryant, B.R., Larsen, S.C., & Rivera, D.M. (1995). *Test of Written Expression* (TOWE). Austin, TX: PRO-ED.

McLean, G. (1994). *Teaching keyboarding.* Little Rock, AK: Delta Pi Epsilon.

McNaughton, D., Hughes, C., & Clark, K. (1997). The effect of five proofreading conditions on the spelling performance of college students with learning disabilities. *Journal of Learning Disabilities, 30,* 643–651.

McNaughton, D., Hughes, C., & Ofiesh, N. (1997). Proofreading for students with learning disabilities: Integrating computer use and strategy use. *Learning Disabilities Research and Practice, 12,* 16–28.

Menyuk, P., & Chesnick, M. (1997). Metalinguistic skills, oral language knowledge, and reading. *Topics in Language Disorders, 17*(3), 75–87.

Merritt, D.D., & Culatta, B. (Eds.). (1998). *Language intervention in the classroom.* San Diego: Singular Publishing Group.

Michaels, S. (1981). Sharing time: Children's narrative styles and differential access to literacy. *Language in Society, 10,* 423–442.

Michaels, S. (1991). The dismantling of narrative. In A. McCabe & C. Peterson (Eds.), *Developing narrative structure* (pp. 303–352). Upper Saddle River, NJ: Lawrence Erlbaum Associates.

Miller, J.F. (1981). *Assessing language production in children: Experimental procedures.* Austin, TX: PRO-ED.

Miller, J.F. (1991). Quantifying productive language disorders. In J.F. Miller (Ed.), *Research on child language disorders* (pp. 211–220). Austin, TX: PRO-ED.

Miller, J., & Chapman, R.S. (2000). *Systematic analysis of language transcripts (SALT)* [Computer program; A. Nockerts, Programmer]. Madison, WI: Waisman Center on Mental Retardation and Human Development, Language Analysis Laboratory.

Miller, L., Gillam, R., & Peña, E. (in press). *Dynamic assessment and intervention of children's narratives.* Austin, TX: PRO-ED.

Mirenda, P. (1999). Augmentative and alternative communication techniques. In J.E. Downing, *Teaching communication skills to students with severe disabilities* (pp. 119–138). Baltimore: Paul H. Brookes Publishing Co.

Moats, L. (1983). A comparison of the spelling errors of older dyslexic and second-grade normal children. *Annals of Dyslexia, 33,* 121–139.

Moats, L. (1995). *Spelling: Development, difficulty, and instruction.* Baltimore: York Press.

Montague, M., & Graves, A. (1993). Improving students' story writing. *Teaching Exceptional Children, 25*(4), 36–37.

Montague, M., Maddux, C., & Dereschiwsky, M. (1990). Story grammar and comprehension and production of narrative prose by students with learning disabilities. *Journal of Learning Disabilities, 23,* 190–197.

Morris, N.T., & Crump, W.D. (1982). Syntactic and vocabulary development in the written language of learning disabled and non-disabled students at four age levels. *Learning Disability Quarterly, 5,* 163–172.

Muschla, G.R. (1993). *Writing workshop survival kit.* West Nyack, NY: The Center for Applied Research in Education.

Musselman, C. (2000). How do children who can't hear learn to read an alphabetic script? A review of the literature on reading and deafness. *Journal of Deaf Studies and Deaf Education, 5*(1), 9–31.

Myers, M. (1985). *The teacher-researcher: How to study writing in the classroom.* Urbana, IL: National Council of Teachers of English.

National Business Education Association. (1992). *Elementary/middle school keyboarding strategies guide.* Reston, VA: National Business Education Association.

Nelson, K. (1974). Concept, word, and sentence: Interrelationships in acquisition and development. *Psychological Review, 77,* 257–273.

Nelson, N.W. (1986). What is meant by meaning (and how can it be taught)? *Topics in Language Disorders, 6*(4), 1–14.

Nelson, N.W. (1989). Curriculum-based language assessment and intervention. *Language, Speech, and Hearing Services in Schools, 20,* 174–184.

Nelson, N.W. (1990). Only relevant practices can be best. In W. Secord (Ed.), *Best practices in school speech-language pathology* (Vol. 1, pp. 15–27). San Antonio, TX: Psychological Corporation.

Nelson, N.W. (1992). Performance is the prize: Language competence and performance among AAC users. *Augmentative and Alternative Communication, 8,* 3–18.

Nelson, N.W. (1994). Curriculum-based language assessment and intervention across the grades. In G.P. Wallach & K.G. Butler (Eds.), *Language learning disabilities in school-age children and adolescents* (pp. 104–131). Boston: Allyn & Bacon.

Nelson, N.W. (1995). Scaffolding in the secondary school. In H. Winnitz (Series Ed.) & D. Tibbits (Vol. Ed.), *Language intervention: Beyond the primary grades* (pp. 375–419). Austin, TX: PRO-ED.

Nelson, N.W. (1998). *Childhood language disorders in context: Infancy through adolescence* (2nd ed.). Boston: Allyn & Bacon.

Nelson, N.W., Bahr, C.M., & Van Meter, A.M. (2002, Dec.). *Writing Lab Outreach Project: Final report.* Available as an ERIC document.

Nelson, N.W., & Van Meter, A.M. (2002). Assessing curriculum-based reading and writing samples. *Topics in Language Disorders, 22*(2), 35–59.

Nelson, N.W., & Van Meter, A. M. (2003, June). *Measuring written language abilities and change through the elementary school years.* Poster session presentation at the Symposium of Research on Child Language Disorders, Madison, WI.

Nelson, N.W., Van Meter, A.M., & Bahr, C.M. (2002, November). *Written language changes for students in inclusive classroom intervention.* Poster session presented at the Annual Convention of the American Speech-Language-Hearing Association, Atlanta, GA.

Nelson, N.W., Van Meter, A.M., Chamberlain, D., & Bahr, C.M. (2001). The speech-language pathologist's role in a writing lab approach. *Seminars in Speech and Language, 22*(3), 209–220.

Newell, A.F., Booth, L., Arnott, J., & Beattie, W. (1992). Increasing literacy levels by the use of linguistic prediction. *Child Language Teaching and Therapy, 8,* 138–187.

Nippold, M.A. (Ed.). (1998a). *Later language development: The school-age and adolescent years.* Austin, TX: PRO-ED.

Nippold, M.A. (1998b). The literate lexicon. In M. Nippold (Ed.), *Later language development, ages nine through nineteen* (pp. 29–48). Austin, TX: PRO-ED.

Nippold, M.A. (2000). Language development during the adolescent years: Aspects of pragmatics, syntax, and semantics. *Topics in Language Disorders, 20*(2), 15–28.

Odom, S.L., McConnell, S.R., & McEvoy, M.A. (Eds.). (1992). *Social competence in young children with disabilities: Issues and strategies for intervention.* Baltimore: Paul H. Brookes Publishing Co.

O'Donnell, R., Griffin, W., & Norris, R. (1967). *Syntax of kindergarten and elementary school children: A transformational analysis* (Research Report No. 8). Champaign, IL: National Council of Teachers of English.

Olson, D.R. (1970). Language and thought: Aspects of a cognitive theory of semantics. *Psychological Review, 77,* 257–273.

Paley, V.G. (1979). *White teacher.* Cambridge, MA: Harvard University Press.

Paley, V.G. (1981). *Wally's stories: Conversations in the kindergarten.* Cambridge, MA: Harvard University Press.

Paley, V.G. (1990). *The boy who would be a helicopter: The uses of storytelling in the classroom.* Cambridge, MA: Harvard University Press.

Paley, V.G. (1994). Every child a storyteller. In J.F. Duchan, L.E. Hewitt, & R.M. Sonnenmeier (Eds.), *Pragmatics: From theory to practice* (pp. 10–19). Upper Saddle River, NJ: Prentice Hall.

Palincsar, A.S., Brown, A.L., & Campione, J.C. (1994). Models and practices of dynamic assessment. In G.P. Wallach & K.G. Butler (Eds.), *Language learning disabilities in school-age children and adolescents* (pp. 132–144). Boston: Allyn & Bacon.

Patterson, J.L. (1994). A tutorial on sociolinguistics for speech-language pathologists: An appreciation of variation. *National Student Speech Language Hearing Association Journal, 21,* 14–30.

Paul, R. (1991). Profiles of toddlers with slow expressive language development. *Topics in Language Disorders, 11*(4), 1–13.

Paul, R. (1996). Clinical implications of the natural history of slow expressive language development. *American Journal of Speech-Language Pathology, 5*(2), 5–21.

Paul, R. (1997). Understanding language delay: A response to van Kleeck, Gillam, & Davis. *American Journal of Speech-Language Pathology, 6*(2), 40–49.

Paul, R. (2000). "Putting things in context": Literal and discourse approaches to comprehension assessment. *Seminars in Speech and Language, 21,* 247–255.

Paul, R. (2001). *Language disorders from infancy through adolescence: Assessment and intervention* (2nd ed.). St. Louis: Mosby.

Paul, R., & Smith, R.L. (1993). Narrative skills in 4-year-olds with normal, impaired, and late-developing language. *Journal of Speech and Hearing Research, 36,* 592–598.

Payne, R.K. (2001). *Framework for understanding poverty* (2nd ed.). Highlands, TX: aha! Process.

Pebly, M., & Koppenhaver, D.A. (2001). Emergent and early literacy interventions for students with severe communication impairments. *Seminars in Speech and Language, 22,* 221–232.

Perera, K. (1984). *Children's writing and reading: Analysing classroom language.* Oxford, England: Blackwell.

Perera, K. (1986). Grammatical differentiation between speech and writing in children aged 8 to 12. In A. Wilkinson (Ed.), *The writing of writing* (pp. 90–108). London: Falmer Press.

Peterson, C., & McCabe, A. (1983). *Developmental psycholinguistics: Three ways of looking at children's narratives.* New York: Kluwer Academic/ Plenum Publishers.

Pinker, S. (1994). *The language instinct: How the mind creates language.* New York: William Morrow & Co.

Pisha, B. (1989). Typing for children with learning disabilities: A new solution, or a new problem? Unpublished qualifying paper, Harvard University Graduate School of Education. Cited in Pisha, B. (1993). *Rates of development of keyboarding skills in elementary school aged children with and without identified learning disabilities.* Retrieved December 15, 2002, from http://www.cast.org/udl/index.cfm?i=1761

Praisner, C.L. (2003). Attitudes of elementary school principals toward the inclusion of students with disabilities. *Exceptional Children, 69,* 135–145.

Prelock, P.A., Miller, B.L., & Reed, N.L. (1995). Collaborative partnerships in a language in the classroom program. *Language, Speech, and Hearing Services in Schools, 26*, 286–292.

Pressley, M., & Wharton-MacDonald, R. (1997). Skilled comprehension and its development through instruction. *School Psychology Review, 26*, 448–466.

Quill, K.A. (2000). *Do-watch-listen-say: Social and communication intervention for children with autism.* Baltimore: Paul H. Brookes Publishing Co.

Rapin, I., & Allen, D.A. (1983). Developmental language disorders: Nosologic consideration. In U. Kirk (Ed.), *Neuropsychology of language, reading, and spelling* (pp. 155–184). San Diego: Academic Press.

Read, C. (1971). Preschool children's knowledge of English phonology. *Harvard Educational Review, 41*, 1–34.

Read, C. (1986). *Children's creative spelling.* London: Routledge & Kegan Paul.

Records, N.L., Tomblin, J.B., & Freese, P.R. (1992). The quality of life of young adults with histories of specific language impairments. *American Journal of Speech-Language Pathology, 1*(2), 44–53.

Redmond, S.M., & Rice, M.L. (1998). The socioemotional behaviors of children with SLI: Social adaptation or social deviance? *Journal of Speech, Language, and Hearing Research, 41*, 688–700.

Rescorla, L. (1989). The language development survey: A screening tool for delayed language in toddlers. *Journal of Speech and Hearing Disorders, 54*, 587–599.

Rhodes, L., & Dudley-Marling, C. (1988). *Readers and writers with a difference: A holistic approach to teaching learning disabled and remedial students.* Portsmouth, NH: Heinemann.

Rice, M., & Oetting, J. (1993). Morphological deficits of children with SLI: Evaluation of number marking and agreement. *Journal of Speech and Hearing Research, 36*, 1249–1257.

Rice, M., & Wexler, K. (1996). Toward tense as a clinical marker of specific language impairment in English-speaking children. *Journal of Speech, Language, and Hearing Research, 39*, 1239–1257.

Richardson, K., Calnan, M., Essen, J., & Lambert, L. (1976). The linguistic maturity of 11-year-olds: Some analysis of the written composition of children in the National Development Study. *Journal of Child Language, 3*, 99–115.

Robinson-Zanartu, C. (1996). Serving Native American children and families: Considering cultural variables. *Language, Speech, and Hearing Services in Schools, 27*, 373–384.

Roblyer, M.D., Edwards, J., & Havriluk, M.A. (1997). *Integrating educational technology into teaching.* Columbus, OH: Merrill.

Rogers-Adkinson, D., & Griffith, P. (Eds.). (1999). *Communication disorders and children with psychiatric and behavioral disorders.* San Diego: Singular Publishing Group.

Rollins, P.R., McCabe, A., & Bliss, L. (2000). Culturally sensitive assessment of narrative skills in children. *Seminars in Speech and Language, 21*, 223–234.

Roth, F.P. (2000). Narrative writing: Development and teaching with children with writing difficulties. *Topics in Language Disorders, 20*(4), 15–28.

Roth, F.P., & Spekman, N.J. (1986). Narrative discourse: Spontaneously generated stories of learning-disabled and normally achieving students. *Journal of Speech and Hearing Disorders, 51*, 8–23.

Roth, F.P., & Spekman, N.J. (1989). The oral syntactic proficiency of learning disabled students: A spontaneous story sampling analysis. *Journal of Speech and Hearing Research, 32*, 67–77.

Scardamalia, M., & Bereiter, C. (1986). Research on written composition. In M.C. Wittrock (Ed.), *Handbook of research on teaching* (pp. 778–803). New York: Macmillan/McGraw-Hill.

Scardamalia, M., & Bereiter, C. (1994). Computer support for knowledge-building communities. *Journal of the Learning Sciences, 3*, 265–283.

Schairer, K.S., & Nelson, N.W. (1996). Communication possibilities of written conversations with adolescents who have autism. *Child Language Teaching and Therapy, 12*(2), 164–180.

Schleper, D.R. (1996). Write that one down: Using anecdotal records to inform our teaching. *The Volta Review, 98*(1), 201–210.

Schuler, A.L., & Wolfberg, P.J. (2000). Promoting peer play and socialization: The art of scaffolding. In S.F. Warren & J. Reichle (Series Eds.) & A.M. Wetherby & B.M. Prizant (Vol. Eds.), *Communication and language intervention series: Vol. 9. Autism spectrum disorders: A transactional developmental perspective* (pp. 251–277). Baltimore: Paul H. Brookes Publishing Co.

Scott, C.M. (1984). *What happened in that?: Structural characteristics of school children's narratives.* Paper presented at the Annual Convention of the American Speech-Language-Hearing Association, San Francisco.

Scott, C.M. (1988a). Producing complex sentences. *Topics in Language Disorders, 8*(2), 44–62.

Scott, C.M. (1988b). Spoken and written syntax. In M. Nippold (Ed.), *Later language development: Ages nine through nineteen* (2nd ed. pp. 49–95). Austin, TX: PRO-ED.

Scott, C.M. (1994). A discourse continuum for school-age students: Impact of modality and genre. In G.P. Wallach & K.G. Butler (Eds.), *Language learning disabilities in school-aged children and adolescents* (pp. 219–252). Boston: Allyn & Bacon.

Scott, C.M. (1999). Learning to write. In H.W. Catts & A.G. Kamhi (Eds.), *Language and reading disabilities* (pp. 224–258). Boston: Allyn & Bacon.

Scott, C.M. (2000). Principles and methods of spelling instruction: Applications for poor spellers. *Topics in Language Disorders, 20*(3), 66–82.

Scott, C.M., & Stokes, S. (1995). Measures of syntax in school-age children and adolescents. *Language, Speech, and Hearing Services in Schools, 26*, 301–319.

Scott, C.M., & Windsor, J. (2000). General language performance measures in spoken and written narrative and expository discourse of school-age children with language-learning disabilities. *Journal of Speech, Language, and Hearing Research, 43*, 324–339.

Silliman, E.R., Jimerson, T.L., & Wilkinson, L.C. (2000). A dynamic systems approach to writing assessment in students with language learning problems. *Topics in Language Disorders, 20*(4), 45–64.

Silliman, E.R., & Wilkinson, L.C. (1994). Discourse scaffolds for classroom intervention. In G.P. Wallach & K.G. Butler (Eds.), *Language learning disabilities in school-age children and adolescents* (pp. 27–52). Boston: Allyn & Bacon.

Simon, C.S. (1987). Out of the broom closet and into the classroom: The emerging SLP. *Journal of Childhood Communication Disorders, 11*, 41–66.

Simonson, M.R., & Thompson, A. (1997). *Educational computing foundations* (3rd ed.). Columbus, OH: Merrill.

Singer, B.D., & Bashir, A.S. (1999a, November). *Authentic assessment of writing: Approaches that inform instruction and intervention.* Paper presented at the Annual Convention of the American Speech-Language-Hearing Association, San Francisco.

Singer, B.D., & Bashir, A.S. (1999b). What are executive functions and self-regulation and what do they have to do with language-learning disorders. *Language, Speech, and Hearing Services in Schools, 30*, 265–273.

Smitherman, G. (1994). "The blacker the berry, the sweeter the juice": African American student writers. In A.H. Dyson & C. Genishi (Eds.), *The need for story: Cultural diversity in classroom and community* (pp. 80–101). Urbana, IL: National Council of Teachers of English.

Snow, C.E., Burns, M.S., & Griffin, P. (Eds.). (1998). *Preventing reading difficulties in young children.* Washington, DC: National Academy Press.

SPSS, Inc. (1999). *SPSS 9.0 for Windows.* Chicago, IL: Author.

Stanovich, K.E. (1986). Matthew effects in reading: Some consequences of individual differences in the acquisition of literacy. *Reading Research Quarterly, 21*, 360–407.

Stanovich, K.E. (1988a). *Children's reading and the development of phonological awareness.* Detroit, MI: Wayne State University Press.

Stanovich, K.E. (1988b). The right and wrong places to look for the cognitive locus of reading disability. *Annals of Dyslexia, 38*, 154–177.

Starr, L. (2001). *Teaching keyboarding—When? Why? How?* Retrieved January 3, 2003, from http://www.education-world.com/a_tech/tech072.shtml

Stein, N., & Glenn, C. (1979). An analysis of story comprehension in elementary school children. In R. Freedle (Ed.), *New directions in discourse processing* (Vol. 2, pp. 53–120). Westport, CT: Ablex Publishing.

Stein, N., & Glenn, C. (1982). Children's concept of time: The development of story schema. In W. Freeman (Ed.), *The developmental psychology of time* (pp. 255–282). San Diego: Academic Press.

Sternberg, R.L., Okagaki, L., & Jackson, A.S. (1990). Practical intelligence for success in school. *Educational Leadership, 48*(1), 35–39.

Stinson, M.S., & Whitmire, K.A. (2000). Adolescents who are deaf or hard of hearing: A communication perspective on educational placement. *Topics in Language Disorders, 20*(2), 58–72.

Stoddard, B., & MacArthur, C.A. (1992). A peer editor strategy: Guiding learning disabled students in response and revision. *Research in the Teaching of English, 27*, 76–103.

Sturm, J.M., & Koppenhaver, D.A. (2000). Supporting writing development in adolescents with developmental disabilities. *Topics in Language Disorders, 20*(2), 73–96.

Sturm, J.M., & Nelson, N.W. (1997). Formal classroom lessons: New perspectives on a familiar discourse event. *Language, Speech, and Hearing Services in Schools, 28*, 255–273.

Sturm, J.M., Rankin, J.L., Beukelman, D.R., & Schutz-Muehling, L. (1997). How to select appropriate software for computer-assisted writing. *Intervention in School and Clinic, 32*, 148–161.

Sturm, J.M., & Rankin-Erikson, J.L. (2002). Effects of hand-drawn and computer-generated concept mapping on the expository writing of middle school students with learning disabilities. *Learning Disabilities Research and Practice, 17*(2), 124–139.

Sulzby, E. (1996). Roles of oral and written language as children approach conventional literacy. In C. Pontecorvo, M. Orsolini, B. Burge, & L.B. Resnick (Eds.), *Children's early text construction* (pp. 25–46). Mahwah, NJ: Lawrence Erlbaum Associates.

Sutton-Smith, B. (1986). The development of fictional narrative performances. *Topics in Language Disorders, 7*(1), 1–10.

Swoger, P.A. (1989). Scott's gift. *English Journal, 78,* 61–65.

Tabors, P.O. (1997). *One child, two languages: A guide for preschool educators of children learning English as a second language.* Baltimore: Paul H. Brookes publishing Co.

Tattershall, S. (2002). *Adolescents with language and learning needs: A shoulder to shoulder collaboration.* San Diego: Singular Publishing Group.

Templeton, S. (1992). Theory, nature, and pedagogy of high-order orthographic development in older students. In S. Templeton & D.R. Bear (Eds.), *Development of orthographic knowledge and the foundations of literacy* (pp. 253–277). Mahwah, NJ: Lawrence Erlbaum Associates.

Templin, M. (1957). *Certain language skills in children.* Minneapolis: University of Minnesota Press.

Thal, D., & Bates, E. (1988). Language and gesture in late talkers. *Journal of Speech and Hearing Research, 31,* 115–123.

Thal, D., Tobias, S., & Morrison, D. (1991). Language and gesture in late talkers: A 1-year follow-up. *Journal of Speech and Hearing Research, 34,* 604–612.

Tharp, R.G., & Gallimore, R. (1989). *Rousing minds to life: Teaching, learning, and schooling in social context.* New York: Cambridge University Press.

Thorndyke, P.W. (1977). Cognitive structures in comprehension and memory of narrative discourse. *Cognitive Psychology, 9,* 77–110.

Tiegerman-Farber, E. (1997). Autism: Learning to communicate. In D.K. Bernstein & E. Tiegerman-Farber (Eds.), *Language and communication disorders in children* (pp. 524–573). Boston: Allyn & Bacon.

Tomblin, J.B., Records, N.L., Buckwalter, P., Zhang, X., Smith, E., & O'Brien, M. (1997). Prevalence of specific language impairment in kindergarten children. *Journal of Speech, Language, Hearing Research, 40,* 1245–1260.

Torgesen, J.K. (1999). Assessment and instruction for phonemic awareness and word recognition skill. In H.W. Catts & A.G. Kamhi (Eds.), *Language and reading disabilities* (pp. 128–153). Boston: Allyn & Bacon.

Torgesen, J.K, & Bryant, B.R. (1994). *Test of Phonological Awareness (TOPA).* Austin, TX: PRO-ED.

Treiman, R., & Bourassa, D. (2000a). Children's written and oral spelling. *Applied Psycholinguistics, 21,* 183–204.

Treiman, R., & Bourassa, D.C. (2000b). The development of spelling skill. *Topics in Language Disorders, 20*(3), 1–18.

Troia, G.A., Graham, S., & Harris, K.R. (1999). Teaching students with learning disabilities to mindfully plan when writing. *Exceptional Children, 65,* 235–252.

Tully, M. (1996). *Helping students revise their writing.* New York: Scholastic Professional Books.

Twachtman-Cullen, D. (2000). More able children with autism spectrum disorders: Sociocommunicative challenges and guidelines for enhancing abilities. In S.F. Warren & J. Reichle (Series Eds.) & A.M. Wetherby & B.M. Prizant (Vol. Eds.), *Communication and language intervention series: Vol. 9. Autism spectrum disorders: A transactional developmental perspective* (pp. 225–249). Baltimore: Paul H. Brookes Publishing Co.

Ukrainetz, T.A. (1998). Stickwriting stories: A quick and easy narrative representation strategy. *Language, Speech, and Hearing Services in Schools, 29,* 197–206.

U.S. Department of Education, Office of Educational Research and Improvement (OERI). (1996). Can students benefit from process writing? *NAEP Facts: A news publication of the National Center for Education Statistics, 1*(3), 1–6.

U.S. Office of Education. (1977, December 29). Assistance to the states for education of handicapped children: Procedures for evaluating specific learning disabilities. *Federal Register, 42*(250), 65,082–65,085.

van Kleeck, A. (1994). Metalinguistic development. In G.P. Wallach & K.G. Butler (Eds.), *Language learning disabilities in school-age children and adolescents* (pp. 53–98). Boston: Allyn & Bacon.

van Kleeck, A., Gillam, R.B., & Davis, B. (1997). When is "watch and see" warranted?: A response to Paul's 1996 article, "Clinical implications of the natural history of slow expressive language development." *American Journal of Speech-Language Pathology, 6*(2), 34–39.

Vaughn, S., Klingner, J., & Hughes, M. (2000). Sustainability of research-based practices. *Exceptional Children, 66,* 163–171.

Vygotsky, L.S. (1978). *Mind in society: The development of higher psychological processes* (M. Cole, V. John-Steiner, S. Scribner, & E. Souberman, Eds. and Trans.). Cambridge, MA: Harvard University Press.

Wallach, G.P., & Butler, K.G. (1984). *Language and learning disabilities in school-age children.* Philadelphia: Lippincott Williams & Wilkins.

Wallach, G.P., & Butler, K.G. (1994). *Language and learning disabilities in school-age children and adolescents: Some principles and applications.* Boston: Allyn & Bacon.

Watkins, R.V. (1994). Specific language impairments in children: An introduction. In S.F. Warren and J. Reichle (Series Eds.) & R.V. Watkins & M.L. Rice (Vol. Eds.), *Communication and language intervention series: Vol. 4. Specific language impairments in children* (pp. 1–16). Baltimore: Paul H. Brookes Publishing Co.

Watkins, R.V., & DeThorne, L.S. (2000). Assessing children's vocabulary skills: From word knowledge to word-learning potential. *Seminars in Speech and Language, 21*, 235–245.

Watkins, R.V., Kelly, D.J., Harbers, H.M., & Hollis, W. (1995). Measuring children's lexical diversity: Differentiating typical and impaired language learners. *Journal of Speech and Hearing Research, 38*, 1349–1355.

Watkins, R.V., & Rice, M.L. (Vol. Eds.). (1994). Specific language impairments in children. In S.F. Warren & J. Reichle (Series Eds.), *Communication and language intervention series* (Vol. 4). Baltimore: Paul H. Brookes Publishing Co.

Weaver, C. (1982). Welcoming errors as signs of growth. *Language Arts, 59*, 438–444.

Wells, G. (1986). *The meaning makers: Children learning language and using language to learn.* Portsmouth, NH: Heinemann.

Westby, C.E. (1984). Development of narrative language abilities. In G.P. Wallach & K.G. Butler (Eds.), *Language learning disabilities in school-age children* (pp. 103–127). Boston: Allyn & Bacon.

Westby, C.E. (1990). Ethnographic interviewing: Asking the right questions to the right people in the right ways. *Journal of Childhood Communication Disorders, 13*, 101–111.

Westby, C.E. (1994). The effects of culture on genre, structure, and style of oral and written texts. In G.P. Wallach & K.G. Butler (Eds.), *Language learning disabilities in school-age children and adolescents* (pp. 180–218). Boston: Allyn & Bacon.

Westby, C.E. (1999a). Assessing and facilitating text comprehension problems. In H.W. Catts & A.G. Kamhi (Eds.), *Language and reading disabilities* (pp. 154–223). Boston: Allyn & Bacon.

Westby, C.E. (1999b). Assessment of pragmatic competence in children with psychiatric disorders. In D. Rogers-Adkinson & P. Griffith (Eds.), *Communication disorders and children with psychiatric and behavioral disorders* (pp. 177–258). San Diego: Singular Publishing Group.

Westby, C.E., & Clauser, P.S. (1999). The right stuff for writing: Assessing and facilitating written language. In H.W. Catts & A.G. Kamhi (Eds.), *Language and reading disabilities* (pp. 259–324). Boston: Allyn & Bacon.

Wetherby, A.M., & Prizant, B.M. (Eds.). (2000). Autism spectrum disorders: A transactional developmental perspective. In S.F. Warren & J. Reichle (Series Eds.), *Communication and language intervention series* (Vol. 9). Baltimore: Paul H. Brookes publishing Co.

Wetzel, K. (1985). Keyboarding skills: Elementary, my dear teacher? *The Computing Teacher, 12*(9), 15–19.

Whitmire, K.A. (2000). Adolescence as a developmental phase: A tutorial. *Topics in Language Disorders, 20*(2), 1–14.

Wilkinson, L.C., & Milosky, M. (1987). School-age children's metapragmatic knowledge of requests and responses in the classroom. *Topics in Language Disorders, 7*(2), 61–70.

Windsor, J., Scott, C.M., & Street, C.K. (2000). Verb and noun morphology in the spoken and written language of children with language learning disabilities. *Journal of Speech, Language, and Hearing Research, 43*, 1322–1336.

Wong, B.L. (1994). Instructional parameters promoting transfer of learned strategies in students with learning disabilities. *Learning Disability Quarterly, 17*, 100–119.

Wong, B.Y.L. (2000). Writing strategies instruction for expository essays for adolescents with and without learning disabilities. *Topics in Learning Disorders, 20*(4), 29–44.

Wong, B.Y.L., Butler, D.L., Ficzere, S.A., & Kuperis, S. (1996). Teaching low achievers and students with learning disabilities to plan, write, and revise opinion essays. *Journal of Learning Disabilities, 29*(2), 197–212.

Wood, L.A., Rankin, J.L., & Beukelman, D.R. (1997). Word prompt programs: Current uses and future possibilities. *American Journal of Speech-Language Pathology, 6*, 57–65.

Worden, M.R., & Hutchinson, T.A. (1992). *Writing Process Test.* Itasca, IL: Riverside Publishing.

Ylvisaker, M., & DeBonis, D. (2000). Executive function impairment in adolescence: TBI and ADHD. *Topics in Language Disorders, 20*(2), 29–57.

Yoshinaga-Itano, C., & Downey, D.M. (1992). When a story is not a story: A process analysis of the written language of hearing-impaired children. *The Volta Review, 94*, 131–158.

Yoshinaga-Itano, C., & Downey, D.M. (1996). Analyzing deaf or hard-of-hearing student's written metacognitive strategies and story-grammar propositions. *The Volta Review, 98*(1) [monograph], 63–64.

Yoshinaga-Itano, C., Snyder, L.S., & Mayberry, R. (1996a). Can lexical/semantic skills differentiate deaf or hard-of-hearing readers and nonreaders. *The Volta Review, 98*(1) [monograph], 63–64.

Yoshinaga-Itano, C., Snyder, L.S., & Mayberry, R. (1996b). How deaf and normally hearing students convey meaning within and between written sentences. *The Volta Review, 98*(1) [monograph], 9–38.

Zeni, J. (1990). *Writing lands: Composing with old and new writing tools.* Urbana, IL: National Council of Teachers of English.

Zhang, X., & Tomblin, J.B. (2000). The association of intervention receipt with speech-language profiles and social-demographic variables. *American Journal of Speech-Language Pathology, 9,* 345–357.

Zigmond, N. (1993). Learning disabilities from an educational perspective. In G.R. Lyon, D.B. Gray, J.F. Kavanagh, & N.A. Krasnegor (Eds.), *Better understanding learning disabilities: New views from research and their implications for education and public policies* (pp. 251–272). Baltimore: Paul H. Brookes Publishing Co.

Zorfass, J., Corley, P., & Remz, A. (1994). Helping students with disabilities become writers. *Educational Leadership, 51,* 62–66.

Index

Page numbers followed by *f* indicate figures; those followed by *t* indicate tables.